From Trauma to Healing

This updated edition of *From Trauma to Healing* is a comprehensive and practical guide to working with trauma survivors in the field of social work.

Since September 11th and Hurricane Katrina, social workers have increasingly come together to consider how traumatic events impact practice. This text is designed to support the process, with a focus on evidence-based practice that ensures professionals are fully equipped to work with trauma. Highlights of this new edition include brand new chapters on practitioner bias and vulnerability, standardized assessment methodologies, and crisis management, as well as a focus on topics crucial to social workers such as Trauma Informed Care (TIC) and Adverse Childhood Events (ACEs). The text also offers additional resources including chapter practice exercises and a sample trauma course syllabus for educators.

With fresh examples and discussion questions to help deal with traumatic events in practice, including interventions that may be applicable to current and future 21st century world events, such as the coronavirus pandemic, *From Trauma to Healing,* 2nd edition remains an essential publication on trauma for students and social workers alike.

Ann Goelitz, PhD, LCSW, is a social work educator and trauma psychotherapist who has done extensive public speaking, published numerous academic articles, and co-authored an award-winning resource directory for caregivers.

"From Trauma to Healing provides a wealth of trauma information for social workers. Easy to read, informative, and full of helpful tips and case examples, it portrays in a sensitive and authentic manner the process of experiencing, coping with, and recovering from trauma."

–Lisa M. Najavits, Ph.D.,
director of Treatment Innovations and adjunct professor,
University of Massachusetts Medical School,
author of *Seeking Safety: A Treatment Manual for PTSD and Substance Abuse* and *Finding Your Best Self. Recovery from Addiction, Trauma, or Both.*

"Social workers – more than other class of helping professionals – are major contributors to trauma recovery: at the scene, in the hospital and community, and providing therapy. Goelitz's comprehensive, and highly usable guide will be gratefully received by all. It is so important, I truly hope it will become required reading in all university and licensure programs. A must-have for every social worker's bookshelf."

–Babette Rothschild,
M.S.W., author of *The Body Remembers*,
Volumes 1 & 2, and 8 *Keys to Safe Trauma Recovery.*

"Dr. Goelitz presents an extremely well-organized resource for social workers and related healthcare professionals on the basics of trauma and resilience. This work fills a necessary gap in graduate training and is a helpful resource for those new to the field. For experienced practitioners, this books issues a vital challenge for those of us who work with trauma to better take care of ourselves and each other."

–Jamie Marich, Ph.D.,
LPCC-S, LICDC-CS, REAT, RYT-500, author of *Trauma and the 12 Steps: An Inclusive Guide for Enhancing Recovery, Trauma Made Simple, EMDR Made Simple, Process Not Perfection, Dancing Mindfulness,* and *EMDR Therapy and Mindfulness for Trauma-Focused Care.*

From Trauma to Healing

A Social Worker's Guide to Working with Survivors

Second Edition

Ann Goelitz

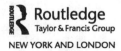

Routledge
Taylor & Francis Group

NEW YORK AND LONDON

Second edition published 2021
by Routledge
52 Vanderbilt Avenue, New York, NY 10017

and by Routledge
2 Park Square, Milton Park, Abingdon, Oxon, OX14 4RN

Routledge is an imprint of the Taylor & Francis Group, an informa business

© 2021 Taylor & Francis

First edition published by Routledge 2013

Library of Congress Cataloging-in-Publication Data
Names: Goelitz, Ann, author.
Title: From trauma to healing : a social worker's guide to working with survivors / Ann Goelitz.
Identifiers: LCCN 2020024450 (print) | LCCN 2020024451 (ebook) | ISBN 9780367029241 (hbk) | ISBN 9780367029258 (pbk) | ISBN 9780429001130 (ebk)
Subjects: LCSH: Psychiatric social work. | Mentally ill–Services for. | Psychic trauma–Treatment.
Classification: LCC HV689 .G64 2021 (print) | LCC HV689 (ebook) | DDC 362.2/0425–dc23
LC record available at https://lccn.loc.gov/2020024450
LC ebook record available at https://lccn.loc.gov/2020024451

ISBN: 978-0-367-02924-1 (hbk)
ISBN: 978-0-367-02925-8 (pbk)
ISBN: 978-0-429-00113-0 (ebk)

Typeset in Garamond
by KnowledgeWorks Global Ltd.

Dedication

This book is dedicated to survivors of trauma and the social workers who work with them.

Contents

PART IV
Healing Trauma on a Micro Level   181

PART V
Healing Trauma on a Macro Level   237

Figures and Tables

Foreword

Traumatic life events signify intense emotional reactions and severe losses. These events include: natural disasters, such as hurricanes; genocide and other historical trauma, such as the Holocaust, slavery and the massacres of American Indians; traumas experienced through war and torture; and personal traumas – arising, for example, from sexual abuse, rape, physical assault, bullying or the unexpected death of a child. While these and other traumatic events are experienced as disastrous and overwhelming, they also do provide opportunities for transformation – for growth and mastery. In this updated edition of *From Trauma to Healing: A Social Worker's Guide to Working with Survivors*, Dr. Goelitz creatively uses theory and practice experiences to provide specific guidelines for the social work practitioner and student. These practical guidelines are insightful and clearly explicated.

Throughout the book, the author provides practical information about: Various types of trauma and their differential impact; the societal and cultural contexts for trauma; creating safe environments; secondary trauma and self-care and practical tools for surviving trauma. This updated edition also covers topics crucial to social workers such as practitioner bias and vulnerability, Trauma Informed Care (TIC), Adverse Childhood Events (ACEs), standardized assessment instruments, practice exercises and questions and a sample trauma course syllabus. Educators will find the latter additions particularly helpful.

The book's reader-friendly style and clear explanation of complex processes make it especially useful to both practitioners and educators. Readers will be reassured by its specificity and unencumbered style and are likely to gain confidence in their own abilities to help people suffering from trauma. I want to convey my appreciation and respect for Dr. Goelitz's ability to present rich ideas without professional and academic jargon and instead with directness and clarity. I thank her for her gift to the profession's literature.

Alex Gitterman, Professor of Social Work
School of Social Work, University of Connecticut

Acknowledgments

First and foremost, I want to acknowledge the co-author of the first edition of *From Trauma to Healing*, Abigail Stewart-Kahn. We shared a vision for the book and it came to fruition despite her busy life. The book has undergone extensive changes with the second edition which she was unable to be a part of but her imprint remains.

Carol Morrison has also been instrumental. Originally asked to be co-author of the first edition, she was unable to do so, but was actively involved throughout, reading chapters, suggesting changes and supporting me along the way. Her expertise has been invaluable. She also did the artwork for the first edition book cover.

Finally, I want to thank my mother, Sydney Wright, who started me reading very early in life. Our Christmas tree was always full of books, and reading in bed under the covers with a flashlight was unofficially endorsed. She instilled in me a love of reading and the desire to be a writer myself. Without her, this book would not have happened. I am most excited when giving *her* each of my new publications and consider them offerings of love.

There are numerous others I would like to thank who helped along the way – experts who read all or portions of the manuscripts, those who endorsed or reviewed the books, Alex Gitterman who wrote the books' forewords and all those who read the books or use them as a texts in their classes. Of course I would be remiss if I did not acknowledge those at Routledge who helped along the way, without whom this would not have been possible. I so appreciate you all.

Ann Goelitz, 2020

Introduction

The world is witnessing a whole new level of trauma. Examples range from multiple onslaughts of hurricanes in Puerto Rico, mass shootings, the coronavirus and strife in the Middle East. Social work leaders, along with many other professional disciplines, have joined together to understand the impact of trauma in a new light and to consider the ways in which trauma experiences are both similar and unique. This book was planned as a guide to the field of trauma for new and experienced social workers to address this growing awareness of the impact of trauma on our clients and on helping professionals. It includes an overview of potentially traumatic events and treatment approaches and uses case examples to assist readers in applying concepts to real situations. Topics that distinguish social work's ecological approach are also covered.

As an experienced social worker in the trauma field, I remember questions and feelings that arose when I encountered trauma issues. This was true as I began my path in social work and as new trauma-related issues emerged later in my career. I remember often having no idea where to begin. This updated edition of *From Trauma to Healing: A Social Worker's Guide to Working with Survivors* addresses this, integrating theoretical principles and practice guidance and responding to questions I often had, such as: What exactly is trauma? What types of trauma exist, and how do they affect people differently? Where should I begin treatment? How do social workers specifically approach trauma? What should I do with the feelings that come up in me as I work with trauma survivors?

ABOUT THE BOOK

The target audience for this book is manifold: new social workers, students, recent graduates, social workers and supervisors in agencies and mental health settings; school social workers; professors teaching courses in social work and related fields; and social workers in private practice. The book is written with pride for social workers and is meant to be a support as they care for one of the most vulnerable populations we encounter. Other health and mental health practitioners who work with trauma will also find it useful.

WHY IS THERE A NEED FOR THIS BOOK?
WHAT'S NEW IN THIS BOOK?

When the first edition of this book was written, we spoke with experts in the field who concur that while some social workers take an interest in trauma early in their careers, many more never study its impact on clients or how to address it. A brief review in 2008 of the ten top social work schools revealed that few offered trauma courses. Although many more trauma courses are now available, as well as trauma certifications, graduates often continue to feel underprepared to address trauma issues in their practice, and this, combined with the fact that trauma material can be difficult for therapists at all levels of training to discuss (Belicki & Cuddy, 1996; Goelitz, 2001b), supports the need for trauma resources among social workers.

Social workers in mental health settings, agencies, schools and universities, private practice, substance abuse settings and many others all encounter survivors of various forms of trauma. Trauma, which is defined by the *Social Work Dictionary* (Barker, 1999, p. 492) as "an injury to the body or psyche by some type of shock, violence, or unanticipated situation," can be experienced first-hand or witnessed and includes war, torture, child abuse and other domestic violence, life-threatening illness, serious accidents and violent crimes, among others.

In attempting to understand how many individuals struggle with these experiences, both exposure to trauma and post-traumatic stress disorder (PTSD) are considered. PTSD has a lifetime incidence of 10% for women and 5% for men among those who experience trauma (Najavits, 2002). The incidence of trauma is even higher as 61% of men and 51% of women experience trauma at some point in their lives – more than half of the overall population (Najavits, 2002). While many do not suffer from psychological issues or come forward for help, many do. These data indicate that social workers' caseloads are, and may increasingly be, filled with clients who have experienced trauma.

Despite the incidence of trauma and many social workers' discomfort with the material, few texts exist to guide them. This book helps fill that gap, providing social workers with a new resource for both practice and education, as it helps them draw connections and make distinctions between varied types of trauma and their impact. It was designed with the intent of providing social workers with the means to approach survivors of trauma with confidence, experience and care.

As social workers, we are required to be experts on an enormous range of subjects. Guides provide us with both a place to start learning about new practice areas and a source of tools to develop expertise. This updated edition of *From Trauma to Healing: A Social Worker's Guide to Working with Survivors* supports the field's movement toward evidence-based practice coupled with the growing need for social workers to be equipped to work with trauma. It does so in the practical guide format already proven to be compelling to social work students, educators and practitioners.

Acknowledging the importance of evidence-based practice, as a social worker, I also understand the need to balance this with other social work concepts such as strength-based work, ethics, a whole-client or ecological approach and client self-determination. This book attempts to strike that balance and meet the needs of both evidence-based practice and social work ethics and principles.

HOW TO USE THE BOOK

One of the goals was to make the book as accessible, clear and easy to follow as possible. Realizing that there are many good books detailing specific clinical approaches, I saw no need to re-create these in this updated edition of *From Trauma to Healing: A Social Worker's Guide to Working with Survivors*. Instead, I have worked to build a framework for our work with trauma survivors, outlining approaches, providing case examples and letting readers know where to find more information.

The book is designed for each chapter to stand alone so that topics of interest can be explored without reading preceding chapters. For ease of use, definitions are included in each chapter, and tips for working with survivors are also interspersed throughout the book. Both are presented in boxed text to make them easy to find and use. Finally, each chapter ends with resources, practice exercises and questions and a one-page sheet that summarizes key points covered. A sample syllabus for a trauma course is also provided in the appendix.

The book begins in Part I with a focus on us. The first chapter explores how we are affected by the work. The second, a chapter new to this edition, goes deeper, looking at what we bring to the work we do with survivors and how this impacts our interactions. These are chapters I encourage everyone to read and to refer to as needed. They are topics we need to keep in mind to ensure we keep ourselves whole as we work. Even reading the material in the book can be traumatizing, and this is addressed along with the importance of making self-reflection and awareness our first priority when working with survivors.

Part II discusses a sampling of various types of trauma. A new chapter on war and terrorism is in this edition, as well one on family abuse and neglect that incorporates material from chapters in the first edition and addresses abuse/neglect of the elderly and disabled. How culture and vulnerable populations interact with trauma are also considered at the end of the section. These topics, which are familiar for social workers, are looked at here through a trauma lens.

Part III turns the lens to safety, stressing the importance of making this our first priority when working with survivors. Coping skills essential to survivors' recovery are also explored, as well as safe relationships. Then, in Part IV, an overview of interventions available for working with survivors is provided. A chapter on some of the alternative methodologies available is included. A new chapter on assessment has also been added to this edition, introducing readers to assessment methodologies and standardized assessment instruments.

Finally, in Part V, program development, advocacy, prevention and community organizing are discussed. These chapters, of particular interest to social workers, explore topics essential to generating the kind of change that can reduce trauma's impact on society. It is hoped that this book will be not only a resource for social workers, but that it will also help them to have an impact on systems, such as families and communities, ultimately enacting societal change.

SELF-CARE

Trauma is not easy to work with. I cannot emphasize enough the importance of self-care both as you read this book and work with survivors. Refer often to the chapter on this topic, discuss cases with colleagues and work with a supervisor you trust who can guide you in the process. Enjoy the work, which is rewarding as well as difficult. The good news is that when survivors get appropriate help, dramatic healing can occur. Watching this transformational process, like seeing a flower bloom, can be awe-inspiring.

Part I

First Things First

Preparing to Work with Trauma

Chapter 1

You can be Affected too: Secondary Trauma

It can be hard to listen to or even contemplate trauma survivors' stories. Emotions engendered by trauma are painful. Simply sharing space with that engulfing raw emotion can be overwhelming. These feelings can seem too big to hold, and yet, as a part of our job, as social workers, we must help contain them. Trauma-related terror, anger, helplessness, sadness, shame and disgust are often so intense that they feel out of control. Pandora's Box opened wide, releasing pure evil without a ray of hope.

Even reading survivors' stories can affect us. In end-of-life-care classes, students have difficulty with stories of death and dying. Some have their own experiences that intervene. Others become emotional without these personal references.

Repeated reading can numb us. During a research study that involved cataloging trauma dreams and coding the emotions they contained, a research assistant became inured to the stories she coded. She saw no trauma material in a woman's response to her fear of a man raping her in a dream, even though the woman's response was to hold a flame under the rapist's penis (Goelitz, 2009).

Because of the difficulty of trauma work, it is important for us to note our responses as we work. The emotion-laden trauma material can affect professionals as well as survivors, so that attending to its impact can protect us from harm. To this end, in this chapter we discuss how to (1) recognize the signs of secondary trauma; (2) understand situations that make us more vulnerable to this condition; (3) utilize skills to lessen the effect of survivors' trauma on us; and (4) practice ways to take care of ourselves when we experience the symptoms of secondary trauma.

TUNE IN TO SELF

Only with self-awareness prior to and during time spent with survivors can we avoid negative effects of trauma survivors' experiences. Self-reflection after encounters is also important. This holds true in individual, group and family work and for less direct routes such as reading the case reports shared in this book.

> **Tips**
>
> • *Tune in to self* – Do a quick check for any physical, emotional and cognitive discomfort. Try to identify the source. Breathe into it or use other means to relax and nurture yourself. If the discomfort remains, remember you are carrying it with you so that it will not cause difficulty later.

While working in an outpatient trauma clinic, I supervised case managers who assisted survivors with concrete services, such as housing referrals and social service applications. These staff often got the brunt of survivors' pain and needed to attend to secondary trauma. When survivors discussed with case managers their need for help, for instance, they often began to cry or to share their experiences.

This is one example of how we witness trauma as we work with survivors. Although the witnessing can heal survivors, it can harm us. One way to prevent this is to be clear about our thoughts, emotions and physical states prior to meeting with survivors. Tuning in allows us to observe tiredness from staying up late the night before, slight uneasiness at meeting a new client or one we know has struggled lately, hunger for the lunch we will eat after this meeting, worry over paperwork to do before going home or fear for a sick relative. While tuning in, it can also help to think about past losses, anticipating the possibility of these feelings coming up.

Focusing in on all these sensations allows us to own them and to acknowledge their presence so that they do not creep up during our time with survivors, distracting us and causing discomfort. Knowing our feelings also helps in another way. If emotions arise during sessions, we can then check back and consider whether they belong to us or to the survivor. If fear comes up, for example, it may relate to the survivor and/or to some reminder of our own worries and fears. Either way, we can focus on our own sense of personal safety as an antidote to the difficult emotions, note and accept our reactions and bring them into the foreground rather than hiding and forgetting them.

> **Definitions**
>
> • *Safety* – State essential to trauma recovery and unique to each individual, in which (1) risky behaviors, unhealthy relationships and negative emotions are reduced and (2) a sense of well-being, trust, calm and positive coping are increased.

Unrecognized and forgotten feelings can cause trouble. Taking time after encounters or at the end of the day allows us to review what transpired internally as we encountered survivors. In the process, we may uncover new sensations, including worries about our children after hearing a survivor reflect on childhood trauma; anxiety and a racing heart after being with a client who was overwhelmingly anxious; deep sadness for no apparent reason after sitting with a survivor who could not utter a word; or pain in the chest after meeting with a survivor with somatic symptoms.

Identifying these sensations means we can let them go rather than continue to carry them. We can do this in many ways such as taking a shower and washing them off, meditating and lighting incense to clear our senses, exercising to sweat out what we have retained or talking about our day. We can even imagine letting go as we wash dishes or shoot hoops after a hard workday. Each time we get the ball in the basket can represent a survivor's experience that we took home with us and now let go. Each dish we wash turns another emotion from negative to positive, brightening our day after hearing so many difficult stories. Noting our responses as we work not only safeguards us but also improves the therapeutic alliance and allows us to work more effectively with survivors.

Tips

- *Body scan* – Sit with your back supported and feet flat on the floor. Scan your body starting at the head and working down to the feet. Explore any tension or discomfort you encounter to identify its source as physical, emotional or cognitive. Physical could be a muscle ache, emotional could be sadness due to a pet's death and cognitive could be worries about life stressors or insecurities related to job performance. The scan can also be used for relaxation, breathing into and letting go of the tension when we locate it.

SIGNS OF SECONDARY TRAUMA

We can compare exposure to trauma with exposure to a sick client's germs. Social workers who interact with survivors are exposed to trauma experiences and reactions just as they are exposed to clients' germs when sick. In the same way that we "catch" illnesses from clients, we can also "catch" their intense emotion and distress. We do not always get sick when exposed to germs but can still pass them on to others. By the same token, we can pass on the intense emotion and distress even if it does not affect us directly (Wicks, 2008). Therefore, we need to pay close attention to secondary trauma.

Besides secondary trauma, a number of other terms describe effects on practitioners from working with survivors: vicarious traumatization, secondary traumatic stress, compassion fatigue, countertransference and burnout are also similarly utilized, although each has a distinct meaning. The *Social work dictionary* (Barker, 1999) defines burnout as feeling "apathy or anger as a result of on-the-job stress and frustration," especially as a result of having "more responsibility than control" at work (p. 57). Barker (1999) also defines countertransference as "*conscious* or *unconscious* emotional reactions to a client" provoked by "the social worker's own developmental conflicts" and "projected onto the client," just as transference causes clients to project their issues onto the practitioner (p. 109). Those who care for survivors can have any of these reactions. Burnout and countertransference are, however, related more to work or personal experience than to trauma witnessed as we work with survivors (Hesse, 2002).

Definitions

- *Burnout* – Work-related stress, which can be exacerbated by unsupportive and demanding work environments and leads to cynicism, lack of interest and discouragement.
- *Countertransference* – Responses to clients, stemming from practitioners' own past experiences, that are projected onto clients and cause practitioners to feel affinity with clients and their associated emotions such as guilt and fear of abandonment.
- *Compassion fatigue* – Caused by the stress of thinking about survivor clients, reliving their trauma experiences and having symptoms similar to PTSD as a result.
- *Secondary traumatic stress* – Results from both exposure to traumatic material and compassion for survivors. Symptoms are the same as with PTSD.
- *Post traumatic stress disorder (PTSD)* – A disorder resulting from exposure to traumatic events that causes symptoms lasting at least a month that include emotional responses of fear, horror or helplessness; flashbacks and/or nightmares of events; avoidance of reminders of the event; and increased arousal.
- *Avoidance* – Individuals staying away from people, places or activities even when these are not dangerous because they are reminders of trauma.

In a different vein, Figley (2002) says that compassion fatigue results from secondary traumatic stress. It causes those who witness survivors' suffering to become engrossed with survivors' traumas so that they have trauma symptoms themselves, re-experiencing the event and becoming numb and avoidant when reminded of what the survivor experienced (Figley, 2002). Those with secondary traumatic stress have symptoms of post-traumatic stress disorder (PTSD) just as survivors do (Hesse, 2002).

Unlike secondary traumatic stress, which can occur after one interacts with a survivor, vicarious traumatization results from exposure over time to multiple survivors. Similar to survivors' experiences, vicariously traumatized practitioners become altered internally as their cognitive schemas are disrupted. This attack on their belief system and innate sense of self erodes trust and feelings of personal safety. It can also distort their view of the world, encouraging a negative outlook on life even among optimistic practitioners. In addition, vicarious traumatization affects memory so that social workers take on survivors' trauma memories and/or associated trauma emotions (McCann & Pearlman, 1990b).

Definitions

- *Vicarious traumatization* – Results from repeated exposures to trauma material and causes disruption of cognitive schemas and distortion of memories so that practitioners take on clients' trauma memories and related emotions.
- *Cognitive schemas* – Individuals' beliefs and thoughts about self and life, including faith in the world being a safe place and ideas about right and wrong.

Secondary trauma can therefore result in symptoms of PTSD even if social workers have never directly experienced a trauma themselves. Trauma therapists particularly run this risk (Cunningham, 2003), but working with survivors can affect anyone. As previously mentioned, secondary trauma can even affect students in the classroom (Graziano, 2001; Miller, 2001). In general, between 18% and 60% of those who work with trauma survivors have serious repercussions related to secondary trauma (Figley, 2002; Tehrani, 2007).

These PTSD symptoms can result from secondary trauma: (1) feeling fearful, horrified or helpless in relation to a survivor's trauma; (2) having flashbacks and/or nightmares of the survivor's traumatic event, or preoccupation with thoughts of the survivor and what they experienced; (3) avoiding reminders of the survivor's trauma, including feeling relief when they miss an appointment and consciously or unconsciously moving away from discussions of traumatic events; and (4) feeling anxious and on edge, hypervigilant or emotionally and physically aroused in a way that makes it difficult to fall asleep.

Definitions

- *Flashback* – Intrusive and involuntary re-experiencing of traumatic events through images, emotions or physical sensations.
- *Hypervigilance* – State of increased attention to the environment, in order to detect threat and prevent harm, that can increase anxiety, prevent sleep and cause fatigue.

OTHER SIGNS OF SECONDARY TRAUMA

Other signs of secondary trauma include (1) frustrated, impatient, apathetic, depressed, hopeless and overwhelmed feelings that fall outside the ordinary scope (Wicks, 2008); (2) not returning calls, lateness or missing sessions with survivors (McCann & Pearlman, 1990b); (3) "spacing out" or feeling disconnected, numb or distracted during sessions (McCann & Pearlman, 1990b; Wicks, 2008); (4) developing somatic symptoms such as head or stomach aches after interactions with survivors (McCann & Pearlman, 1990a); (5) not believing survivors' stories or minimizing their severity (Herman, 1992); and (6) changed cognitive schemas so that practitioners no longer feel safe in the world, becoming suspicious and/or losing trust in self and others (Cunningham, 2003).

This example from the literature (McCann & Pearlman, 1990b) shows the impact of secondary trauma on a trauma worker:

> Tom, a married man in his late 20's and father of two young children, was frequently disturbed by intrusive images involving danger befalling loved ones. He became obsessed with safety precautions and was hypervigilant about strange noises in the house. As a result, he often woke up suddenly in the middle of the night, fearing that a prowler was in the house. Despite the absence of evidence of immediate danger, he would lie vigilant in his bed for several hours before finally dropping off to sleep. These recurring feelings of impending danger disrupted his sleep pattern and left him with a pervasive sense of anxiety and vulnerability.
>
> (p. 131)

VULNERABILITIES TO SECONDARY TRAUMA

A variety of issues can contribute to our vulnerability to secondary trauma. Those working with survivors of human-made trauma such as child abuse, intimate partner violence or war have a higher likelihood of suffering from secondary trauma (Cunningham, 2003) because it affects us more pervasively than non-human-made traumas such as life-threatening illness or natural disasters (American Psychiatric Association, 2000). Non-human-made traumas have somewhat less impact, since they lack the intent to cause harm, which can be difficult to reconcile and make sense of, often impeding recovery and the healing process. It has also been found that it is more challenging to work with child survivors (Lahad, 2000). This no doubt contributes to the high rate of secondary trauma among child welfare workers (Dane, 2000).

Tips

• *Decreasing vulnerability* – Create a permeable but protective shield for yourself prior to starting the workday that allows survivors' feelings to enter your consciousness without being absorbed. Imagine putting the shield on as you shower in the morning, being careful to cover yourself thoroughly. Let go of the workday as you remove the shield at night.

Practitioners who are survivors themselves, students, new therapists or those new to working with trauma also have potential vulnerability to secondary trauma (Pearlman & Saakvitne, 1995; Saakvitne, 2002). Social workers who are survivors themselves can have particularly strong countertransference reactions to individuals affected by trauma. These intense emotions can make stories hard to hear, resulting in practitioners focusing on their own needs and disconnecting from survivors. Students, new therapists and those new to trauma work are also more vulnerable because they may tend to lack confidence and experience with countertransference. This is particularly true if they are survivors themselves (Pearlman & Saakvitne, 1995).

We need to know our own limitations when working with survivors. Individuals or situations vary in difficulty (Wicks, 2008; Worden, 2003). Survivors' traumas, for example, stem from such challenging events as the Holocaust and the September 11th disaster. Our identification and empathy are increased by anything – like family members who survived concentration camps or living near the World Trade Center – that links us to survivors' stories. When this occurs, the stories permeate deeper inside us, increasing exposure to secondary trauma (Lahad, 2000).

Stories also permeate deeper when we lack work-related boundaries (Lahad, 2000). This includes meeting clients with no prior intake procedure or in less formal environments such as hospital rooms or survivors' homes. Groups also afford fewer boundaries than traditional meetings with clients in offices that provide safe containers within which to work (Ziegler & McEvoy, 1997–2002). We must take particular care to avoid secondary trauma when practicing in these more vulnerable and less protected settings.

Unmet psychological needs, including safety, trust, self-esteem, independence, power, intimacy and support, can increase the risk of secondary trauma (Tehrani, 2007). Social workers' own stress and losses contribute to unmet needs (Wicks, 2008). We should watch ourselves during times of financial worry, illness, conflict and relationship/familial issues, busy schedules, insufficient food or sleep, life transitions and loss. Loss plays a part in most trauma (Saakvitne, 2002), so working with survivors can increase consciousness of personal loss. This is particularly true with recent or not fully processed losses (Worden, 2003).

TRANSFERENCE AND COUNTERTRANSFERENCE

Countertransference reactions come in many forms, most commonly identification with and avoidance of those affected by trauma (Ziegler & McEvoy, 1997–2002). This includes social workers experiencing survivors' feelings of helplessness, vulnerability, anger and sadness. Feeling helpless can be particularly troubling for practitioners because it not only increases risk of secondary trauma (Wicks, 2008) but can also cause loss of confidence in the ability to help survivors. In addition, while feeling powerless, we may unrealistically strive for perfection and control (van der Kolk, McFarlane, & Weisaeth, 1996). Trauma workers can also experience rescue fantasies. These fantasies represent attempts to reduce feelings of vulnerability, as with this example of a therapist going into savior mode with a survivor:

Ron: I'm really scared and worried about what this will do to my family.

Social worker: What do you think might happen to them?

Ron: They don't have money either but I know they will try to pay for my hospital bills. There's no point in all that. *Wiping away tears.* I'm going to die anyway.

Social worker: But don't you have insurance? If you don't we can help.

Ron: I've tried and can't because I'm a visitor in this country. I'm too sick to go home and get help there and don't have any money. There is no solution. I'm so scared.

Social worker: Of course there's a solution and I will help you find it.

Ron: My family is spending all their money. I'm afraid of what this is doing to us.

Social worker: *Looking at computer.* Let's see. Have you tried...?

The therapist is missing an opportunity to connect on a deep level with Ron, a man with terminal brain cancer. Had she explored the fear he expressed and helped him find ways to deal with it, their relationship would have become a healing force as he gained much-needed coping tools. Instead, she became overwhelmed by the intensity of his emotion. Her fear that she could not help him drove her to become detached, looking at a computer screen instead of at him. Helping with insurance is an important social work function, but it was not what Ron was asking for at that moment.

Transference reactions also vary. Survivors can have conflicting feelings for practitioners. They want to feel connected and secure in relation to them, but also fear being hurt again (Turner, McFarlane & van der Kolk,1996). This can even lead to re-enactment of the abuse and victimization, so that they see the helper (1) as the abuser and a dangerous and/or critical authority, in charge but untrustworthy, who will betray or abandon them; or (2) as the safe caregiver or friend who may even run the risk of being hurt by the survivor when they are feeling out of control and dangerously angry (McCann & Pearlman, 1990a).

Definitions

- *Transference* – Responses to practitioners stemming from clients' own past experiences that are projected onto practitioners and cause clients to relate to practitioners as though they are abusers, family members or other individuals from the clients' often unresolved past experiences.

Groups can have even more potential for transference and countertransference than individual work, because in groups, reactions occur with each group member and also involve family issues unique to group settings (Ziegler & McEvoy, 1997–2002). Other circumstances that make these complicated reactions more likely include trauma work by social workers who are survivors themselves. These practitioners may attribute their own experiences with trauma and recovery to survivor clients, inadvertently lessening the authenticity of the relationship and potentially affecting their objectivity as professionals. Others may project unwarranted views onto clients of what they consider to be their own bad qualities (Pearlman & Saakvitne, 1995).

We need to watch for, recognize and address countertransference. It is in these moments that we move away from survivors and ourselves, not wanting to encounter trauma emotions and our corresponding scars. The therapeutic relationship can then become inauthentic and distant or, if we choose awareness, it can become genuine and allied. Without awareness, we not only sever connection with survivors but also unwittingly encourage them to hide their feelings. If we do not want to encounter their pain, why should they (Bromberg, 2006)?

As an intern, I experienced this while leading a group for caregivers of cancer patients, many nearing death. The group met on Thursday evenings, and I began to notice after doing the group for a few weeks that I felt very sad on weekends. It took me some time to connect the sadness to the group because

I did not feel sad during it, and group sessions did not prompt any emotional memories of past experiences with illness. Eventually I sought help in therapy and realized that the group members' sadness had touched similar feelings in me from my own losses. With this awareness, I no longer felt sad on weekends and became more present during the group sessions.

TRACKING AND PROCESSING EMOTIONS

We can recognize both countertransference and transference reactions by the emotions they engender. Becoming aware of emotion helps to track these reactions. As they provide services, social workers naturally encounter survivors' feelings (Figley, 2002). Therefore, differentiating the causes of our emotion can become a source of confusion. We start the day with some, pick up others from survivors and then emotional reactions come up in response to the work. Attention to and tracking of our emotional states can give us the information we need to identify their sources.

Processing intense trauma emotion also helps. We may, for instance, get angry with the inability of survivors' family members to deal with trauma reactions appropriately because it feels more comfortable than getting mad at the damage caused by the trauma (Ziegler & McEvoy, 1997–2002). Realizing this means that we can use the anger constructively by helping survivors recognize their own anger about what happened.

Tracking our emotions helps us as we function as a "container" for feelings, demonstrating to survivors that trauma emotions are not repugnant or too much to hold (McCann & Pearlman, 1990a). This can be a difficult endeavor, since the emotions often become intense and overwhelming (Ziegler & McEvoy, 1997–2002). As a result, we may avoid trauma material, afraid of being traumatized ourselves (McCann & Pearlman, 1990a). I have encountered this while interviewing practitioners regarding their clients' trauma dreams. Even many who were experienced and skilled with trauma admitted to not wanting to talk about the dreams because they were upsetting.

Use of self is a methodology for working with emotions as well. When not able to quickly identify the source of emotions during encounters with survivors, I use them to explore feelings they may have split off from awareness. For instance, suddenly feeling sad in the midst of discussing how angry a survivor is with her partner, I ask her:

Tips

- *Quick tune in to self* – During meetings with survivors, do a quick check as feelings arise or if you are confused about how to proceed. Try to identify the source of the emotion or confusion. Relax into the feelings and use what you learn as you talk with survivors.

Social worker:	Does it make you sad when you two fight?
Joy:	No, I'm mad at her. She doesn't understand…
Social worker:	Of course you're mad but you could be sad too.
Joy:	What's there to be sad about? Can't you see how mad I am?
Social worker:	You might be sad that she can't hear you just as you were never heard as a child during the abuse.
Joy:	I do hate that she can't hear what I say. *Thinking.*
Social worker:	You have experienced so much loss and this is one more.
Joy:	Why can't she hear me? What do I have to do to make her hear me? No one ever listens to me. *A tear runs down her cheek.*

THE IMPORTANCE OF APPROPRIATE BOUNDARIES

Therapeutic boundaries help reduce the negative effects of transference and countertransference and prevent secondary trauma. This includes finding clarity about the purpose, time and length of meetings, as well as how survivors can contact practitioners or get help between meetings, while carefully defining the therapeutic relationship as limited to the work agreed upon. This process, which requires sensitivity to survivors' vulnerability and flexibility as to their special needs, can pose challenges for social workers (Herman, 1992); for example, having regular appointment times and stressing punctuality, while also allowing for clients who "space out" and lose their sense of direction on the way to a meeting. We have found that it also helps to spend extra time with survivors in crisis even if the allotted time has expired. It is not appropriate, for instance, to let survivors leave and walk out to the street in tears or dissociated. Suggesting splashing water on his or her face, utilizing relaxing aromatherapy or spending time in the waiting room or a few more minutes in session may help to process what occurred during the session.

Definitions

- *Dissociation* – Disconnection from thoughts, memories or emotions that provides internal distance from reminders of traumatic events, but also prevents integration of trauma material and disrupts normal psychological functioning.

Establishing flexible but clear boundaries with survivors can be particularly troublesome for social workers who are survivors themselves. These practitioners may have a higher likelihood of violating therapeutic boundaries, particularly by inappropriately disclosing too much information about themselves

(Pearlman & Saakvitne, 1995). This is one of the pitfalls of intimacy with survivors. Survivor therapists care about their survivor clients; at times, this leads to enmeshment as they inappropriately tell them what to do or try to increase the depth of their connection, leading to inappropriate exchanges and boundary violations (Hesse, 2002).

Without appropriate boundaries, other disruptions to the therapeutic relationship can occur (Herman, 1992). These not only harm survivors (Hesse, 2002) but can also contribute to secondary trauma as social workers take their work home, either literally or figuratively in their thoughts. For example, I had an experience with a cancer patient who insisted she had to meet with me that day, even though I had no time to do so. Relaxing the therapeutic boundary, I met with her against my better judgment. She was very distraught and, as survivors often do, "dumped" all her fears, concerns and anger in an avalanche of feeling. Already tired and stressed, I was overwhelmed by the conversation and unable to hold the intensity of her emotion. This experience left the patient feeling more bereft because she reached out for help and felt like no one was there for her. Waiting to meet felt impossible to her, but it would have prevented such a painful rupture.

AWARENESS, SELF-REFLECTION AND COPING

Working with secondary trauma requires self-reflection (Bromberg, 2006). Bromberg (2006) shares a story he recalled when struggling with what could have been a secondary trauma response to the September 11th disaster had he not dealt with it. He kept thinking of an aggressive cat he knew and hated as a child that he saw attacked and seriously hurt by blue jays. Unsure why this was coming up, he examined it and realized that under his hate for the cat was helplessness he felt while witnessing the presumably invincible cat being overpowered. This was too terrifying to consider as a child because it highlighted a vulnerability he felt then (and also during the September 11th disaster). Without self-reflection, this process and the ensuing healing would not have occurred, potentially impeding Bromberg's work with survivors. As we work with survivors ourselves, keeping a journal of reactions to their traumas can aid this reflection process (Ziegler & McEvoy, 1997–2002).

Enhancing resiliency helps protect social workers from the effects of secondary trauma (Wicks, 2008). This includes developing a program of coping and self-care. Doing so creates a foundation of safety that bolsters us as we work with survivors. Self-care programs call for a balance of work, relaxation and fun (Herman, 1992; Saakvitne, 2002). We need to find meaning in life and a sense of belonging to community as well (Saakvitne, 2002). See Chapter 12 on coping and self-care for tips that apply to us as well as to survivors.

> **Definitions**
>
> • *Coping* – Process of dealing with difficulties, problem solving and adapting to the environment in order to manage stress and conflict effectively.

An adjunct to this general self-care is coping that assists with letting go of survivors and their emotions at the end of the day. To that end, I review my day as I drive home, looking for ways I could have done better or where I felt particularly happy about the work. Then I think about each encounter that day and consciously let go of each individuals and their issues, trying to do so with love and compassion.

Other means of coping that are important to practitioners include participating in psychotherapy, especially for those who are survivors themselves, and exploring and processing personal and work-related losses (Hesse, 2002; Pearlman & Saakvitne, 1995; Worden, 2003). Employing a strengths perspective as a part of a personal coping regime helps. Studies reveal, for instance, less secondary trauma among motivated practitioners who have a sense of fulfillment and competence (Bell, 2003; Tehrani, 2007).

In our experience, these practices benefit not only social workers but also survivors, who are healed by our sense of well-being and safety. Just as survivors' intensity and distress affect us, they can feel and learn to depend on how comfortable we are taking care of ourselves. This helps them in the moment as they struggle with chaotic feelings and gives them hope for a more secure future.

> **Tips**
>
> • *Grief rituals* – Since working with trauma involves grieving, rituals can be beneficial for practitioners who do not have many ways to express their sadness. Doing grief rituals with colleagues at work can be particularly powerful. Put papers into a box with notes about the survivors' losses. Take turns choosing one and reading it aloud. Listen to music and talk about all you have gained from working with survivors despite the sadness.

CLINICAL SUPERVISION

If we think of social workers as "containers" of survivors' trauma emotions and stories (McCann & Pearlman, 1990a), it makes sense that over time the containers will become full. Clinical supervision empties the containers, ensuring they will not overflow and make a mess of our lives. It also inoculates practitioners, protecting them from secondary trauma (Dane, 2000; Lahad, 2000). In addition, supervision provides perspective, a key ingredient of effective coping (Saakvitne, 2002):

Judy: I've been so tired lately.
Supervisor: Any idea why? I know you have a lot going on, but this work can be stressful and [it] may be related.
Judy: You think so? *Thinking*. It does seem worse since I started with John.
Supervisor: I know that case is hard, it would be for anyone (*he was aggressively sexually abused by his mother*). What are you doing to take care of yourself?
Judy: Well I was doing a lot, but sort of forgot. I used to take a walk at lunch, eat outside if the weather's good, and I was doing yoga. Somehow I'm too busy now.
Supervisor: You are busy, but sometimes it feels like we have to work very hard to take care of our clients and that there can't be time for us until everything is fixed.
Judy: *Smiling*. That's exactly how I feel. Doesn't work though, does it?

Despite the advantages to supervision, not many agencies provide it, and paying for it out of pocket can be difficult on a social work salary. In one study, only 55% of social workers utilized supervision as a form of support (Tehrani, 2007). When working with trauma, social workers benefit greatly from supervision and should advocate for agencies to provide it if it is unavailable.

NETWORK OF SUPPORT

A robust network of support helps avoid secondary trauma (Tehrani, 2007). This includes supportive relationships of all kinds: Familial, social, cultural, spiritual, collegial and work (Herman, 1992). Administrative support at work can increase social workers' strengths so that they are resilient. A pleasant work environment, with access to natural light and nature (even in the form of plants), good smells, vibrant yet relaxing colors and seating arrangements conducive to creating connection, is supportive for both staff and survivors (Goelitz & Stewart-Kahn, 2006/2007).

Giving staff constructive feedback provides support, as it contributes to them feeling competent and appreciated (Tehrani, 2007). An administrative assistant at a trauma outpatient clinic needed support due to the effects of secondary trauma. She had fallen behind in her work. I began to set limits, including reviewing her pending work and helping her come up with due dates. When she could not make the dates, we talked about why. When she made her dates, I praised her, and if she was late with good reason, I let her know how much

I appreciated the quality of her work. I also asked her to participate in a redecorating effort to make the environment more supportive of survivors. She enjoyed this and did a good job. She subsequently expressed both how good she felt about her work and how she was being affected by secondary trauma from encounters with survivors. It seems unlikely she would have shared so openly without feeling good about herself as a result of the support she received for her efforts:

Virginia: They really like the way the office looks. *Looking happy and proud.*
Supervisor: You should feel good. You really helped a lot.
Virginia: It was fun, but I feel bad for them.
Supervisor: What do you mean?
Virginia: So many of them have had a bad time of it. Sometimes it makes me sad. I think about it as I lay in bed at night. Not always, but...
Supervisor: It sounds like you're being affected by the work. Let's talk about ways you can take care of yourself so you won't be. I'm glad you told me.

Training is an important support as well, including obtaining skills related to trauma and coping (Cunningham, 2003; Dane, 2000). Social work organizations can also help empower staff through advocacy and social action (Hesse, 2002). These activities counteract the feelings of helplessness engendered by trauma work as they help fight root causes of trauma on a macro level.

Tips

- *Social action* – Working with survivors can cause us to feel helpless and alone. Social action offers a constructive way to fight the wrongs we witness as we work with survivors. Getting a group of survivors or colleagues together to ask legislators to increase funding for cancer research or to fight intimate partner violence is an empowering action that may not only alleviate the impact of trauma in society but also prevent secondary trauma.

Case Study

Andrea was a second-year master's-level social work intern in her 20s. She lived with her fiancé, attended a prestigious college and did well in school. She felt enthusiastic about the competitive internship she procured at an outpatient trauma clinic and raved about the training and peer support available. She looked forward to beginning to provide treatment herself. Her enthusiasm waned with the assignment of her first individual client, a survivor of intimate partner violence who lived with her abuser.

In supervision, Andrea asked if another intern could take her client, saying it was not a good fit. She admitted she did not like the client who was always late, complained about Andrea during sessions and asked Andrea if she could work with someone else. Delving deeper, it became clear that part of the problem was her approach. She described sitting with a notebook in front of her, taking notes and making little eye contact as a result. It almost sounded as though she was hiding from her client.

Andrea also had difficulties co-leading a group. She did not speak up unless assigned something specific to say and delivered these contributions authoritatively with no genuine emotion. As she slowly began to say more, she often made out-of-place comments as though she had missed much of the conversation. She also tended to downplay traumatic stories and the group members' difficulties.

Finally, Andrea shared that she was a survivor herself. She realized it when she learned about trauma and got in touch with how abusive her father was. He hit her mother, and the house was often chaotic and scary. He called Andrea names, telling her she was not as important as she thought she was. Even though he never hit her, she lived in fear, witnessing his aggression and bearing the brunt of his verbal abuse.

Her background made Andrea vulnerable to vicarious traumatization, which started to affect her during the training period and worsened as she began to work with clients. Getting in touch with this allowed her to work on these issues in psychotherapy. As a fortuitous consequence, this realization empowered her to raise awareness of the effects of secondary trauma among other interns.

RESOURCES

Figley, C.R. (1995). *Compassion fatigue: Coping with secondary traumatic stress disorder in those who treat the traumatized*. New York: Routledge.

Pearlman, L.A., & Saakvitne, K. (1995). *Trauma and the therapist: Countertransference and vicarious traumatization in psychotherapy with incest survivors*. New York: WW Norton & Company.

Rothschild, B.A. (2006). *Help for the helper: The psychophysiology of compassion fatigue and vicarious trauma*. New York: WW Norton & Company.

Saakvitne, K., & Pearlman, L.A. (1996). *Transforming the pain: A workbook on vicarious traumatization*. New York: WW Norton & Company.

Wicks, R.J. (2008). *The resilient clinician*. New York: Oxford University Press.

Practice Exercises and Questions

- Observe your emotions and reactions to clients, making note of what may be secondary trauma reactions
- Come up with a list of ways you can begin to take care of yourself and cope
- Institute your new coping regime and observe the results, also noting how you feel when you cope less than planned
- Try different kinds of coping and compare the results
- Role-play a supervision session or an attempt to get help from a supervisor

You can be Affected too: Secondary Trauma Summary

Tune in to Self

- *Be aware of your personal sense of safety*
- *Remember past losses and current stressors*
- *Focus on emotions, thoughts and your physical state*

Watch for Signs of Secondary Trauma

- *Symptoms similar to those of survivors*
- *Intense emotional reactions*
- *Distracted, disconnected, fatigued or bored*

Vulnerabilities

- *Student, new therapist or new to trauma work*
- *Past history of trauma or traumatic loss*
- *Current stressors, including feeling sick, hungry or tired*
- *Insufficient or inconsistent self-care*

Key Practitioner Skills

- *Be aware of transference and countertransference*
- *Track emotions as they occur – yours and those of the survivors*
- *Establish appropriate boundaries*

What Helps

- *Awareness, self-reflection and coping*
- *Clinical supervision*
- *Network of support, including administrative support*
- *Empowerment through social action and advocacy*

Chapter 2

Practitioner Bias and Vulnerability

What practitioners bring to the table as they work with survivors is important to the process. Our biases and vulnerabilities aid or hinder these relationships, depending on our level of awareness and how we work with them. Practitioner cultural heritages and backgrounds create values and beliefs, essentially making us who we are. To truly understand our clients and ourselves, we must be aware of the postures we take toward life, as well as the emotive responses life experiences elicit. These dimensions create incalculable levels of intensity and can encourage a cooperative spirit between us and our clients rather than antagonisms that can jeopardize healing.

A hodgepodge of elements such as our ages, disabilities, religions, ethnicities, sexual orientations, genders, relationship and family statuses, sizes, attractiveness, relationships with violence and trauma and emotional and physical woundedness (Brown, 2009a), among others, lurk in the background as we work with clients. This chapter explores how Trauma Informed Care (TIC) allows us to be effective and genuine practitioners as these factors in us and our clients interact.

TUNE IN TO SELF

Self-awareness, which is key to TIC, entails tuning in to ourselves often and reflecting on what we find (Hammond, 2013). Doing so is helpful before and after meeting with clients and at any time we begin to feel stuck, even if only for a moment during a session. It can also be helpful when experiencing trauma indirectly, such as with reading a book such as this or when witnessing trauma personally or through the media.

While reflecting, note which parts of you (e.g., your age, gender, trauma background) are affected by interactions. Explore these areas as they intersect with survivors so that you can be as clear as possible about what is happening between you as you work, remembering that you are as much a part of this process as are your clients.

> **Tips**
>
> - *Tune in to self* – Do a quick check for any physical, emotional and cognitive discomfort. Try to identify the source. Breathe into it or use other means to relax and nurture yourself. If the discomfort remains, remember you are carrying it with you so that it will not cause difficulty later.

SETTING THE STAGE FOR MULTICULTURALISM AND TRAUMA INFORMED CARE

When I was new to the field and working with a supervisor, he said something that has always stayed with me. He said that he worked as openly and authentically with as much of his inner self exposed as he could, while still maintaining good boundaries. He also said that the balance of this changes with time and circumstances. I have found this to be true, and it has challenged me to be present and authentic with clients, rather than stepping back and observing them from a clinical distance.

This is a part of TIC and involves not just knowing the facts of their histories and current existences but getting to the heart of who they are at the apex of the factors that constitute them, including culture, ethnicity, economic status, physicality, history, current circumstances and other (Brown, 2009a). It also means coming from a place of acceptance and beginning the work as they direct rather than where we think it should (Brown, 2009a). Staying aware of the fact that our ideas and perspectives are socially constructed, just as our clients' are, helps us to accept them as they are and to work with an openness to how they present their lives (Del Rio, 2004).

An example of this is work I did following the sudden death of my mother. I later read about a practitioner who was so affected by the death of a loved one that he stopped working. I now understand why. The vulnerability was intense, and I was often close to tears. Compounding this, I had just returned from a two-week vacation when this occurred and wanted my clients to know that I was taking additional time off for something important so I told them about her death. This knowledge changed therapeutic relationships. One, in particular, was touching. A man who began working with me following his mother's death, proclaimed he was attracted to me and asked me out. In the midst of a discussion about therapeutic intimacy often mistaken for something else, it became clear that this was his way of trying to help. It was an offering to me in my grief and was a beautiful thing that could have easily been misconstrued had I not allowed myself to be open. In this circumstance, I was able to work with this client both openly and authentically with, as my supervisor said, as much of my inner self exposed as possible while still maintaining good boundaries.

HOW SOCIAL WORK PRINCIPLES PERTAIN

The principles of social work are in line with multiculturalism and can guide us in our work. Going where clients are, for instance, and working with them, there is a tenet of social work that includes finding ways to work that fit their individual needs (Brown, 2009a). We tend to gravitate toward approaches and develop techniques that suit us as helping professionals. Making changes to allow for what survivors need stretches us, making us more accessible to them, changing our focus from treatment-centric to client-centric (Jacob, 2013) and ultimately improving treatment outcomes.

We also need to follow the principles of (1) social justice and (2) respect for the dignity and worth of all people, being vigilant about discrimination/bias and the imperative of social workers supporting and promoting their clients' socially responsible self-determination (Del Rio, 2004; Wahler, 2012). This involves understanding who survivors are and striving to see through their lens rather than our own, since ours is colored by who we are and can block us from who they are (Wahler, 2012).

Finally and most importantly, we must do no harm (APA, 2017), remembering that even harm is a social construct, the definition of which varies from person to person based on all that has made them who they are (Wendt, Gone, & Nagata, 2015). The following section discusses potential pitfalls that can lead to inadvertent harm.

PITFALLS OF IGNORING CULTURE

It can be harmful to ignore culture or to be culturally insensitive (Wendt, Gone, & Nagata, 2015). This includes areas we might not ordinarily think about. I recently had a client who described a night of drinking after insisting he did not have an issue with alcohol although his boyfriend said he did. He drank a large amount for him and he was a small man – nine drinks of hard liquor before he lost count, passed out at a stranger's house, woke still feeling drunk and proceeded to drive home. It was an hour's drive, and as he drove, he began feeling sicker and then had a panic attack. He described crying and making multiple phone calls while driving. I was concerned and told him he was lucky to be alive. That was not inappropriate, but what I failed to do was to be with him in the moment, looking at it from his eyes. No matter how right I felt I was, my judgement was not helpful. I failed him in that moment and therefore, in my estimation, did harm. It may have been a wake-up call for him as well but could have been done with acceptance and understanding rather than judgement. How different would his experience have been, for instance, had I said, "I am angry at you for jeopardizing your life and so grateful that you are safe and whole."

Acceptance of survivors as individuals, versus seeing them as traumatized people separate and different from us, enables connection and is an important piece of multiculturalism (Brown, 2008). This may seem simple and natural, since our caring natures led us to trauma work, but in actuality, it can often feel safer and easier to be the experts and to keep ourselves separate by doing so (Sweeney, Filson, Kennedy, Collinson, & Gillard, 2018). The fact that therapists often feel nervous about using TIC treatments – which makes sense, since trauma work can be difficult (Van Minnen et al., 2018), can increase the desire for distance. I like to think of it as me on my throne with my subjects at my feet. I got this analogy from a client who laughed at my new higher-backed chair, playfully calling it my throne. There is always a power dynamic in our relationships with clients. My chair is a metaphor for the hierarchy. Just thinking about it can bring me back to earth and into connection with clients.

Other barriers to connected multicultural care include relationships that are hierarchical, exhibit authority/power over clients or reduce their self-determinism (Sweeney et al, 2018). These snafus can also retraumatize and/or diminish survivors' self-confidence as they trigger memories of perpetrators who also had power over them (Sweeney et all, 2018). Not only this, but some treatment approaches can be ethnocentric – westernized, for instance – and without awareness of this, psychoeducation can become an attempt to change survivors' perspectives so they can see the approaches as we do (Wendt, Gone, & Nagata, 2015). Fortunately, because students can be prone to these mishaps, education in this area is increasing (Wahler, 2012).

PRINCIPLES OF TRAUMA INFORMED CARE AND MULTICULTURALISM

Respect, consideration, seeing beyond individuals' trauma experiences to who they are at their cores and appreciating the attributes found there are all proponents of TIC and of multiculturalism. TIC also demands qualities like "kindness; warmth; empathy; honesty; trustworthiness; reassurance; friendliness; helpfulness; calmness; and humor" (Sweeney, Fahmy, Nolan, Morant, Fox, Lloyd-Evans, et al. , 2014, p. 6), as well as "transparency, collaboration and mutuality, [and] empowerment" (Sweeney et al, 2018, p. 18). These aspects of therapeutic relationships are key to TIC and to trauma recovery (Jacob, 2013).

Multiculturalism goes beyond this to the rich contextual landscape that forms our multifaceted perceptions of all aspects of life in society. Asking questions allows us to explore and gain knowledge of this within both ourselves and survivors (Jacob, 2013). The questions we can ask are numerous and include things like: What is the problem that needs addressing? What caused it? How does it affect you? How bad is it? What's the worst part about it? What scares you the most about it? As we ask these and specific questions about cultural context, we can notice where our thoughts on the questions differ from theirs. This underscores where our beliefs, values and other constructs differ (Del Rio, 2004).

Exploring these differing beliefs engenders trust (Del Rio, 2004), as do the methodologies we utilize. We can, for instance, be like the American television detective, Columbo, who interrogates in an innocent and curious way that is accepting and disarming, but who is also wise and gets to the root causes of things, reminding ourselves that culture changes as social/political contexts change and that multiculturalism requires knowledge of similarities and differences (Del Rio, 2004).

OUR IDENTITIES AND VULNERABILITIES VERSUS SURVIVORS'

As we work with survivors, our combined multicultural identities and vulnerabilities coalesce, complimenting and/or complicating interactions, depending on our levels of awareness and how we work with them. Practitioner vulnerabilities and contexts include our expectations, positive/negative coping, stressors, levels of proficiency and support/supervision, trauma histories and physical/cultural characteristics (Saakvitne & Pearlman, 1996). Survivors' multicultural identities and vulnerabilities include the problems they come in with, limited resources, suffering due to trauma, lack of trust, safety issues, shame and lack of coping skills (Saakvitne & Pearlman, 1996). In addition, societal factors come into play that include judgement about trauma, such as blaming the victim, and organizational milieus that are not trauma informed (Saakvitne & Pearlman, 1996).

Trauma itself also has an identity that is a part of the mix. The emotions that come up for us as we work point to where our wounds are (Brown, 2009a). The effect can be so intense that our positivity can wane (Kaufman, 2014) and life can begin to lose meaning (Hammond, 2013). This can be true even if we do not have trauma histories of our own, but is intensified if we do, especially if we are caught unaware. How trauma impacts the survivors we work with also affects us and can at times not make sense. It is in these moments that we can learn more as we make an effort to see things as they do (Brown, 2008).

INTERSECTION OF SURVIVOR AND PRACTITIONER BIASES

The intersection of survivor/practitioner biases and cultures can weave a tapestry of healing when multiculturalism and TIC are employed, allowing us to see survivors as part of a shared human experience instead of as damaged by trauma. We can then acknowledge them as a part of the same mix we all face. This adds a richness to the experience and aids healing of them, as well as us, because the work we do is in fact a shared experience (Brown, 2008).

Exploring this intersection requires careful attention to identity and cultural norms – theirs and ours – and consciousness of how we differ (Brown, 2009a).

Discovering the nature of their personal metamorphoses and dreams for the future also helps. This is particularly true if we can acknowledge that these supersede the effects of trauma, noting how both relate to our own stories (Brown, 2009a).

Staying closely aligned with the ways we differ from clients is key, keeping in mind cultural, physical, economic, ethnic, emotional and social aspects of selves. This includes remembering that practitioners are automatically at a different level hierarchically (Brown, 2009a), making our efforts to find balance in the relationship crucial. Knowing that identity – ours and theirs – is altered when positivity, resilience, stress and dysfunction are introduced is also important (Brown, 2009a).

ALLOWING CONNECTION AND HEALING BY DROPPING OUR PRACTITIONER MASKS

Working with survivors from this place of intersection enables the removal of our practitioner masks, so that we can connect authentically rather than clinically. Doing so while maintaining appropriate boundaries can be challenging but is well worth the effort. It means utilizing the TIC/human qualities of compassion and acceptance – for ourselves and clients – and the language of us rather than you as we work instead of the classic practitioner neutrality.

Being aware of biases when they come up is also important and helps us work with them. Sharing them with clients can create connection when done in a culturally sensitive way, such as when requesting elucidation of unfamiliar cultural nuances (Brown, 2009a). I, for instance, was conflicted by my first encounter with a polyamorous client. I had a view at the time of infidelity as hurtful and potentially damaging, particularly when clandestine, and had to adjust my thoughts so as to not to put polyamory in this category, as all parties in this type of relationship have knowledge and consent of everyone involved. The process was challenging, since my first polyamorous client believed in the approach but was hurt by her partner not following the practice guidelines. Making an effort to be open, I found that once I learned about the boundaries of this practice, I began to admire how well thought out it is, particularly regarding safety and balance. These excavation processes are multiculturalism (Brown, 2009a).

SELF-CARE AND REFLECTION ARE KEY TO TRAUMA INFORMED CARE

Multiculturalism is not possible without reflection and self-care. This is why TIC core values emphasize self-care for staff and caring environments for organizations (Hales et al., 2019). The three Rs illustrate this – realizing that trauma is prevalent, recognizing signs and symptoms in staff and responding by reflecting this in organizational policies and practices (Kaufman, 2014).

Reflection includes being aware of and nurturing our humanity as we work (Hammond, 2013). This is important because understanding and accepting clients requires self-exploration and healing (Del Rio, 2004). Knowing ourselves, via self-reflection, allows us to be mindfully present with clients as they share horrendous trauma (Rothschild, 2006). In these moments, our connection with ourselves lets us feel compassion rather than our own and our clients' pain (Rothschild, 2006).

A reciprocal transformation occurs when these multicultural TIC practices are employed. Connecting with and learning about clients changes how we look at the world so that we heal and grow. They grow as well, learning from the process about safe relationships and trust – key for healing from trauma (Brown, 2008).

See Chapter 12 for more information on self-care. By building our skills in this area, we boost our abilities as practitioners and improve our personal lives as well.

Definitions

- *Coping* – Process of dealing with difficulties, problem solving and adapting to the environment in order to manage stress and conflict effectively.
- *Safety* – State essential to trauma recovery and unique to each individual in which (1) risky behaviors, unhealthy relationships and negative emotions are reduced and (2) a sense of well-being, trust, calm and positive coping are increased.

Case Study

Something that is not often discussed is the issue of practitioner privacy and what can occur when it is broken. This is an even more interesting question in light of the principles of multiculturalism and TIC, which encourage authenticity, openness and honesty. Of course, following these principles does not mean we have no secrets and inappropriately share our personal information with clients, but it does mean a different way of working with boundaries than how we may have been trained.

Craig was a single man, with a history of childhood sexual abuse, who was lonely and looking for a mate online. While reviewing possibilities, he came upon my profile and mentioned it to me in an offhand way. Although I was single at the time and knew clients might see me online, his comment was unexpected. He made it easy for me, saying, "You know what it's like looking online." He said this with a smile and what looked like relief. I agreed that online dating is difficult and a bit like looking for a needle in a haystack, and he laughed.

Ulman (2001) writes about how experiences like this with clients can create vulnerability. Examples of personal information becoming available to clients include pregnancy, engagement (when wearing a ring), divorce (when ring is no longer worn), being seen in public with or without family or friends and potentially engaged in activities clients could not have known about or dressed in a manner we would not during business hours. There is also the possibility of clients googling us and finding information that way.

Fortunately, vulnerability is not necessarily a bad thing, especially if we have the opportunity to prepare for it ahead of time, such as when we plan for how we will introduce our pregnancy with clients. With awareness and reflection, vulnerability can allow more connection and authenticity into the relationship (Ulman, 2001).

Ulman (2001) also says that we can take advantage of these situations and derive positive outcomes that propel growth. I found this to be true with Craig. We were able to talk about his dating and hunger for a relationship in a more meaningful way after his admission, and I shared more openly as well. I did not share personal information, but he assumed a lot, saying things like, "You know how it is" or "I know you know what it means to be single." And when he noticed I was no longer online, he assumed I was in a relationship and was heartened by that. It seemed to give him hope that he would be too. These are important things for trauma survivors, who often feel alone with their suffering and may have difficulty opening up, trusting and connecting. As Ulman (2001) states, these experiences can help clients connect and feel less alone. That was true with Craig. He felt safer as a result and was able to do Eye Movement Desensitization and Reprocessing (EMDR) work (see chapter 17 for more information) that he had resisted before that, aiding his recovery. This would not have occurred had I not been willing to follow the multiculturalism and TIC principles of authenticity and openness, enabling our relationship to deepen and grow.

RESOURCES

Brown, L.S. (2008). *Cultural competence in trauma therapy: Beyond the flashback.* Washington, D.C.: American Psychological Association.

Brown, L.S. (2009). Cultural competence: A new way of looking at integration in psychotherapy. *Journal of Psychotherapy Integration, 19*(4), 340–353.

Filson, B., Kennedy, A., Collinson, L., & Gillard, S. (2018). A paradigm shift: Relationships in trauma-informed mental health services. *BJPsych Advances*, *24*(5), 319–333.

Wahler, E. (2012). Identifying and challenging social work students' biases. *Social Work Education*, *31*(8), 1058–1070.

Practice Exercises and Questions

- Write all the aspects of who you are, including categories discussed in this chapter
- Think about someone who is different from you, and write down what aspects are different and where you are similar
- Role-play working with a client who is different from you and has aspects you know nothing about. Discuss afterwards any challenges encountered
- Role-play working with a client who is similar to you and discuss afterwards how similarities can throw you off as well. Hint: We can be less vigilant exploring those we think we know because they seem like us

Practitioner Bias and Vulnerability

Setting the Stage for Multiculturalism and Trauma Informed Care: How Social Work Principles Pertain

- *Knowing not only clients' histories and issues but all aspects of who they are*
- *Includes their ages, disabilities, religions, ethnicities, sexual orientations, genders, relationship and family statuses, sizes, attractiveness, hopes and dreams*
- *Follows the social work principles of working where the client is, doing no harm and practicing from a point of view of social justice and respect for the dignity and worth of all people*

Pitfalls of Ignoring Culture

- *Clinical approach in which we see clients as traumatized and other*
- *Relationships with clients that are hierarchical, exhibit authority/power over them or reduce their self-determinism*
- *Treatment approaches that are ethnocentric or otherwise difficult for survivors to relate to*

Principles of Trauma Informed Care and Multiculturalism

- TIC embodies respect, consideration, kindness, warmth, empathy, honesty, trustworthiness, reassurance, friendliness, helpfulness, calmness, humor, transparency, collaboration, mutuality and empowerment
- Multiculturalism goes beyond this to the rich contextual landscape that forms our multifaceted perceptions of all aspects of life in society

Intersection of Survivor and Practitioner Biases

- The intersection of survivor/practitioner biases and cultures can weave a tapestry of healing when multiculturalism and TIC are employed
- Exploring this intersection requires careful attention to identity and cultural norms – theirs and ours – and consciousness of how we differ
- Working with survivors from this place of intersection enables the removal of our practitioner masks, so that we can connect authentically rather than clinically. This process allows reciprocal healing and growth to occur.

Self-Care and Reflection Are Key to Trauma Informed Care

- The three Rs – realizing that trauma is prevalent, recognizing signs and symptoms in staff and responding by reflecting this in organizational policies and practices
- Reflection – including being aware of and nurturing our humanity as we work. Knowing ourselves allows us to be mindfully present with clients.
- Building our self-care skills boosts our abilities as practitioners and improves our personal lives as well

Part II

Understanding Trauma

Chapter 3

Traumatic Events

People who fear for their own or others' safety can have difficulty processing traumatic events; at times, this can lead to post-traumatic stress disorder
(PTSD). The *Diagnostic and Statistical Manual of Mental Disorders* (DSM-IV-TR)
(American Psychiatric Association, 2000) specified these events as (1) military
combat; (2) violent personal assaults (physical attacks, robberies, muggings and
sexual assaults, including developmentally inappropriate sexual experiences
without threatened or actual violence or injury); (3) kidnappings; (4) hostage
situations; (5) terrorist attacks; (6) torture; (7) incarcerations as prisoners of
war or in concentration camps; (8) natural disasters; (9) man-made disasters;
(10) severe automobile accidents; or (11) being diagnosed with a life-threatening
illness.

The distressing impact on survivors of these types of events is explored here
and in the following chapters of Part II of the book.

Definitions

- *Post-traumatic stress disorder (PTSD)* – A disorder resulting from
  exposure to traumatic events that causes symptoms lasting at least a
  month that include emotional responses of fear, horror or helplessness; flashbacks and/or nightmares of events; avoidance of reminders
  of the event; and increased arousal.
- *Flashback* – Intrusive and involuntary re-experiencing of traumatic
  events through images, emotions or physical sensations.
- *Safety* – State essential to trauma recovery and unique to each individual in which (1) risky behaviors, unhealthy relationships and negative emotions are reduced and (2) a sense of well-being, trust, calm
  and positive coping are increased.

TUNE IN TO TRAUMA

Tune in to your own experiences of exposure to trauma. As you do so, keep safe in the process, avoiding memories that might distress you and referring to Chapter 12 on self-care and Chapter 1 on secondary trauma if coping with these memories becomes difficult.

If no events within these categories come to mind or if tuning in to these events is too upsetting, focus instead upon secondary trauma from clients with whom you have worked, family or historical trauma such as the Holocaust, media reports or difficult losses. As you focus on a specific event, make note of your responses, paying attention to your thoughts, physical sensations and emotions. This will help you to understand and relate as you read the chapter.

Tips

- *Tune in to self* – Do a quick check within yourself for any physical, emotional and cognitive discomfort. Try to identify the source of any discomfort you find. Breathe into it or use other means to relax and nurture yourself. If it remains, remember you are carrying it with you, so that it will not cause difficulty later.

BACKGROUND INFORMATION

Traumatic events with (1) the fear or reality of bodily harm or victimization for self or others and (2) the feeling that nothing can be done to stop what is happening are horrendous (Reyes, Elhai, & Ford, 2008). When experiences overwhelm survivors to the point where they are unable to make sense of them and feel unsafe as a result, psychological trauma or a trauma response occurs (Giller, 1999).

The incidence of trauma in the United States is high, with about 70% of adults having experienced a traumatic event at least once in their lives, and up to 20% of those developing PTSD. In fact, about 5% of Americans (more than 13 million people) have PTSD at any given time and 8% of adults (1 in 13) will develop PTSD during their lifetime. Estimates show that women are twice as likely as men to develop PTSD, with about one out of ten women in the United States diagnosed with PTSD at some time in their lives (PTSD Alliance, 2001a).

To society, the financial cost of trauma is high. In the United States, survivors with PTSD are among the highest users of healthcare. They report a range of symptoms, generally not identified as resulting from trauma. Treatment related to anxiety disorders costs about US$42.3 billion a year. This includes psychiatric and medical treatment, prescription drugs and indirect workplace and mortality costs. More than half of this expense comes from frequent healthcare for anxiety-related symptoms that look like other physical conditions. Most expenses from anxiety disorders, including PTSD, are direct medical costs, estimated at US$23 billion a year (PTSD Alliance, 2001a).

TYPES OF TRAUMATIC EVENTS

Chapters 4, 5 and 6 discuss several types of traumatic events encountered by social workers' clients: Family abuse/neglect, war and terrorism and life-threatening illness. The magnitude of other potentially traumatic events is in itself overwhelming: Rape and sexual abuse/assault, physical assault, community and school violence, industrial accidents, car accidents, fires, natural disasters, plane/train crashes, sudden deaths (PTSD Alliance, 2001b), growing up with alcoholics or drug addicts (McCann & Pearlman, 1990a), severe and unexpected losses, serious injuries, invasive medical procedures, discrimination and historical trauma (Weingarten, 2004).

For the purpose of discussion in this chapter and the following three chapters, we will categorize events as (1) family traumas; (2) school and organizational traumas; (3) community traumas; (4) disasters; (5) war and terrorism; (6) unexpected events; and (7) other potentially traumatic events.

- Family traumas include child, the disabled and elder abuse/neglect and intimate partner violence; school and organizational traumas include death or suicide, bullying and disasters occurring in these domains; community traumas include violence, stalking, human trafficking and rape; disasters include major accidents and natural disasters; war and terrorism include torture and child soldiering; unexpected events include severe losses such as sudden death; and other potentially traumatic events include discrimination and historical trauma. This chapter does not discuss severe injuries and invasive medical procedures, but they share characteristics of life-threatening illness and sudden unexpected losses.

Definitions

- *Post-traumatic stress disorder (PTSD)* – A disorder resulting from exposure to traumatic events that causes symptoms lasting at least a month that include emotional responses of fear, horror or helplessness; flashbacks and/or nightmares of events; avoidance of reminders of the event; and increased arousal.

FAMILY TRAUMA

Family trauma, which is discussed in the following chapter, is complicated by the fact that those who should provide safety and protection are the perpetrators. It is also generally a chronic issue rather than a one-off occurrence, and repeated traumatic events have been found to have a more harmful and enduring impact (Courtois, 2010).

Incest (sexual abuse by family members) harms survivors in a number of ways that include emotional dysregulation, a distorted and often negative sense of self, physical issues such as chronic pain and somatic preoccupation, sexual promiscuity or withdrawal and orgasmic disorders, interpersonal difficulty relating to and trusting others and social isolation or compulsive over involvement. Incest can also confuse survivors because most are coerced by people they know and love who tell them they are having normal, pleasurable and even educative sexual acts. Perpetrators generally tell children that the incest is a secret, not to be shared with others. And incest often has apparent benefits that attract children: Closeness to and special attention from a family member they love and look up to; favors and gifts; and sexuality that can be both pleasant and scary for children not developmentally prepared for the stimulation (Courtois, 2010).

The cultural practice of female circumcision has been termed a form of sexual abuse as well. Sadly, the practice is not uncommon, with approximately 130 million victims. At least 2 million girls a year (or 5,500 a day) are likely to have their genitals cut, usually with no anesthesia. Many have chronic pain and infection; difficulties with sexual intercourse, urination and childbirth; and psychological reactions as a result. Some even die from bleeding or infection. One survivor talked about being ridiculed and called a coward when she refused to have it done. She also described cruelty during the procedure, having the knife waved in her face before being cut and her wound being pried at after being cut (Gathanju, 2006). Studies have found that circumcised women have significantly more PTSD and other mental illness than the general population (Behrendt & Moritz, 2005).

Substance abuse is another family issue that can have traumatic effects. It is harmful because it is often accompanied by emotional, physical and sexual abuse. Furthermore, the insecurity of unmet needs and of never knowing what to expect in households with substance abuse teaches children to be rigorously self-sufficient, promoting difficulty with trust and limiting their abilities to find intimacy with others (McCann & Pearlman, 1990a).

Reactions to family traumas can be severe and are often not treated until survivors become adults out on their own. When possible and safe, family treatment can be particularly helpful. Groups are also healing. See Chapters 15 and 16 on these modalities for more information.

Definitions

- *Intimate partner violence (IPV)* – Emotionally, physically, sexually, economically or psychologically violent behavior used to exert power and control in the context of intimate or formerly intimate relationships.
- *Neglect* – Failure to provide for a dependent individual's basic needs, including physical, educational and emotional needs.
- *Physical abuse* – Behavior that includes a pattern of hitting, kicking, shaking, burning or otherwise physically harming an individual.
- *Sexual abuse* – Coercive use of an individual for sexual gratification and/or other sexual purposes. With the elderly, disabled and children, this includes any unlawful sexual act even if coercion is not involved.

SCHOOL AND ORGANIZATIONAL TRAUMA

School and organizational trauma includes death or suicide, bullying and disasters occurring in these domains. These should be safe places with authorities such as teachers, bosses, medical practitioners and government officials protecting those for whom they are responsible. The betrayal of not being protected can contribute to survivors' difficulty in recovering, especially if they do not get good post-trauma care.

A variety of traumas happen in schools, including the death or suicide of a student or staff member, accidents, fires and disasters in the community. In order to deal with these events, schools have developed crisis plans that include ensuring safety and security, communicating information about the event to those involved and providing psychological support and referrals when needed (Newgass & Schonfeld, 2005).

Bullying, often a school issue, can also occur in organizations, even with adults. Victims become increasingly vulnerable when bullied, and this worsens if it continues over time. It traumatizes many children, particularly if their pain goes unrecognized or is misunderstood by others (Mishna, 2007). If teachers, for instance, see bullying and do nothing to stop it, children become more distressed (Weingarten, 2004). The results of this potentially traumatic experience can be lethal. A factor contributing to the Columbine High School shooting in 1999 was that the perpetrators were bullied (Mishna, 2007). At least one adolescent boy, Eric, has even committed suicide as a result of bullying (James, 2009).

How management and other authorities respond to traumatic events truly matters because (1) a caring response is the right thing to do for humane reasons; (2) workers who are taken care of and feel safe are more productive; and (3) it makes sense from a legal point of view (Klein & Alexander, 2011). One of the ways in which workers can be supported after a disaster is by management helping them to build their resilience. Human services organizations utilizing the Sanctuary Model® have done so successfully. This is an evidence-based methodology in which staff commit to open communication, growth as an organization, nonviolence, emotional intelligence, social learning, democracy and social responsibility (Bloom, 2011).

COMMUNITY TRAUMA

With community violence, residents need to feel that those in charge will protect and care for them. Community trauma includes assault, stalking, human trafficking and rape. It has far-reaching effects, disturbing many individuals and families in a variety of ways, including causing feelings of danger or potential danger and loss of lives, homes and security (Klingman & Cohen, 2004). This is true whether an individual or a group directly experiences a traumatic event, since individual traumas in the community are upsetting for its members. For instance, when someone stabbed a social work student to death on her way home from her internship, it reverberated throughout the social work school, traumatically impacting staff and students.

Stalking terrifies individuals, even leading to paranoia when it is long term. Survivors feel unable to maintain the safety of their personal space, losing their freedom and solitude. Some must relocate, leaving those they love, in order to escape the stalker, but they often remain afraid even after the move (Knox & Roberts, 2005).

Sexual assault and rape in the community can shock and overwhelm, particularly when enacted by a peer whom they considered safe. Survivors are at risk for PTSD and need to find a way to feel secure after the event. This trauma deepens in complexity when cultural beliefs lead to shame and secrecy about what occurred. Survivors often even blame themselves (Briere & Scott, 2006).

Definitions

- *Human trafficking* – Occurs when services are obtained fraudulently, coercively, forcefully or from children under 18 years old, leading to involuntary performance of sexual acts, servitude or slavery.

Poor, immigrant, young, isolated and female individuals are most vulnerable to human trafficking, another form of community trauma. The phenomenon generally occurs when individuals are born into slavery, hoodwinked, kidnapped, sold or physically forced. Similar to victims of intimate partner violence, those affected cannot escape because they are afraid, isolated, physically and psychologically restricted and unable to get help. These marginalized survivors need resources and outreach (Logan, Walker, & Hunt, 2009).

As with many trauma survivors, survivors of mass murder in the community require special care, including access to mental healthcare providers as needed when in crisis due to intense nightmares, flashbacks or other trauma symptoms. In addition, these survivors tend to become angry when in session with practitioners because of intense emotions related to their trauma experience (Roberts, 2005b).

During and after a community trauma, it is crucial that community members are cared for, with public officials ensuring they are kept from harm; offered support and medical care if needed; and provided with food, clothing, water and shelter (Roberts, 2005b). Community outreach is needed to access survivors who often do not seek help. Many rape victims, for instance, never seek assistance despite the high incidence of PTSD and other trauma reactions. When large numbers of community members are affected directly, outreach is even more important (McCann & Pearlman, 1990a). Parents, for example, often need assistance because they can have difficulty being there for their children when they themselves are traumatized (Weingarten, 2004).

DISASTER

Disaster includes major accidents and natural disaster. With large-scale transportation accidents, fires and natural disasters, survivors' needs for support, comfort, medical treatment, food, water, clothing and shelter must be attended to. Even car accidents traumatize individuals and can be complicated by (1) injuries such as head trauma and (2) self-blame, particularly if someone else was hurt or killed (Briere & Scott, 2006).

Large-scale fires and house fires also traumatize. Loss of lives, homes and belongings adds to the resulting distress. Burns, scars, disfigurement and chronic pain compound traumatic effects, making it difficult for survivors to move on from the event (Briere & Scott, 2006). This dream from a survivor illustrates the horror:

> What I recall is an absolutely terrifying nightmare in which the fire had developed an organic consciousness. It was the embodiment of evil. It hid itself very well up on the hill in a pile of brush where it waited for all the fire departments to leave. Then it came back to get the houses it had missed. Somehow it had marked these houses with a fire seed and all it had to do was pass by the fire seeds for the house to ignite. I woke up screaming because I saw our "fire seed" begin to swell. In the dream, I was alone in the house.

Natural disasters tend to be widespread, affecting whole communities and leading to loss of lives, homes, jobs, schools, hospitals and utilities. The perpetrator of the events is nature, which can be difficult (Weingarten, 2004). Instead of nurturing, nature seems to become malevolent, which can feel like a betrayal and loss of security. This dream of a survivor shows the disbelief and shock with this type of event:

> I am in a remote jungle-like region. I am holding the hand of a 4-year-old girl. I know that a volcano is going to erupt, but no one will believe me. I continue to warn people of the impending danger, yet no one will believe me. I have to get to the top of the mountain, to the very edge of the volcano. It is very difficult to climb, the trail is steep and slippery. It is too hard for the little girl, so I have to put her on my back. There is a feeling of doom if I don't get to the top. It is so steep and difficult that I have to crawl on my hands and knees, still carrying the child. At the top of the mountain, the volcano starts to blow…

With some natural disasters, such as Hurricane Katrina in 2005, survivors face multiple traumas. With Katrina, this included the hurricane, flooding, loss of loved ones and community violence. The impact was seen with reports of 31% of children having PTSD symptoms (Jaycox et al., 2007). Others who were vulnerable included those with physical disabilities and mental illness (Rosen, Matthieu, & Norris, 2009).

During disasters, familiar surroundings and belongings are often lost; children, who depend on these things for their security, find this difficult. The loss of a cherished blanket or stuffed animal can be harder for a child than not knowing when food will be available. Validating these concerns and letting children know they are understood after a trauma are important. Comforting them and helping them to relax are also essential (Brooks & Siegel, 1996).

UNEXPECTED EVENTS

Unexpected events include severe losses like sudden death and divorce. Loss of life is most likely to traumatize when the person who dies is someone close to the survivor. It can also be traumatic when caused by a traumatic event or if it triggers past trauma or loss memories (McBride & Johnson, 2005).

The experience of a woman who was very upset by the death of her husband's co-worker illustrates the traumatic triggering of past losses. She did not know the co-worker well, but his death reminded her of her brother's sudden death and the loss of control she felt as a result. Trauma can also be triggered by the inability to locate the bodies of loved ones, as with many deaths caused by the September 11th disaster; and the combination of multiple losses/stressors and stage-of-life issues, as was the case for a 13-year-old girl whose father was an alcoholic. Her parents divorced a year before the death of her much-loved grandmother. The death traumatized her because of the combined stressors and losses (McBride & Johnson, 2005; O'Halloran, Ingala, & Copeland, 2005). Grief in these instances can be complicated and difficult to process if the traumatic impact is not addressed.

Ramona, who came to a bereavement group mourning the sudden death of her father, offers an example of grief complicated by trauma issues. Her father collapsed on the street near his home and died, with no known medical issues and at a time of life when he was not expected to die. The sudden and unexpected nature of his death made it difficult for her to process it. She was unable to do so until she got help in applying trauma theory and found a safe place within herself through extensive coping.

Definitions

* *Coping* – Process of dealing with difficulties, problem solving and adapting to the environment in order to manage stress and conflict effectively.

Divorce can be complicated by extenuating circumstances as well, triggering a traumatic response. This was true for the man who came home to find his wife having sex with two men and for the woman infected with genital herpes resulting from her husband having sex with their neighbor (Granvold, 2005). Unexpected disturbing details complicated both events.

In order to protect children from a traumatic impact related to death or divorce, we need to work with them to establish safety. Inviting and helping them to tell and/or write their own story of what happened is beneficial. Children have a difficult time grasping the concept of death. Because they often think their parent will return after they die, children need help understanding how the death will change their lives. We should prepare them for times when they will feel their loss more; for example, on parents' night at school (Brooks & Siegel, 1996).

With divorce, it is crucial for parents to share with children how hard it was to decide to take this step and that it had nothing to do with them, being as age-appropriately honest with them as possible, not blaming either spouse and continually reassuring them. Letting them know about all the things that will not change – such as their home, school and the custodial parent – helps them to create structure and safety (Brooks & Siegel, 1996).

OTHER POTENTIALLY TRAUMATIC EVENTS

Other potentially traumatic events include discrimination and historical trauma. Survivors of trauma not getting assistance can also be traumatizing, such as with teachers watching and not intervening when a child is being bullied. This can traumatize not only the child but also teachers who do not know how to respond because their superiors did not prepare them (Weingarten, 2004).

Discrimination against classes of individuals includes negative or inaccurate portrayals of them in the media, denial of services and making them the target of bias-related attention or violence. For members of the lesbian, gay, bisexual, transgender and questioning community, for example, discrimination complicates decision-making and creates stress about (1) when or how to "come out" at work and with friends and family and what it will mean and (2) life decisions such as having children, getting married or otherwise making a partnership union official (Kaplan, 2007). The combination of stressors and discrimination can be traumatic.

Historical trauma or intergenerational trauma – such as slavery, slaughter and mistreatment of Native Americans and the Holocaust – can be passed on through families or cultural groups. "Historical unresolved guilt" (Brave Heart, 2007, p. 178) often accompanies this, along with related symptoms of self-harm, substance abuse, depression, anxiety, anger, difficulty coping with emotion, poor self-image, survivor guilt, intrusive trauma images, feeling affinity with the pain of those traumatized in the past, somatic symptoms and higher mortality rates. Awareness of the past loss and restoration of forgotten cultural beliefs and practices can help heal this type of trauma. For Lakota families with intergenerational trauma, for instance, restoring the tradition of tiospaye (networks of families supporting each other) has been found to be central to recovery (Brave Heart, 2007).

THE #METOO MOVEMENT

Public awareness of other trauma can also aid survivors' healing, as with awareness of sexual assault being increased by Tarana Burke's 2006 effort to help survivors. She called the movement "Me Too" to show solidarity, and in 2017, actress Alyssa Milano sent it viral when she tweeted survivors to use the hashtag "#MeToo" to further demonstrate the prevalence of sexual abuse (Evans, 2018; Hostler & O'Neil, 2018).

This global movement has been important not only because of how it has brought the problem to the forefront, empowering survivors and exposing perpetrators, but also because it has helped reframe the problem as one of systems rather than individuals. Prior to the movement the pathology of sexual abuse, when recognized, lay with individual perpetrators. Post #MeToo, it has come to be recognized as a pathology of the systems that allow perpetration to continue, leading to initiatives like Time's Up, which connects survivors to legal and public relations assistance and purports to be "a 'first step' toward ending the systemic inequities that underlie sexual violence" (Hostler & O'Neil, 2018).

Case Study

I formed a short-term (12 sessions) support group after the September 11th disaster to help New Yorkers cope. The members came from a diverse cross-section of the city. Many of them had previous trauma histories:

Social worker:	We have almost reached the end of the group, so I wanted to talk about how to end. *Pause.* Is there anything special you'd like to do the last time we meet?
Lindy:	I don't want the group to end. Does it have to?
Social worker:	This group will be ending, but I can bring in information about other groups if you are interested. *Several members nod.* Is it hard to think about ending?
Linda:	We have talked about so much. So many feelings have come up.
Jeanie:	It really got me in touch with my sexual abuse. That has been healing.
Ginny:	Me too. It was painful, but good too.
Jim:	It made me think about when I got beaten a while back. It wasn't that bad. *He said quickly.* But I had a lot of feelings about it.
Lois:	Watching everyone's feelings was painful too.
Social worker:	We all had feelings about this trauma [September 11] because it's our city. That made it easy to understand the feelings, but scary too. *Nods from members.*
Jeanie:	It was scary when Jim blew up in group.
Jim:	It was scary for me too, but you all helped me.
Social worker:	Their support helped you cope. How else did you learn to cope?
Jim:	My writing helps. *Tearful.*
Linda:	You're writing again?
Jim:	I have been. *Seeming to forget he had talked about not being able to.*
Jeanie:	Going out of the city and being in nature has helped me.
Ginny:	Swimming has been so good.
Social worker:	That's great. Anything else?
Jim:	*Wiping his tears away.* Maybe we could write a poem together the last day, about all our feelings and what we have been through.
Social worker:	We could do that. What do you think? *Nods around the room.*
Jim:	I could write what people say and put it together. *Demonstrating his own healing (being able to write again) and his willingness to help others.*

The large number of survivors in the group was notable. Those with past trauma histories have greater risk from current trauma. These members must have felt more need for support after the disaster as a result. This also meant that the group could contribute to healing previous trauma as well as trauma from the current disaster, as demonstrated by Jim talking about being beaten, grieving the event and helping others as a way of healing himself. In order for this healing to happen, it was necessary for the facilitator to establish and ensure safety, particularly when previous traumas or intense emotions were shared, such as when Jim "blew up" in group. Ensuring safety at moments like this creates a healing environment for recovery.

RESOURCES

Briere, J., & Scott, C. (2006). *Principles of trauma therapy: A guide to symptoms, evaluation, and treatment*. Thousand Oaks, CA: Sage Publications.

Bussey, M. (Ed.). (2007). *Trauma transformed: An empowerment response*. New York: Columbia University Press.

Tehrani, N. (Ed.). (2001). *Managing trauma in the workplace: Supporting workers and organisations*. New York: Routledge.

ONLINE RESOURCES

International Society for Traumatic Stress Studies: http://www.istss.org/Home.htm
The PTSD Alliance: http://www.ptsdalliance.org

Practice Exercises and Questions

- Explore why it is important to take care of ourselves as we learn about trauma and hear/read survivors' stories
- Discuss ways to help communities heal from trauma
- Talk about the example in the chapter of teachers witnessing bullying, exploring why they did not intervene and possible ramifications
- What makes unexpected events traumatizing?
- Role-play talking with survivors about their perspectives on the #MeToo movement, keeping in mind the importance of maintaining safety during the discussion

Experiencing Trauma Directly Summary

Family Trauma

- Verbal/sexual/physical abuse, neglect and substance abuse
- Perpetrators should be providing safety and protecting survivors

School and Organizational Trauma

- Includes death, suicide, disaster and bullying
- How authorities respond is crucial to survivors' recovery

Community Trauma

- Mass murder, assault, stalking, rape, human trafficking
- Effects are far-reaching, disturbing security in a variety of ways

Disaster

- Includes major accidents and natural disasters
- Security is shattered as survivors lose jobs, homes and belongings

War and Terrorism

- Traumatic response is more pronounced when trauma is human-caused
- Children are more vulnerable to atrocities and enslavement

Unexpected Events

- Includes severe losses such as sudden death and divorce
- Treating trauma can help prevent complicated grief issues

Other Potentially Traumatic Events

- Discrimination and historical trauma such as the Holocaust
- The #MeToo movement
- Authorities not caring for trauma victims is also traumatizing

Chapter 4

Family Violence, Abuse and Neglect

Family members hurting each other, and in particular children, is unthinkable and yet there are more than three million reports of child abuse in the United States per year (US Department of Health and Human Services, 2008), with children generally hurt by people they know, such as parents or other family members (US Department of Health and Human Services, 2009). Intimate partner violence (IPV), also pervasive, is globally one of the most common forms of human-made trauma and can negatively impact on survivors' physical, mental, sexual and reproductive health (World Health Organization, 2005).

In this chapter, incidence, impact, history and response to family violence, abuse and neglect are reviewed. Best-practice responses and resources for further reading are also highlighted, as unique indicators of family trauma, practice considerations and evidence-based interventions are explored.

TUNE IN TO FAMILY VIOLENCE, ABUSE AND NEGLECT

In order to support survivors of family abuse, first try tuning in to related experiences in your life. Ensure you are feeling safe enough to consider potentially upsetting memories, and if you are, ask yourself these questions: Have you ever felt scared of someone you cared about? Has a friend or partner ever attempted to exert too much control over you? What does it feel like when your boss doesn't listen to you and demands obedience?

And how does it feel to have these experiences as a child? Remember your life at five years old, for example, including how the world around you looked and felt, who was most important to you and what you were afraid of. If you have difficulty with this, try tuning in to children around you. What might be hurtful to this child? Keep this in mind throughout your day, noticing children's height and the emotions on their faces. You will know you have succeeded in getting their perspective when you experience how big and simultaneously exciting and bewildering the world is to them.

Now consider having these feelings either as an adult partner or a child and imagine what it would be like to feel unsafe or lack attention or food. Keep this sense of vulnerability in mind as you read this chapter. Also note your reactions as you read because stories of family violence, abuse and neglect can be upsetting. Consider reading the chapter gradually and using self-care techniques as needed. For more information, see chapters 1, 10 and 12 on secondary trauma, safety and coping.

FAMILY VIOLENCE, ABUSE AND NEGLECT DEFINED

Family abuse comes in many forms including coercive control, emotional abuse, physical abuse, sexual abuse and neglect. Those who are children, elderly, disabled or dependent (including financially) are particularly vulnerable and therefore at risk for abuse and neglect. Isolation from the world outside the family is also a risk factor as evidenced by Westover's experience living with family members' mental illness and abusive behavior. In her book, *Educated: A Memoir* (2018), she shares about finally coming to realize just how abusive her home life was when she left for college after rarely being separated from her family as she grew up. And her experience included not only neglect and emotional abuse but also debilitating physical abuse.

Definitions

- *Coercive control* – Physical/sexual violence, emotional/economic abuse, threats and other techniques used to gain dominance over individuals, eroding their sense of agency, liberty and/or personal power
- *Emotional abuse* – Patterns of behavior toward individuals that impair their emotional development or sense of self-worth, including constant criticism, threats, rejection and exposure to familial violence
- *Intimate partner violence (IPV)* – Emotionally, physically, sexually, economically or psychologically violent behavior used to exert power and control in the context of intimate or formerly intimate relationships
- *Neglect* – Failure to provide for a dependent individual's basic needs, including physical, educational and emotional needs
- *Physical abuse* – Behavior that includes a pattern of hitting, kicking, shaking, burning or otherwise physically harming an individual
- *Sexual abuse* – Coercive use of an individual for sexual gratification and/or other sexual purposes. With the elderly, disabled and children, this includes any unlawful sexual act even if coercion is not involved

---

There are several forms of child abuse and neglect. Often collectively referred to as "child maltreatment," child abuse and neglect include physical, sexual and emotional abuse and neglect. Increasingly, children's exposure to violent and controlling tactics associated with Intimate Partner Violence (IPV) is also recognized as a form of maltreatment since exposure to violence can have a traumatic impact (Evans, Davies, & DiLillo, 2008; Foster & Brooks-Gunn, 2009; Fowler & Chanmugam, 2007; McAlister Groves, 2002). For more information see chapter 7 on witnessing trauma.

These violent and controlling IPV relationships exhibit a pattern of aggressive behavior within the context of intimate or formerly intimate relationships. The aggression may be emotional, physical, sexual or economic, with coercive control creating an environment of fear and further traumatization as survivors' liberties and sense of agency are compromised (Mahoney, Williams, & West, 2001; Stark, 2009).

Many experiencing IPV are traumatized by more than one form of abuse in a relationship. For example, Maria was a 35-year-old woman with depression and suicidal thoughts. She had recently left her husband who violently raped her almost every night. When she said she was going to leave, he threatened to kill her mother – her only source of support in the United States. The violence in this relationship was pervasive – physical and sexual plus emotional in the form of threats. Maria said that she felt locked in a trap with the choice of either continuing to be raped nightly or risking her mother's death.

The elderly and disabled are also at risk. Cultural considerations can increase risk for the disabled even more. According to Wikipedia, for instance, Tanzanian individuals with Albinism have been attacked by witchcraft practitioners who were after their organs (Wikipedia contributors, 2019, February 21). And infanticide of disabled children exists in some cultures (Disability Rights International, 2018). For the elderly and disabled, abuse takes forms which may be difficult to ascertain including caregivers refusing to help them obtain healthcare, medication, assistive devises and help with bathing or using the toilet. These vulnerable individuals are also susceptible to other forms of abuse and neglect including physical, emotional and sexual abuse.

Incidence of Family Violence, Abuse and Neglect

The incidence of abuse and neglect is high. This is particularly true for children with one in four adults reporting physical abuse as children and an estimated 41,000 child homicides a year plus one in five women and one in thirteen men reporting sexual abuse as children, worldwide (World Health Organization, 2016). In the United States, 3.5 million reports of child maltreatment were made in 2017. The most common forms of abuse reported were neglect (74.9%) and physical abuse (18.3%). In addition, it is estimated that 1,720 children died the same year due to abuse and neglect (US Department of Health & Human Services, 2019).

The incidence of IPV is also high with 30% of women worldwide reporting IPV and 38% of women's murders attributed to intimate partners (World Health Organization, 2017). In the US, one in three women and one in four men report IPV, with nearly 20 people abused by intimate partners each minute – 10 million per year. Additionally, almost half of all men and women in the United States are emotionally abused by intimate partners (Social Solutions, 2018).

The statistics for abuse of the elderly and disabled are similarly high. One in six older adults (60 and over) worldwide experienced abuse in 2017 and it is estimated that this number will increase from 900 million in 2015 to about 2 billion in 2050 (World Health Organization, 2018). Among the disabled incidence is even higher with 70% of survey respondents reporting abuse, 90% reporting multiple occurrences of abuse and 73% reporting bullying (Baladerian, Coleman, & Stream, 2013).

UNDERREPORTING OF FAMILY VIOLENCE, ABUSE AND NEGLECT

Despite high incidence of reported abuse, there is reason to believe the numbers are even higher. Only one in 24 cases of elder abuse, for instance, are reported (World Health Organization, 2018) and about two thirds of disabled abuse cases are not reported (Baladerian, Coleman, & Stream, 2013). Most cases of IPV are not reported and while it is true that 85% of IPV is perpetrated by men against women (US Department of Justice, Bureau of Justice Statistics, 2005), there is a growing understanding that the incidence of IPV perpetrated by women against men is underreported and thus under the radar (Tjaden & Thoennes, 2000).

In 2005, the Surgeon General of the United States identified child abuse as the number one public health crisis in the country (Carmona, 2005). While only one in three million annual reports of child abuse are substantiated, population surveys indicate that the actual rates of child abuse and neglect may be as much as 40 times higher than official numbers (Theodore et al., 2005), indicating underreporting in this area as well.

Traumatic Impact of Family Violence, Abuse and Neglect

It is important to note that although this abuse and neglect could be traumatizing, not all victims have adverse reactions (Gil, 2006). For example, what leads to one child's long-term struggle with the after-effects of trauma versus another's being ultimately resolved in a healthy way is an area of inquiry and debate (Carlson, Furby, Armstrong, & Shlaes, 1997; Gil, 2006; Mabanglo, 2002; Margolin & Vickerman, 2007; Putnam, 2003). The nature and duration of abuse; availability of stable caregivers and institutions; age, gender, cognitive abilities, internal resiliency, coping strategies and temperament – all play a role in how children respond (Gil, 2006; McAlister Groves & Zuckerman, 1997; Putnam, 2003). This variation in response supports Gil's (2006) advice for clinicians to carefully assess for both the existence of an abuse history and the nature of its traumatic impact.

Tips

- When working with a child who has been abused, get the abuse history from the child and adults in the child's life. Ask yourself, have this child's experiences led to a traumatic impact? This question helps us to avoid concluding that a child is experiencing an adverse reaction to trauma simply because the history of abuse is horrifying

---

HISTORY OF FAMILY VIOLENCE, ABUSE AND NEGLECT

Central themes in the historical fight to protect children from maltreatment are society's advancing understanding of the concept of parental ownership of children (Gelles, 1993). Prior to the 20th century, when children were viewed as miniature adults rather than as children with unique developmental objectives, it was difficult to protect them from abuse (Laird & Hartman, 1985). Similarly, even when their maltreatment began to be recognized, it remained difficult to protect them, as they were viewed as the property of their parents and government involvement in family life was rare (Pleck, 2004).

There have been crucial cases and social movements that have influenced the response to child abuse. Perhaps the most famous case is Mary Ellen Connolly (Costin, 1991). Born in 1864 against the backdrop of the Women's Rights Movement of the 1870s, she was removed from her foster home after neighbors told a charity worker, Etta Wheeler, about her nightly screams. Ms. Wheeler went to the home and found 10-year-old Mary Ellen, brutally abused and neglected, but had no means to remove her. Eventually, she engaged the support of Henry Bergh, head of the American Society for the Prevention of Cruelty to Animals. He argued in court that she should not be returned to her abusive foster home. Mary Ellen testified in court, her foster mother was prosecuted and convicted and she was placed in a different foster care setting.

This case highlighted the inability of the courts or police system to respond to issues of maltreatment and played a role in the formation of the New York Society for the Prevention of Cruelty to Children, the first society of its kind.

Soon after, similar societies formed across the United States and internationally to advocate for child protection (Finkelhor, 1986). Since that time, society has advanced its understanding of maltreatment. Research as early as the mid-1980s began to document its impact (Finkelhor, 1986) and, more recently, child traumatic stress began to be recognized.

Violence against women by intimate partners has also been evident throughout history (Pleck, 2004) although it has taken several social movements for it to be seen as traumatic. As recently as the 1920s, the view was common that women drove their husbands to beat them and that their fragile natures and "hysteria" caused their issues rather than abuse (Herman, 1992; Pleck, 2004). Most physical violence in the household is now considered a crime in the United States. That said, while sexual and physical violence are generally illegal, other forms of aggression, such as tactics of economic control, are more difficult to prove and prosecute.

These advances in understanding of IPV are tied to social movements (Herman, 1992), such as the revitalized Women's Movement and the Anti-rape Movement in the 1970s, which led to the Battered Women's Movement (later renamed the Domestic Violence Movement). This movement began with spare bedrooms in women's homes used as safe havens for battered women and became a network of agencies, crisis lines, legal services, therapeutic interventions, children's services and consciousness-raising non-profit organizations, as well as federal, state and local government entities whose shared mission is to protect survivors of violence and fight to end IPV in society (Pleck, 2004).

In the United States, the passage of the Violence Against Women Act in 1994 was key, creating federal funding and oversight and raising the profile of this issue (Boyer, 2001). Similar legislation exists in many other countries, and in 2008, the United Nations launched the UNiTE to End Violence Against Women campaign – a multiyear effort aimed at preventing and eliminating violence against women and girls in all parts of the world (UNiTE, 2010).

Abuse of individuals with disabilities has a long history as well, dating back as far as prehistoric times. Despite this, it has only begun to be acknowledged as a problem in the last 20–30 years. Hallmarks of this process include adoption by the United Nations of the *Declaration on the Rights of Disabled Persons* in 1975 and of the *Convention of the Rights of the Child* in 1989 in order to safeguard adults and children with disabilities. These *Rights* extol the necessity of ensuring the disabled are treated with dignity and respect without discrimination or abuse (Thornberry & Olson, 2005).

Finally, elder abuse was first referred to in the literature as "granny battering" in 1975 but, according to the World Health Organization, has existed since ancient times (Krug, Dahlberg, Mercy, Zwi, & Lozano, 2002). Research and enactment of protective measures began in the United States but existed soon after in multiple locals throughout the world (Krug et al., 2002). Key efforts in the United States were 1950's "protective service units," alleged to be starting points for state legislation, and federal policy that began with the 1965 Older Americans Act and included the establishment of adult protective services units in the 1970's, the Omnibus Budget Reconciliation Act providing rights for elder's in nursing homes in the 1980's, amendments to the Older Americans Act in the 1990's and the Elder Justice Act in 2010 (Blancato, 2012). This is an area of work that will be more important as the over 60 years old population grows worldwide, with estimates that by 2025 it will more than double (Krug et al., 2002).

Unique Signs of Trauma

Just as children react differently to life events that their adult counterparts, their reactions to trauma also differ (Margolin & Vickerman, 2007). Since there are numerous unique impacts of potentially traumatizing incidents, the focus here will be on a few central concepts. For more information see the Resources section.

Definitions

- *Post-traumatic stress disorder (PTSD)* – Caused by exposure to traumatic events and leading to symptoms that last at least a month and include emotional responses of fear, horror or helplessness; flashbacks and/or nightmares of events; avoidance of reminders of events; and increased arousal
- *Hyperarousal* – Heightened emotionality that can lead to agitation, anger, difficulty sleeping and/or hypervigilance
- *Hypervigilance* – State of increased attention to the environment, in order to detect threat and prevent harm, that can increase anxiety, prevent sleep and cause fatigue

---

There is increasing evidence that exposure to chronic trauma can affect a child's developing brain (Finkelhor, 2008). Demonstrating this, 3-year-old Angela, who was exposed to chronic physical abuse and IPV, presented with depressive symptoms. She could not make eye contact and teachers reported she played aggressively. After a comprehensive assessment, social workers determined she existed in a constant state of hyperarousal in which she perceived all people as a potential threats. She was unable to attach and lashed out at other children whom she thought would hurt her.

Traumatized children are often brought to see healthcare professionals due to aggressive or regressed behaviors. Parents are concerned when their 6-year-old begins to wet the bed, for example. Developmental tasks most recently mastered are the most susceptible to regression (Rutter, 1988).

> **Tips**
>
> - When working with a child who has experienced abuse and has regression or aggression issues, be sure to assess other children in the home who may be manifesting reactions to their abuse experiences in less noticeable ways

Among the most troubling impacts of childhood trauma is sexualization due to sexual abuse (Finkelhor, 2008; Letourneau, Schoenwald, & Sheldow, 2004). For example, young survivors are more likely to act in sexually inappropriate or aggressive ways toward other children, thus perpetuating the abuse; and teenage girls may experience reduced sexual inhibition, putting them at risk for further trauma, early pregnancy or sexually transmitted diseases (Putnam, 2003).

Anxiety is a common effect of all forms of trauma in all age groups and PTSD was categorized as an anxiety disorder in the 4th edition of the *Diagnostic and statistical manual of mental disorders* (American Psychiatric Association, 2000). Anxiety in children can manifest as behavioral problems and may cause somatic complaints (National Child Traumatic Stress Network, n.d.b). Children can also experience more typical anxiety symptoms, but social workers should be on the alert for atypical presentations.

Another unique sign of child abuse relates to issues of trust and attachment. A fundamental goal of child development is healthy attachments (Ashford, Lecroy, & Lortie, 2001) and abuse can interrupt this process, especially if perpetrated by a trusted caregiver (National Child Traumatic Stress Network, n.d.b). Child survivors may have difficulty trusting caregivers or other children, or they may assume new people they meet are going to hurt them. Gil (1991) provides an example of a girl who, after determining that her new therapist cared about her, brought in a paddle and handed it to the therapist to hit her with. The child believed that anyone who cared about her would hurt her. These disrupted attachments can impact children, potentially leading to the development of relationships with antisocial peers and, without intervention, continuing on to unhealthy adult relationships (Finkelhor, 2008).

Survivors of IPV also struggle with reactions common to all forms of traumatic experience, such as anxiety, depression and PTSD. The nature of IPV may lead to unique signs, such as fearing new relationships or jumping into them quickly in an attempt to avoid memories of previous pain.

Many survivors feel guilt and shame about their experiences. Even as they begin to heal and intellectually understand it was not their fault, it may take years for them to believe it on an emotional level. This is both because it is common for batterers to blame victims for the violence and because society's response to victims, once they ask for help, also often involves blame (Mahoney, Williams, & West, 2001). For example, Jessica spent five years in a violent relationship, in which her boyfriend worked to convince her that if she were a better cook, he would not "have" to hit her:

Social worker:	So he told you that he hit you because you weren't a good cook?
Jessica:	Yes, at first I remember thinking it was ridiculous. I was a pretty terrible cook, but it wasn't so bad I should be hit. Over time, I started to believe him … I don't know how it happened. He said I shouldn't be allowed to cook for my son and that my son's illnesses came from my cooking. I was so worried about my son's health … *silence.*
Social worker:	You began to believe him. It sounds like he chose the points in your life where you were most vulnerable, like your son's health, and used them against you.
Jessica:	I don't know how I could have been so stupid as to believe him.

This narrative highlights the manipulation often used by batterers to terrorize partners. It also demonstrates that even having escaped the violence, they can face an uphill emotional and psychological battle to understand batterers' efforts to control them.

As is often true for survivors of all human-made traumas, it is not unusual for survivors of IPV to struggle with people in authority. In addition, the experience of a partner attempting to control one's every move may heighten sensitivity to perceived attempts for control in the future. One survivor struggled with her relationship with her father after a violent relationship. He was worried about her and became very involved in her life. Interpreting his support as controlling, she rebuffed his offers of help rather than risk another abusive relationship.

Tips

- Social workers are in positions of power when working with clients. Because survivors of IPV are understandably mistrustful of power and authority, tune in to these issues when working with them. Before a meeting with a survivor of IPV, spend one minute thinking about how you are a gatekeeper to things the survivor needs – healing; referrals to shelters, attorneys and other services; advocacy and knowledge. Also, remember to bring issues of power and authority to clinical supervision and case conferences or in-service training

Unique signs of trauma for the disabled and elderly can also involve changes in mood and behavior such as increased anxiety, depression, withdrawal or aggression. Appearance can change with abused/neglected individuals appearing disheveled, tired due to poor sleep/diet or health issues, displaying bed sores or other signs of their health/self-care not being properly monitored. Compounding this, these signs can be downplayed when ascribed to their age or disability. Or they can aggravate existing conditions such as dementia and high blood pressure, decreasing the likelihood of the abuse/neglect being detected and acted upon (Baladerian, 2013; National Institute on Aging, 2016).

Special Populations/Considerations

IPV and other family violence are often related to gender, racism, anti-immigrant, agism and lesbian, gay, bisexual and transgendered oppression. Just as batterers often use gendered slurs as part of their violent behavior, those in same-sex relationships often use homophobic insults (National Coalition of Anti-violence Programs, 2009). This combination of IPV and oppression can be noxious.

Survivors of IPV, for example, who are also immigrants can face challenges, such as batterers using threats of deportation or restriction of access to legal immigration to control them. Dutton, Orloff, and Hass (2000) found that 72.3% of battered Latinas surveyed in their study reported spouses never filed immigration petitions for their wives, even though 50.8% were eligible. Further, immigrant survivors are often fearful of contacting the police due to their legal status (Shetty & Kaguyutan, 2002). In addition to control of immigration status and threats of deportation, immigrant victims often cannot legally work, allowing batterers further control over finances and economic freedom (Shetty & Kaguyutan, 2002).

Research indicates that IPV occurs in same-sex relationships at rates similar to opposite-sex relationships (Haurgrud, Gratch, & Magruder, 1997; Greenwood et al., 2002) and can be connected to societal oppression of lesbian, gay, bisexual and transgendered (LGBT) individuals. And there are some aspects of IPV that are unique to same-sex relationships. Examples include societal and police response to IPV in same-sex relationships, with many LGBT survivors experiencing harassment and even brutality at the hands of the police when they attempt to report the violence they have experienced. Additionally, services available to survivors of IPV in same-sex relationships are limited, potentially increasing the isolation of LGBT (National Coalition of Anti-violence Programs, 2009).

Another area of increasing focus is the incidence of violence among teens. Davis (2008) reported that approximately one in three adolescent girls in the United States is a victim of physical, emotional or verbal abuse from a dating partner; and, one in five tweens say their friends are victims of dating violence (Teenage Research Unlimited, 2008). The impact is devastating; research indicates that teen survivors of physical date violence are more likely to smoke, use drugs, engage in unhealthy diets, take part in risky sex and attempt or consider suicide (Silverman, Raj, Mucci, & Hathaway, 2001).

Dynamics in violent teen relationships can be different than with adults. For example, teens in their first serious relationship who are being controlled by their partners may have no point of comparison and thus connect control with love. In addition, the developmental task of adolescence is to form one's own identity. In the context of an abusive relationship, this process is complicated. Teens face an additional disadvantage because rocky, roller-coaster relationships are often considered normal for this age range; making it difficult to differentiate a healthy, albeit dramatic, teen relationship from one that is controlling or dangerous, especially for survivors of a violent relationships. Teens often need additional support from adults to understand what makes relationships healthy. Survivors can also experience oppression in the form of agism. Specifically, teens seeking help may struggle in their interactions with police, schools and caregivers, many of whom do not take teen IPV seriously (Davis, 2008).

Finally, while not often discussed, many survivors of IPV struggle with substance abuse issues. These issues may have developed as unhealthy coping with the trauma or as a part of the coercive control tactics used by the batterer (Nurius & Norris, 1996). One survivor reported an addiction to crack cocaine. She had never wanted to use it, but when her partner began dealing, he made her "test" the drug before he sold it, or risk severe physical punishment.

Tips

- Assess survivors of IPV for additional trauma histories and possible substance abuse. Many survivors have experienced childhood traumas or abuse and, while the IPV may be the most recent in their experience, it is important to consider how the layers of trauma may interact to impact on survivors' sense of safety and healing

---

Child maltreatment similarly poses special considerations. Finkelhor (2008), for instance, points out that child survivors can be vulnerable to future trauma, noting that, for some, victimization is more of a "condition than an event" (p. 36), with many experiencing multiple traumas such as sexual abuse at home and bullying at school. When working with victims of family violence, attention to this possibility is crucial.

> ## Tips
>
> • When working with a child survivor of child abuse, consider other ways in which the child may be vulnerable due to their abuse experience. Ask the child about interactions with peers at school to assess victimization at school, and work on self-esteem and self-advocacy through role-play or other methods in order to protect the child from future trauma.

Impact on Physical and Mental Health

Family violence may lead to mental health challenges. The emotional effects of abuse – isolation, self-blame, fear and an inability to trust – can translate into lifelong consequences, including low self-esteem, depression and relationship difficulties (Child Welfare Information Gateway, 2008; Dominguez, Nelke, & Perry, 2006; Herman, 1992). Anxiety disorders such as PTSD are also common.

Witnesses of family violence can also be harmed. Research indicates that 15.5 million children in the United States reside in households with at least one occurrence of IPV in the previous year (Whitfield, Anda, Dube, & Felittle, 2003). Family violence can interrupt developmental processes and, in some cases, particularly where there is chronic abuse, impact structural development of their brains, creating complex trauma reactions that make it difficult for them to self-regulate, concentrate, learn or maintain stable mental health (Perry, 2001).

In addition to the trauma of being exposed to violence, parents and other caregivers are often not emotionally available. The combined traumas can contribute to children (Bogat, DeJonghe, Levendosky, Davidson, & von Eye, 2006; Lang & Smith Stover, 2008; McAlister Groves, 2002): (1) having difficulty forming social relationships; (2) regressing to earlier forms of development; (3) becoming aggressive as they model the behavior they see at home; (4) becoming withdrawn or struggling with depression and anxiety or (5) developing risk-taking behavior.

Experiencing child abuse and other trauma can also affect long-term physical health (Hussey, Chang, & Kotch, 2006). Research indicates that abused/neglected children's immune system functioning, for example, may be impaired, and that they may have higher risk as adults of issues such as alcoholism, depression, drug abuse, eating disorders, obesity, sexual promiscuity, smoking, suicide and certain chronic diseases (Centers for Disease Control and Prevention, 2006; Edwards et al., 2005; Sachs-Ericsson, Plant, Blazer, & Arnow, 2005; Shirtcliff, Coe, & Pollak, 2009; Springer, Sheridan, Kuo, & Carnes, 2007; Swan, 1998).

Tips

- Since survivors of abuse are at risk of long-term physical health issues, ensure referrals for holistic medical care with providers adept in trauma work

Cost to Society

On a societal scale, family violence correlates with increased use of public and private resources. Expenditures accrue in areas such as child welfare, public mental health, early intervention and education, juvenile delinquency and criminal justice, public welfare and health. Examples include the cost of child abuse/neglect to the United States – $103.8 billion annually, $284 million per day in combined hospitalization, healthcare, mental healthcare, child welfare, law enforcement, judicial, special education, juvenile delinquency and productivity costs (Wang & Holton, 2007). Another study found that the long-term impacts of childhood maltreatment include higher rates of unemployment, poverty and use of social services as adults (Zielinksi, 2009). The costs of IPV are also immense. It has been estimated that in 2004, IPV cost the United States over $5.8 billion in lost work time and associated medical and mental health costs (Max, Rice, Finkelstein, Bardwell, & Leadbetter, 2004). Estimates of elder abuse/fraud costs in the United States are high as well, from $2.9 to $36.5 billion a year (National Coalition of Anti-violence Programs, 2009).

PRACTICE CONSIDERATIONS

Our understanding of child maltreatment and other family violence is changing (Laird & Hartman, 1985). While previously focused on child protection and parental punishment, the field of child welfare now focuses on supporting parents and keeping families together whenever possible. Indeed, the Centers for Disease Control and Prevention, Division of Violence Prevention is currently promoting the development of "stable and nurturing" relationships with adult caregivers as the best means for helping children heal from abuse and preventing further incidents of maltreatment (Centers for Disease Control and Prevention, 2008). This reaffirms what social workers have understood for some time: That the best way to help a child is to work with the family. This concept applies to caregivers of the disabled and elderly as well.

If family violence has occurred or is suspected, it is critical to build supports for caregivers and provide educational opportunities so they can have a better understanding of developmental processes and the nature and impact of abuse.

Education about appropriate disciplinary skills is particularly important. For example, parents often lament that their children are lying to them, necessitating discipline – but these parental complaints come *before* most children are even *capable* of lying, according to current developmental beliefs (Bronson & Merryman, 2009). Another example is Jessica, who read in parenting books that rocking can help babies settle when crying. She was not properly educated about the fragility of a child's neck and brain and moved in a way that shook her child, causing permanent brain damage.

Abuse may also occur when appropriate disciplinary techniques fail and caregivers, exhausted or embarrassed by their charge's behavior, feel harsher discipline is required. Education about positive and productive discipline techniques can help empower caregivers of children, the elderly and disabled, thus deterring future abuse.

Tips

- When working with a caregiver you suspect may be at risk of abusing a family member, ask the family member privately what gets them "in trouble" with the caregiver and what the consequences are. Answers to these questions can help social workers determine the caregiver's developmental understanding, level of stress and disciplinary techniques

---

SAFETY PLANNING

There are some special practice considerations when working with survivors of family violence and in particular IPV. First, is the difficulty finding safety from violence in the home. Safety planning, i.e., creating a plan that will help keep survivors safe, is a tool designed to not only create safety, but more importantly, engage a survivor's cognitive resources, empowering him/her to consider ways in which s/he has kept safe in the past and can work to stay safe in the future.

Definitions

- *Safety planning* – Empowers survivors as they learn to create or enhance existing protective strategies related to specific situations or time periods

---

See resources section at the end of the chapter for information that includes sample safety plans. Drawing from these examples is important, but it is essential to ensure that a plan works for specific situations by developing it with the survivor. Finally, once a safety plan has been used to successfully escape a violent incident, it cannot be relied on in the future because it is no longer secret. Thus safety planning requires consistent attention on the part of the social worker and the survivor, offering new opportunities to build empowerment each time a new plan is conceived.

Tips

- When working with a survivor regarding safety planning, ask open-ended questions before getting to the specific plan. For example, ask the survivor how he or she knows when violence is about to occur. Next, ask what has worked in the past in terms of staying safe from the abusive partner. These questions empower as they communicate the understanding that the survivor has always worked to stay safe and can continue to do so

---

Good coping is an essential part of safety and recovery for all survivors of family violence, as discussed in chapter 12. Survivors need healthy coping skills in order to manage the emotional impacts of trauma and increase confidence. Teaching coping skills also supports those who, in the therapeutic context, are beginning to address traumatic experiences in order to make sense of what occurred.

Tips

- To teach young children calming breathing, use bubbles or a pinwheel. Children need to learn to control their breath to blow bubbles successfully, and the joy in creating the bubbles will help children stay focused on the task

---

Processing Trauma

Once survivors have learned sufficient coping skills and caregivers are receiving support and education, decreasing the risk of abuse in the household, social workers can begin working with them to process the abuse. Twenty years ago, experts believed that non-directive, insight-oriented play therapy was the best approach when working with abused children (Gil, 1991). Researchers are increasingly advocating for cognitive behavioral approaches or approaches that combine directive and non-directive techniques (Cohen, Deblinger, Mannarino, & Steer, 2004; Gil, 2006; Lieberman & Van Horn, 2004). Non-directive approaches remain important because they allow the child, who has often experienced a lack of control, to control the therapy process, guiding the therapist to their key issues. This is a core play therapy concept – children communicate through play rather than conversation. Some examples of this include creating a book or a series of sand trays about the traumatic experience (Gil, 2006).

Utilizing these approaches, social workers actively assign tasks that support the child as he or she revisits the abuse. The social worker and the child can then identify emotions and reactions to these experiences. The social worker can also provide the child with psychoeducation about violence in the home, revisiting coping skills often, consistently reinforcing the need for them and supporting the child. For example, Carlos, a 6-year-old whose mother suspected sexual abuse, developed coping skills with his social worker that included relaxation and deep breathing before addressing potential abuse. During the first conversation about sexual abuse, Carlos read a story about a child who had been sexually abused. Here is the interaction between Carlos and the social worker:

Carlos:	*Tentatively.* The boy in this book was touched by his father.
Social worker:	I wonder if you have anything in common with the boy in this book?
Carlos:	Well … *Pausing for a long time.* My stepdad used to touch me when I was in the bathtub.
Social worker:	Oh. Can you tell me more about when your stepdad touched you?
Carlos:	He would take the wash cloth to clean my pee pee, but then he stopped using the wash cloth and rubbed my pee pee up and down like this. *Demonstrating a motion on his finger.* One time, my mother tried to come in when he was rubbing me, but he locked the door. She was yelling from the outside.
Social worker:	So you and the boy in the book do have something in common. Can you remember how you were feeling when your [step]father was touching your pee pee?
Carlos:	*Shrugging, looking away, unable to make eye contact.*
Social worker:	The boy in the book said he felt lots of things. Scared and mad and also that it felt good sometimes.
Carlos:	Yeah. I felt kind of scared and mad. Why couldn't my Mom come in? *Beginning to look extremely upset, with tears in his eyes.*
Social worker:	Carlos, you are so brave for talking about this with me. I'd like us to talk about it more, but first I wonder if you can tell me how you are feeling in your body right now?
Carlos:	My tummy doesn't feel good.

Social worker:	I was wondering about that because you are showing me in your face that this is hard to talk about. Do you remember some of the things we've learned that you can do when your tummy is feeling bad?
Carlos:	*Brightening.* Yes! I can blow bubbles!
Social worker:	Great job! Let's try that now together!

Another critical way in which children process the abuse is called traumatic play or traumatic re-enactment. Utilizing this process, social workers look for re-enactment of trauma in children's play. While the actual trauma, such as a child acting out sexual abuse with dolls this is sometimes observed, often children act out scenes that feel similar to the abuse. For example, a sexually abused child might use play to depict a little girl who is trapped under something heavy and whose mother cannot hear her. Traumatic play also tends to be repetitious. The child, who seems stuck in the play, often expresses no emotion despite the disturbing content and is unable to obtain resolution without support and intervention (Association for Play Therapy, 2007; National Child Traumatic Stress Network, n.d.c). Seasoned play therapists have developed techniques to work with children who demonstrate this kind of traumatic re-enactment. See the resources section at the end of the chapter for further reading.

Definitions

- *Traumatic play or traumatic re-enactment* – Symptom of trauma in which children act out scenes related to the traumatic event. There is no resolution to the trauma, emotion is often constricted and children can appear transfixed by the process

---

EVIDENCE-BASED AND BEST PRACTICES

Stover, Meadows, and Kaufman (2009) and others advocate for increased use of evidence-based substance abuse treatment, couples therapy and trauma-focused interventions when working with family trauma survivors.

Definitions

- *Trauma-informed interventions* – Designed with understanding of trauma's impact and often including utilization of psychoeducation, relaxation and coping prior to delving into trauma history

---

One-stop shopping is one such evidence-based approach. Survivors of trauma have complex needs and often rely on multiple support systems. Retelling their stories combined with the anxiety involved in finding new provider locations, meeting new people and taking the risk to trust providers may impede healing. Support models that comprehensively meet survivors' needs, such as one-stop shopping models, decrease the likelihood of this occurring.

Definitions

- *One-stop shopping* – Service models that work to meet the comprehensive needs of clients by co-locating essential concrete support services under one roof or through agency connections and agreements

---

Empowering survivors is also important. Perhaps the most traumatizing aspect of experiencing family trauma is the sense of powerlessness and lack of control (Stark, 2009). Creating a sense of empowerment through legal action, restraining orders, support groups, counseling, education or other methods is a critical aspect of healing.

In addition, family trauma survivors often feel disempowered by how alone they are with their experience. Reducing isolation and rebuilding survivor's support networks, support groups that provide psychoeducation and develop mutual aid are a common and important part of healing for many (Lee & Swenson, 2005). More information can be found in chapter 16.

Definitions

- *Psychoeducation* – Process of teaching about the nature and incidence of physical and mental illness, its impact, consequences and approaches to healing

---

A central theoretical framework for IPV recovery that is rooted in the feminist movement is the Duluth Model (Pence & Paymar, 1993). It focuses on the concept that IPV is generated by men's attempts to gain power and control over their partners and presents IPV as a social and political construct connected to male power and privilege, providing an alternative to interpretations that blame the victim. It recommends a multifaceted and coordinated response to prevent IPV, combining interventions for batterers with criminal justice, shelters and support services for battered women (Sullivan & Gillum, 2001). The Power and Control Wheel is a Duluth Model tool. It defines IPV, gives examples of battering and highlights the importance of power and control in IPV. See the Resources section at the end of the chapter for more information.

Definitions

* *Duluth Model* – Feminist approach to IPV which postulates that abuse is a method men utilize to control women. The approach advocates for a coordinated and preventative response that includes shelter and support services for victims and a variety of batterer interventions

---

While the Duluth Model and shelters, counseling, legal, hotline and other related services that draw from this perspective have changed the way society views IPV, divergent opinions have emerged that challenge the methodology and call attention to the fact that very little empirical evidence exists to support its efficacy (Ehrensaft, 2008; Stover, Meadows, & Kaufman, 2009).

Child-focused home visitation programs have existed throughout the child protection movement (Laird & Hartman, 1985). One such evidence based program, SafeCare®, has been found to help reduce the incidence of neglect/physical abuse with at-risk families or in families where abuse/neglect has already occurred. SafeCare is an 18- to 20-week program. Trained staff visit homes, teaching parents: (1) to plan developmentally appropriate activities with children; (2) parenting skills related to the child's health; (3) time-management skills and (4) how to utilize reinforcement/reward and behavioral understanding/consequences with children. The visits, which also include the child, often focus on the demonstration of skills with parents. Home visitors also observe and provide feedback as parents attempt new parenting skills (Edwards & Lutzker, 2008; Gershater-Molko, Lutzker, & Wesch, 2002). For example, a SafeCare-trained home visitor provided an activity card for George, asking him to practice the activity with his 3-year-old child, June. The home visitor noted that he became competitive with June and admonished her for being unable to follow the activity's rules. She intervened and worked with George by discussing the initial goals of the activity (e.g., to have a positive interaction between parent and child), reviewing June's developmental age, thus reminding George about June's ability to comprehend and follow instructions.

Trauma-focused Cognitive Behavioral Therapy (Cohen, Deblinger, Mannarino, & Steer, 2004) is a highly structured, evidence-based model that includes the following components: (1) psychoeducation; (2) learning to recognize the relationship between thoughts, feelings and behaviors; (3) relaxation skills; (4) processing of the abuse once sufficient relaxation and coping have been taught; (5) joint parent–child sessions and (6) training to help parents address children's behavioral issues. This treatment modality was designed for children who were sexually abused, but evaluations of the model have demonstrated its effectiveness with other populations.

The field of child maltreatment has seen an increase in consistently evaluated programs designed to treat trauma in a counseling/therapy context. Child–Parent Psychotherapy is one such model (Lieberman & Van Horn, 2004). Developed and evaluated by Lieberman and Van Horn (2004), this model targets young children exposed to IPV. The treatment approach is a 52-week model that includes focusing on the mother–child dyad with the goal of improving parenting and communication and reducing trauma symptoms in the family.

Another evidence-based model in the area of child maltreatment is Parent–Child Interaction Therapy (PCIT). It involves two components, Parent-directed Interaction and Child-directed Interaction, in which the trained therapist functions as a parenting "coach." The coaching efforts focus on teaching effective parenting skills. In both components – one in which the parent learns to follow the child's lead; and the other in which the parent learns to take the lead when necessary – the parent is provided with coaching by the therapist, who watches the session through a one-way mirror and talks to the parent through a microphone in the parent's ear. This trauma-informed intervention has demonstrated reduction in incidents of child maltreatment and in children's trauma symptoms (Boggs et al., 2004; Schuhmann, Foote, Eyberg, Boggs, & Algina, 1998). Eye movement desensitization and reprocessing (EMDR) is also an evidence-based treatment that, although originally designed for adults, is increasingly used with traumatized children with encouraging results. Because the treatment is verbally guided rather than play-focused, it has been applied to and tested with older children, school-aged and above (Chemtob, Nakashima, Hamada, & Carlson, 2002; Shapiro, 2001). For more information on EMDR, see chapter 17 on other trauma interventions.

Case Study

A 6-year-old, Janice, was brought to a medical clinic by her mother, Sue, with complaints of stomach pain. When medical issues were ruled out, they were referred to a social worker who determined Janice was being physically abused by her mother's boyfriend. The mother, who was also being abused, was afraid of losing her daughter to Child Protective Services (CPS) but did not know how to protect her. The social worker made a report to CPS and gave Sue resources for shelters and domestic violence services that she did not utilize. Two weeks later, the social worker followed-up and learned CPS had determined there was no abuse although the violence had escalated. Sue said she was ready to take action to protect her child, despite anger about the CPS report.

Janice was referred for therapy, where she learned skills to keep herself as safe as possible during violence in the home, including coping that addressed her stomach pain. A validated assessment tool, the Child PTSD Symptom Scale (Foa, 2001), revealed she was experiencing nightmares, hyperarousal and intrusive thoughts, making her anxious and likely creating the stomach pain.

In the following months, Janice's behavior worsened while they lived in a shelter. Unable to manage Janice's tantrums and outbursts, Sue worked with Janice's social worker, learning healthy discipline techniques such as setting house rules, providing her daughter with clear warnings when her behavior was not okay, and with "time outs" to help her regroup when her behavior escalated. She and Janice also learned coping skills such as playing games for distraction, age-appropriate relaxation exercises and drawing to manage what often felt like out of control emotions.

When Janice's behavior improved, she agreed to make a book outlining her abuse story, with notes about her understanding of why he hurt her, saying for example that, "it's not OK what he did to me and he needs to get help so he doesn't hurt other little kids." Though considerable future work was necessary to support this mother and daughter, Janice was on the path to healing and her mother was healing as well, exemplifying how individuals can recover from family violence.

RESOURCES

Courtois, C.A. (2010). *Healing the incest wound: Adult survivors in therapy* (2nd ed.). New York: WW Norton & Company.

Finkelhor, D. (2008). *Childhood victimization: Violence, crime and abuse in the lives of young people.* New York: Oxford University Press.

Gil, E. (2006). *Helping abused and traumatized children: Integrating directive and nondirective approaches.* New York: Guilford Press.

Pleck, E. (2004). *Domestic tyranny: The making of American social policy against family violence from colonial times to the present.* Chicago: University of Illinois Press.

Renzetti, C.M., Edleson, J.L., & Bergen Kennedy, R. (2001). *Sourcebook on violence against women.* Thousand Oaks, CA: Sage Publications.

ONLINE RESOURCES

Includes tip sheets and information on assessment and intervention of child survivors: http://www.apa.org/pi/families/resources/task-force/child-trauma.aspx

Agency for Persons with Disabilities (APD) Cares website. Signs and Symptoms of Abuse/Neglect of the disabled: http://apd.myflorida.com/zero-tolerance/common-signs/#/

Child Welfare Information Gateway. Signs and Symptoms of child Abuse/Neglect: https://www.childwelfare.gov/pubPDFs/whatiscan.pdf

HelpGuide. Signs and Symptoms of Domestic Violence: https://www.helpguide.org/articles/abuse/domestic-violence-and-abuse.htm/

HelpGuide. Signs and Symptoms of Elder Abuse/Neglect: https://www.helpguide.org/articles/abuse/elder-abuse-and-neglect.htm

Information on child trauma issues, assessment tools, treatment, research and new developments in the field: http://www.nctsnet.org

Power and Control Wheel developed by the Domestic Violence Intervention Project in Duluth, Minnesota: http://www.theduluthmodel.org

Safety Planning – This website provides safety plans and planning tools. Assess for appropriateness. Consider further web research for safety plans that best fit your client's situation. http://www.ncdsv.org/publications_safetyplans.html

---

Practice Exercises and Questions

- What are the types of family violence and how are they different?
- How do children, adults, the elderly and the disabled react differently to family violence?
- What makes individuals vulnerable to trauma?
- Role-play talking with a survivor as she/he comes in for the first time, seeking assistance

---

Family Violence, Abuse and Neglect Summary

Tune in to Family Violence, Abuse and Neglect

- *Remember a time you were controlled or coerced*
- *Observe mistreatment around you such as bullying of individuals who are different and parents disciplining their children by yelling, slapping or ridiculing*

Incidence, History and Impact of Family Violence, Abuse and Neglect

- *Family Violence, Abuse and Neglect, including IPV, child abuse/neglect, elder abuse and abuse of the disabled, are common today*
- *Many are hurt by someone close to them*
- *Despite the abuse, individuals may not experience a trauma reaction. Assess for PTSD and other impacts. Also assess for safety and the ability to cope*
- *Consider the history of the Family Violence, Abuse and Neglect prevention movements and stay up-to-date on emerging evidence-based practices*

Look for the Signs of Trauma Unique to Each Population

- *Reactions to trauma may look very different in children than in adults and among the elderly and disabled*
- *Regression, aggression, tantrums, acting out, anxiety, depression, withdrawal, sexualized behavior and issues with attachment and trust are not uncommon reactions for survivors of familial abuse*

Attend to Each Population's Special Needs

- *Remember that abuse can impact survivors' long-term physical health. Ensure they receive adequate medical care*
- *Work to support the whole family including parents and other caregivers. Teach parenting/caregiver skills as needed and increase understanding of appropriate child/adult development as well as ways to increase safety*
- *Teach survivors coping before processing trauma. Discuss safety plans and provide resources/referrals to ensure reduction in vulnerability and isolation*

Chapter 5

War and Terrorism

War and terrorism destroy safe environments essential for healthy development, creating helplessness and despair. The media can contribute to this process by broadcasting graphic images and descriptions that unsettle and instill fear. Healing requires making sense of what happened and finding a new safety, in many cases even in the midst of continued unrest.

> **Definitions**
>
> - *Safety* – State essential to trauma recovery and unique to each individual, in which: (1) risky behaviors, unhealthy relationships and negative emotions are reduced and (2) a sense of well-being, trust, calm and positive coping are increased

TUNE IN TO WAR AND TERRORISM

Tune in to yourself, noting how you are now at your baseline. Notice your thoughts, emotions and how your body feels. Then recall a time you had a brush with war or terrorism. This could have been a personal experience, a loved one's or even a reaction to news reports or fictionalized accounts. Stay in the memory for a moment and then check in again on how you are, noting what's changed in your body, thoughts and feelings. Do not be surprised if your mood has changed because these are difficult events to think about. Do some self-care – deep breathing, a hot cup of tea or stretching are possibilities – and file away your reaction. It will help you tune in to this chapter and to individuals you work with who have similar experiences.

BACKGROUND INFORMATION

The traumas of war and terrorism include torture, combat and child soldiering. Because the response to trauma is more serious when caused by human beings, these events can be especially damaging (Goelitz, 2009; Klingman & Cohen,

2004). Here are some of the factors that engender soldiers' responses to war, for instance: (1) psychosocial status prior to enlistment; (2) experiences while in combat and (3) the state of society and its responsiveness when they return home. The greatest effect seems to stem from the degree of combat experienced by soldiers. Many have difficulty with relationships, adjusting to society and developing successful careers post combat and these difficulties are impacted by their trauma experience and reaction (Rosenheck & Fontana, 1995).

Child soldiers have a particularly hard time with war. Longing to flee the aggression, these children must instead become aggressors themselves at a time in their lives when they would normally be learning to regulate violent urges. Most also witness atrocities as they soldier. Contrary to their youthful training, many survivors do not want to be soldiers in the future, but rather wish for peace and think about ways they can help others (Shaw & Harris, 1995).

Refugees of war and terrorism are also at risk. Although a high percentage have experienced torture, this piece of their histories is often not shared with mental health practitioners who do not think to ask about it, even when refugees have fled their countries because of persecution (Briere & Scott, 2006). The harm to individuals from torture is impacted by day-to-day safety factors. Holocaust survivors' extent of psychological harm, for example, was found (Roberts, 2005b) to be related to their: (1) quality of life; (2) ability to cope and (3) housing situation prior to and after the event.

Tips

- Assess survivors of war and terrorism thoroughly, taking particular care with refugees. These vulnerable individuals have survived a traumatic event, been uprooted from their homes and communities and may have experienced torture as well

---

Reactions to disasters related to terrorism have been found to be even worse than reactions to natural disasters. These features of the traumatic event increase survivors' difficulty (Dziegielewski & Sumner, 2005): (1) happening unexpectedly; (2) jeopardizing current safety and the ongoing security of society and (3) revealing a terrifying path of destruction, creating disorder and feelings of lost control and helplessness.

Evidencing reactions like these, Saul, a survivor of the September 11th disaster, was anxious and unable to relate well to his family after the event. He worked in the area, lost his job as a result and witnessed calamity on the day of the attack. He also had a brother in Afghanistan and began watching footage of the war obsessively after the attack, in an attempt to understand what was going on there and magically thinking it would somehow keep his brother safe. As a result, his anxiety increased.

Healing is necessary after traumatic events and community members reaching out to survivors can be healing. After the September 11th disaster, a Maasai village wanted to give a gift to comfort survivors. They made a presentation of 14 cows, their most precious commodity, and it helped survivors who were touched by their compassion and humanity. Another example of this kind of empathic healing support is a 12-year-old non-Muslim girl who fasted during Ramadan for those affected by the war in Afghanistan (Weingarten, 2004).

IMPACT AND INCIDENCE

War and in particular combat are traumatic and can cause tremendous stress (Callahan, 2010). This is true not only for soldiers but also for their loved ones who may not live in a war zone. The incidence of mental health disorders and of suicide among survivors of combat, affects these family members as well, causing stress and even at times leading to secondary trauma. The Mental Health Advisory Team (MHAT), a group established by the US Army in July 2003 after a marked increase in survivor suicides and mental health disorders, found that combat stressors leading to these issues include thoughts about killing, multiple and/or lengthy combat deployments, combat injuries, being shot at, seeing comrades injured and encountering dead bodies. Exemplifying this, in 2004, when the combat intensity was less in Afghanistan, the Post-Traumatic Stress Disorder (PTSD) rate for US service men and women there was 6% as compared to 12% in Iraq, where combat intensity was higher (Callahan, 2010).

Definitions

- *Post-traumatic stress disorder (PTSD)* – A disorder resulting from exposure to traumatic events that causes symptoms lasting at least a month that include emotional responses of fear, horror or helplessness; flashbacks and/or nightmares of events; avoidance of reminders of the event and increased arousal
- *Flashback* – Intrusive and involuntary re-experiencing of traumatic events through images, emotions or physical sensations

---

According to research findings from Afghanistan, the Balkans, Cambodia, Çhechnya, Iraq, Israel, Lebanon, Palestine, Rwanda, Sri Lanka, Somalia and Uganda, children are even more vulnerable than adults to stress of war and terrorism (Murthy & Lakshminarayana, 2006), with reactions that include PTSD and mood disorders as well as somatization and acting out and often disruptive behaviors (Shaw, 2003). This vulnerability is increased by issues such as refugee status and being forced to be a child soldier. Adolescents have been found to be particularly at risk. Other vulnerable groups include women, the elderly and the disabled (Murthy & Lakshminarayana, 2006).

The effects of war and terrorism take their toll on both individual survivors and society as a whole. This impacts many areas that include individual and societal well-being as well as finances. War-related stressors, for instance, emotionally and physically wear down combat survivors, often causing confusion as old ways of thinking and being no longer work, potentially resulting in personality changes if not addressed. These effects can also worsen over time as seen with the Vietnam War where 10–20 years after service, prevalence in the United States of PTSD increased from 15% among men and 8% among women to 30% for men and 25% for women, according to the National Vietnam Veterans Readjustment Study (Callahan, 2010). This incidence of PTSD and other mental health disorders increases the cost of supporting veterans, approximately 300,000 of whom have come home with Major Depressive Disorder (MDD) or PTSD (as compared to National Institutes of Health estimates that 3.6% of the US population aged 18–54, have PTSD). Based on the probability that about 30% of combat veterans will suffer from PTSD, MDD and Traumatic Brain Injury, disability payments and medical care are projected to total more than $600 billion (Callahan, 2010).

Tips

- Check in with yourself periodically while reading this material, continuing to practice self-care as needed. War and terrorism, which are caused by humans and often have horrific results, can be even more difficult to fathom and process than other traumas

---

UNIQUE SIGNS OF A TRAUMATIC RESPONSE

There are unique signs of the stress caused by war and terrorism. Both are human-made traumas and involve mass destruction. Tick (2005), for example, describes the effects of combat trauma as similar to that of a concentration camp survivor – chain smoking, unable to sleep and having nightmares when s/he does, hiding from light, not practicing basic self-care including cleanliness and isolating from family and friends. The truth of the matter, as he so eloquently describes, is that hearts must be changed by war in order for soldiers to be able to kill as it necessitates. A change in life perspective is required, particularly with child soldiers who are even more vulnerable to war's effect on the heart.

Each of us has a sense of identity that includes our perspective on good and evil and which helps form our moral principles. Tick (2005) reminds us that we are improved by choosing good and that when forced to choose evil, such as with killing during war, something is destroyed and soldiers are "spiritually poisoned" (Tick, 2005, p. 113) by their own destructiveness. As this unfolds, they experience loss of self and the sense they cannot trust themselves anymore, fluctuating between being drawn to and even addicted to the violence of war to being horrified by it – similar to how parachute jumpers go from being scared to feeling exhilarated (van der Kolk, 2014). Many cannot tolerate the betrayal of their ethical codes and suffer as a result (Tick, 2005).

But war is also an initiation of sorts and embracing this experience of being a spiritual warrior allows combat veterans to recapture their "good" selves thru healing and become true warriors who exhibit "decency, honesty, kindness, compassion, cooperation, strength, courage, clear mindedness, vision, wisdom, ethics" (Tick, 2005, p. 199). Combat survivors also learn to heal through telling their stories, facing their destructive actions, allowing themselves to feel the betrayal of their ethics; rebuilding dignity and restoring peace in the process (Tick, 2005). Although many hesitate to remember what happened, learning to tamp down on their pain; facing the past and beginning to accept what occurred helps them acknowledge that the violence is in the past. This makes it possible for them to see the world differently and to begin to heal as they find a relatively safe place in it (van der Kolk, 2014).

SPECIAL CONSIDERATIONS

As with all types of trauma, vulnerable populations experiencing terrorism and war are more at risk than most. This includes the elderly, disabled, physically/mentally ill, children and those with prior trauma or barriers to care (Gallow-Silver, 2004).

Vulnerability is increased by the impact of mass trauma which can also lead to social upheaval. Countries in flux, like Northern Ireland, are particularly vulnerable. And stable countries are reminded of their vulnerability when calamity occurs such as with the September 11th terrorist attacks occurring in three US Locations and instilling fear in many. War, especially if widespread and long-term, has an even greater impact (Webb, 2004). Both war and terrorism and are limited not only to victims but also to (1) loved ones, (2) individuals who perceive themselves to also be in danger even if not directly affected and (3) to caregivers who experience trauma secondhand as they witness victims' distress. Hospital workers, for instance, were greatly affected by victims' loved ones asking about and posting photos of those missing after the World Trade Center September 11th attack (Gallow-Silver, 2004).

Children's vulnerability and subsequent difficulty coping with trauma is apparent in the following cases. Bobby was 7 years old when his father was missing after the World Trade Center September 11th attack. He began waking in tears from disturbing dreams. The timing coincided with a memorial service for his father that was conducted after his finger, the only body part recovered, was found. Bobby would go to his mother's bed at night where she was often crying. Around this time, he began missing school due to stomach aches. He was confused and scared about his father's missing body parts and his mother's tears and worried that his schoolmates knew his father was in pieces (Webb, 2004).

Mary, who was also 7 at the time, was trapped in an elevator with her classmates at the World Trade Center during the 1993 bombing. Not only that but she was visiting relatives at the time of the Oklahoma City bombing. Due to developmentally emotion based reasoning, Mary came to the illogical conclusion that she caused both events and would cry if she heard bombs mentioned (Webb, 2004).

Another Mary, aged 9 at the time of the September 11th World Trade Center attack, had headaches and nightmares after the event and exhibited fear. Her symptoms worsened when she studied earthquakes months later and remembered relatives in Taiwan who had lost their home in an earthquake. Her family, Chinese Americans with possible cultural barriers to care, did not seek help despite referrals being made until her grades suffered and the school got involved when her fears escalated with worry about earthquakes and terrorists, hypervigilance and fear of the dark and of sleeping alone (Fang & Chen, 2004).

Definitions

- *Coping* – Process of dealing with difficulties, problem solving and adapting to the environment in order to manage stress and conflict effectively
- *Hypervigilance* – State of increased attention to the environment, in order to detect threat and prevent harm, that can increase anxiety, prevent sleep and cause fatigue

---

In each of these cases, children made connections that were not easily recognized by adults caring for them. The connections were made based on a child's undeveloped reasoning and made sense to them. Bobby was worried his schoolmates would find out his father was in pieces and this embarrassed him. Seven-year-old Mary blamed herself for the World Trade Center and Oklahoma City bombings. Nine-year-old Mary's fears were compounded as she linked them to both the World Trade Center Attack and earthquakes in Taiwan (Fang & Chen, 2004; Webb, 2004).

Tips

- Assess survivors of war and terrorism for skewed thinking and/or other potentially risky reactions, taking special care with any who are vulnerable and/or marginalized. Examples include children, the elderly, the disabled, those who are in need of financial support, the mentally or physically ill and culturally disenfranchised groups

PRACTICE CONSIDERATIONS

Strong emotions related to terrorism and war can make processing and recovering from them difficult. Feelings of anger and shame about what they did and of revenge for dead comrades, for instance, can become so intense that their behavior appears to be psychotic with combat veterans reporting things like hearing babies crying and seeing burned and bloodied bodies of babies. They think these are current memories, but they are actually flashbacks from past combat. Separating themselves from what occurred can be challenging with these kinds of emotional reminders (van der Kolk, 2014).

This influx of emotions happens because extremely violent events are not processed by the brain like other memories. The events are not integrated or remembered in a cogent narrative form because the pre-frontal cortex is not able to make sense of them, making it difficult for survivors to adapt and re-enter the reality of their everyday lives (Bragin, 2014).

Tips

- To understand what it is like to have memories that are not integrated, imagine a romantic breakup that occurred unexpectedly and for no apparent reason. Think about how your brain would have difficulty letting go of this experience because it could not make sense of it

---

Adaptation to emotional overflow includes survivors finding ways to separate from the pain, for instance, by not talking about it or the events that caused it. Not talking about what happened is even encouraged at times by practitioners who may be overwhelmed themselves, unsure how to deal with it or afraid the emotions are unsafe for survivors (Tick, 2005). This can increase isolation and potentially hinder recovery.

Tips

- Remember that it is always important for survivors to talk about what occurred in a safe way. Safety includes being listened to and accepted when they talk, providing assistance with modulating emotion if needed, helping them to find hope in what might seem like a hopeless situation, educating about the effects of trauma and how to cope and working with them to cope by encouraging them to stay in the moment and to ground themselves it they dissociate

---

Intensity and duration of emotional trauma experiences are important determinants of psychological outcomes as is the degree of vulnerability involved in both the experience and in survivors' lives post-trauma. In all instances, supportive care, including through spirituality and cultural activities, have been found to mitigate the effects (Murthy & Lakshminarayana, 2006). This is true not only for individuals but also for families and communities, both as victims themselves and as loved ones of victims.

Unfortunately, barriers to supportive care often exist. Statistics reflect this. One study showed that only 50% of veterans seeking it found adequate care and that others did not even seek it mainly due to concern for side effects, harm to career or loss of security clearance (Callahan, 2010). Cultural barriers can also exist. Outreach and education can assist with barriers to care (Fang & Chen, 2004).

A form of supportive care that has been found to be efficacious with survivors of terrorism and war is the utilization of creative arts including storytelling. Zlata, for instance was a 11-year-old survivor of the Sarajevo war who recorded her thoughts, feelings and experiences in a diary in the same way Anne Frank did while hiding with her family from the Nazis. Zlata began to come to terms with what happened as she wrote (Webb, 2004).

Writing was advantageous for a family that experienced trauma in Northern Ireland as well. They lived near a "peace wall" dividing a Protestant community from their Catholic one. Stones and missiles were thrown at their home from over the wall. The children were scared and their mother was on medication for her anxiety. Writing about their experiences as a part of therapy helped them to process this and to begin to heal. Margaret, one of the children, continued writing even into peaceful times, completing a memoir. She exemplified the healing by saying that "Writing about the bad is good" (Reilly, McDermott, & Coulter, 2004, p. 320).

Drawing can also help heal emotions stirred up by trauma. Five-year-old Noam's picture of a traumatic event demonstrated this. He drew a trampoline he said would save those who fell, if a plane flew into the World Trade Center again. Drawing it helped him after he and his classmates watched from their classroom as the September 11th disaster occurred (van der Kolk, 2014). A post September 11th mural project was healing for New York City children as well. Participating in the mural helped survivors as it provided social support for the community and encouraged resilience (Mapp & Koch, 2004).

EVIDENCE-BASED PRACTICE

Not only is supportive care helpful for survivors' recovery from war and terrorism but it can also lower the cost of treatment as exemplified with US veterans. Estimates from one study showed that evidence-based care would pay for itself in 2 years, reducing lifetime disability compensation and other costs related to

PTSD and MDD. This was without taking into account costs resulting from family issues, homelessness and substance abuse, which are prevalent with veterans. The study also found that suicides decreased and productivity improved with evidence-based care of veterans (Callahan, 2010).

Evidence-based approaches include pharmacotherapy, psychosocial support and community based prevention and healing. Although the selective serotonin reuptake inhibitor (SSRI) medications sertraline (Zoloft) and paroxetine (Paxil) are the only pharmacological approaches approved in the US for PTSD treatment (Alexander, 2012), studies suggest that "off-label" administration of propranolol may help prevent PTSD (Callahan, 2010). Osteopathic manipulative treatments and other mind body and alternative approaches such as meditation, creative therapies and yoga are not evidence based but with further use and study, may be found to be efficacious as well (Callahan, 2010).

In terms of psychosocial support, the US Departments of Veterans Affairs and Defense recommends cognitive restructuring techniques, EMDR, stress inoculation and narrative therapy, among others (2017). The Institute of Medicine (US) Committee to the Psychological Consequences of Terrorism also recommends Psychological First Aid immediately following these types of traumas (2003). Both pharmacotherapy and the psychosocial approaches are recommended utilizing methods of care that include monitoring for adverse effects by providers that treat the patients regularly.

Tips

• Closely monitor survivors as they are treated. Watch for signs of dissociation and decompensation caused by inadvertent triggers related to violent memories of war and terrorism

---

Multiple studies have found wider spectrum approaches that take a systemic view to be key. Ecological Systems Theory, for example, looks at protective factors, risk and resilience and recommends tiers of care that address: (1) basic needs and security; (2) supportive care including for children, first responders, teachers and parents and (3) specialized care for those deemed to be most at risk such as the seriously mentally ill (Bragin, 2014). Institute of Medicine (US) Committee to the Psychological Consequences of Terrorism (2003) also recommends special attention for those most at risk as well as the development of additional evidence based techniques and training/education targeting societal responses to terrorism. The preparatory training would be geared to mental health, primary care and school based professionals and to developing workplace guidelines (Institute of Medicine (US) Committee to the Psychological Consequences of Terrorism, 2003).

Preventative community-based approaches have also been found to be efficacious for veterans. Israelis, for example, stress preventative- and resiliency-based training not only as part of military training but also for communities at risk where resiliency centers that teach PTSD prevention and self-regulation techniques to individuals, communities and leaders have been developed (Callahan, 2010). In the United States, the Kansas National Guard Resiliency Center incorporates Israeli techniques. Its Flash Forward resiliency instruction program focuses on pre-deployment readiness and offers the "Warfighter Diaries," a social networking site where the military and their families can post and review information about resiliency issues they encounter (Callahan, 2010). These approaches utilize systemic methodologies that fit social work's lens and offer hope for society as they prepare communities with the goal of alleviating both immediate distress and long term repercussions of war and terrorism.

Take a moment and check in with yourself as you digest the material in this chapter and prepare to move on to the following case study. As previously mentioned, many find war and terrorism particularly difficult to comprehend and make sense of. Use self-care if needed to modulate your reactions and come to terms with what you have read.

Case Study

Martina grew up in Milan, Italy during World War II. There were frequent air raids and air raid sirens that sent her and her family to shelters with their neighbors. Homes were blacked out at night so that house lights would not invite attack. Martina was too young to understand about war but she picked up the anxiety around her. Fear was particularly prevalent in her mother and caused her to be afraid too. She associated the noise of the attacks with thunderstorms and developed a fear of them also. Her anxiety became so intense that even signs of rain could make her afraid.

She moved to the United States as a newlywed and was happy for a time until her husband died unexpectedly after the birth of her son. This increased her anxiety as did her son's cancer diagnosis in his early 20s. It reached crisis proportions while she was away on vacation and she went to the emergency room there, was diagnosed with anxiety and put on medication. Later, when new health related stressors emerged, her anxiety worsened again and she sought help through psychotherapy.

As she engaged in therapy, it became clear that she was hypervigilant and scared much of the time. Worry for her was a way of life and was hard on those around her, especially her son and close friends. It was because of them that she decided to try therapy but she did not believe it would really help and constantly asked when it was going to get better.

Through the use of hypnosis, EMDR and cognitive restructuring in therapy; meditation, physical exercise, deep breathing and cognitive behavioral techniques at home and adjustments to her medication regime, her anxiety began to recede. Psychoeducation also helped as it clarified how her brain used anxiety to try to keep her safe and protect her because it was still caught in the loop of her past trauma. She began to understand that she no longer needed to worry. The danger had passed. This process was not easy for her. She got caught back in the trauma loop often but became better and better at recognizing what was happening and taking care of herself instead of worrying, allowing healing and peace to reside where there had been fear and alarm.

RESOURCES

Bragin, M. (2014). Clinical social work with survivors of disaster and terrorism. In J. Brandell (Ed.), *Essentials of clinical social work* (pp. 366–401). London: SAGE Publications. https://www.cswe.org/getattachment/ac73b154-b499-4d52-aa40-0a479141afd6/Clinical-Social-Work-in-Situations-of-Disaster-(1).aspx

Tick, E. (2005). *War and the soul*. Wheaton, IL: Quest Books.

Webb, N. (Ed.). (2004). *Mass trauma and violence*. New York: The Guilford Press.

ONLINE RESOURCES

National Child Traumatic Stress Network, & National Center for PTSD. (2005). *Psychological First Aid: Field operations guide*. https://learn.nctsn.org/course/index.php?categoryid=11

Practice Exercises and Questions

- Become conscious of your reactions to media reports on war and terrorism and observe your emotions as you do, making note of what may apply when working with these populations
- If/when you have emotional responses to the media reports, try various ways of coping, noting this as well so that you can recommend similar approaches for survivors you work with
- List some of the unique signs of trauma and special considerations when working with survivors of these types of trauma
- Review the practice considerations and evidence-based practice sections, selecting methodologies you think would be helpful for your clients. Explain why you made these choices

- Role-play from your practice experience with this population or from one of the cases noted in the chapter. When determining how to approach the client you choose to role-play, consider not only care for your client but also impact on loved ones and community members

War and Terrorism

Tune in to War and Terrorism

- *Check inside and notice your current thoughts, emotions and physical sensations*
- *Take a moment to remember/reflect on experiences you have had with war and/or terrorism, including media reports*
- *Note your reactions to the memories. This will help you to tune in to survivors' experiences. Do self-care to calm emotions roused by the memories*

Background Information

- *The fact that war and terrorism – including combat, child soldiering, torture and refugee status – are caused by human beings, makes them more difficult to deal with and heal from*
- *Human made traumas such as these engender intense emotional reactions – fear, helplessness, sadness, hopelessness, shame and anger – that can be difficult to cope with*
- *Not only do the long-term results of these emotions impact mental health – often leading to PTSD, MDD or even psychosis – but they have financial costs to society as well*

Special Considerations

- *Vulnerabilities such as being elderly, a child, disabled or otherwise disenfranchised, increase risk of negative mental health outcomes*
- *Isolation and inability to acknowledge and process intense trauma emotion is also an issue*
- *Barriers to care can make it difficult for survivors to seek and receive help*

Practice Considerations

- *Duration/intensity of trauma experiences are key determinants of outcome*
- *Supportive care is effective and helps quell strong emotions*
- *Creative therapies such as with art, writing and music can offer effective support, helping survivors process emotions and memories*

Evidence-Based Interventions That are Effective with This Population

* *Financial costs to society can be curtailed when evidence-based treatments are utilized*
* *Approaches include pharmacotherapy, psychosocial support and community based prevention and healing*
* *Specific approaches include CBT techniques such as EMDR, Ecological Systems Theory, stress inoculation and medications such as Propranolol*

Chapter 6

Life-Threatening Illness

Life-threatening illness has become more prevalent than in the past. As populations age and medicine extends lives, the incidence of individuals living with incurable disease increases. According to a report by the Centers for Disease Control and Prevention (2003), for instance, the life expectancy of Americans reached a high of 77.2 years in 2001 and the number of deaths attained an all-time low. For example, cancer has become so common that half of all men and one-third of all women in the United States will have it at some time in their lives. Despite this, only about half will die from it (Glajchen et al., 2002). Furthermore, although about one-third of these cancer patients are at risk psychosocially, only 15% to 25% of them seek help from professionals with their difficulties in adjusting to being ill (Cwikel & Behar, 1999). Therefore, determining appropriate psychosocial screening, assessment and treatment options for this growing population of trauma survivors has become a significant endeavor.

TUNE IN TO ILLNESS AND THE POSSIBILITY OF DYING

Many social workers have had personal experience with illness. This includes having loved ones who are sick, being diagnosed with life-threatening illness or thinking about the possibility of poor health. As a result, when working with individuals and families who face life-threatening illness, it is important to be mindful of the ways our own histories may affect both our work and well-being.

To tune in to what survivors of life-threatening illness experience, get in touch with your feelings about sickness. Finding a safe place first will anchor you and allow feeling fear of pain and death, anger at having life cut short or changed by illness and grief related to losing the ability to work and live life as in the past. Tolerating and accepting these feelings is crucial when working with individuals who are sick. Many people do not know what to say to those diagnosed with serious illness, and either stay away from them or tell them it will be okay when it may not be. Having someone who can just be with them, bearing witness to their suffering related to illness, can be healing in itself for survivors of life-threatening illness.

> **Tips**
>
> • *Accessing a safe place* – A safe place must be very low-stress and positive. Examples include a beach or other place in nature, a spiritual location or a happy memory. If you cannot think of a place, use your imagination to create one with characteristics that make you feel safe and happy. Use all your senses to bring the safe place alive in your mind until you feel it strongly. This exercise can be used with survivors as well

HISTORY OF LIFE-THREATENING ILLNESS BEING RECOGNIZED AS A TRAUMA

Recognition of illness-related trauma took time. Hospitals first acknowledged the need for psychosocial attention to illness, utilizing social workers to facilitate care when they saw that sickness impacted individuals socially as well as physically. This process started in England and progressed to the United States between 1905 and 1915 when 100 social workers were hired in American hospitals. The field of oncology has been one of the leaders in recognizing psychological issues related to illness. Ida Cannon, a major facilitator of this movement, switched careers from nursing to social work after hearing Jane Addams speak. Between 1905 and 1945, Cannon proceeded to develop an approach to patient care that included a medical, social and psychological focus (Fobair et al., 2009).

Consultation liaison psychiatry began in the 1960s and the field of psycho-oncology, which addresses psychosocial issues related to cancer, was established in 1975, further facilitating an integrative model when treating the medically ill (Holland, 2002). In 1967, about the same time as psycho-oncology emerged in the United States, Dame Cicely Saunders, a social worker, nurse and physician, established the first hospice, St. Christopher's in London (Raymer & Reese, 2004). Her work with a terminally ill Polish Jew who had escaped from Poland during World War II inspired this project. Traditional Western care had not helped him address spiritual and psychosocial issues. Saunders designed a concept (hospice) to fill this gap. Since that time, recognition of the value of social workers has grown, resulting in 1982 in a mandated role for Medicare-reimbursed hospice care in the United States (Raymer & Reese, 2004).

Medical practitioners have become even more aware of the need to address psychosocial issues in recent years, encouraging an increase in holistic care. This perspective led to the discovery that illness is not only stressful, but can also be traumatic. Consequently, life-threatening illness was included as a cause of post-traumatic stress disorder (PTSD) in the 1994 edition of the *Diagnostic and Statistical Manual of Mental Disorders* (DSM-IV).

Definitions

- *Post-traumatic stress disorder (PTSD)* – A disorder resulting from exposure to traumatic events that causes symptoms lasting at least a month that include emotional responses of fear, horror or helplessness; flashbacks and/or nightmares of events; avoidance of reminders of the event and increased arousal

---

INCIDENCE OF TRAUMATIC RESPONSES TO LIFE-THREATENING ILLNESS

Psycho-oncology's founder, Jimmie Holland, studied patients' emotional needs and found that 25% had psychiatric diagnoses, primarily related to anxiety and depression (Rosenthal, 1993). PTSD also exists with the seriously ill, but with less likelihood than from other, more violent, traumatic events. The risk for developing PTSD for those who have experienced rape is about 49%, while the risk for a child diagnosed with life-threatening illness is only about 10.4% (Sidran Traumatic Stress Institute, 1995–2009). Despite this, a review of the literature found that the percentage of cancer patients with PTSD symptoms is as high as 60%, with 15% to 80% reporting symptoms of intrusive cancer-related thoughts and avoidance of cancer reminders in the first month after diagnosis or recurrence, when these symptoms tend to be highest for the medically ill (Kangas, Henry, & Bryant, 2002). Post-traumatic stress disorder (PTSD) and other trauma responses exist with a variety of medical conditions, including post myocardial infarction (MI) (Chung, Berger, Jones, & Rudd, 2008; Tedstone & Tarrier, 2003), cardiac surgery, hemorrhage and stroke, childbirth, miscarriage, abortion, gynecological procedures, intensive care treatment, human immunodeficiency virus (HIV) infection, awareness under anesthesia (Tedstone & Tarrier, 2003) and diagnosis of multiple sclerosis (MS) (Chalfant, Bryant, & Fulcher, 2004). Of 210 patients with HIV, 34% had PTSD and 43%

Definitions

- *Avoidance* – Individuals staying away from people, places or activities, even when not dangerous, because they are reminders of trauma
- *Hyperarousal* – Heightened emotionality that can lead to agitation, anger, difficulty sleeping and/or hypervigilance
- *Hypervigilance* – State of increased attention to the environment, in order to detect threat and prevent harm, that can increase anxiety, prevent sleep and cause fatigue

had an adjustment disorder (Israelski et al., 2007) and in another study, after an MS diagnosis, 75% had PTSD symptoms and 16% had PTSD (Chalfant, Bryant, & Fulcher, 2004).

Despite these indicators of psychosocial vulnerability, many patients in need of support never receive psychosocial care in the course of life-threatening illness (Cwikel & Behar, 1999). Patients often do not realize they need and can get help. In addition, healthcare workers who lack experience detecting psychological distress do not always identify it. Attitudinal and cultural barriers discussed below under "Special Considerations" also prevent some from getting assistance.

UNIQUE SIGNS OF A TRAUMATIC RESPONSE

A literature review on PTSD in cancer patients found documentation for the following differences between cancer and other traumatic stressors. These differences apply to many chronic and potentially life-threatening illnesses: (1) cancer's influence extends from diagnosis to death because of the risk of recurrence (Kangas, Henry, & Bryant, 2002); (2) its potential for recurrence persists as an ongoing stressor; (3) the immediacy and degree of danger from cancer varies at different points in the disease process and (4) there are multiple traumatic events related to the illness (Smith, Redda, Peyserb, Vool, 1999), including diagnosis, surgery, treatment, pain and other symptoms and recurrence.

Other aspects of trauma unique to this population are the fact that the trauma originates internally rather than externally, and that survivors' intrusive focus is on future potential dangers rather than past dangers (Sumalla, Ochoa, & Blanco, 2009). In addition, some characteristics of post-traumatic growth (PTG) are unique to the ill (Sumalla, Ochoa, & Blanco, 2009).

Definitions

- *Post traumatic growth (PTG)* – Condition resulting from exposure to traumatic events that causes symptoms that include the ability to see trauma from positive perspectives, to find benefit in it, to attach meaning to it that makes sense and inspires and to make constructive and helpful behavioral changes as a result

---

Although a literature review noted that medical-illness-related trauma resembles other long-term traumas, no other cause of trauma shared all the aforementioned aspects. Living in a war zone, near a nuclear power plant or in a flood region share many of the same aspects, but not all (Smith, Redda,

Peyserb, & Vool, 1999). Unlike most survivors of trauma who experience PTG, for instance, some with illness see their trauma as a gift because of the positive growth it entails (Hefferon, Grealy, & Mutrie, 2009).

The ongoing nature of life-threatening illness, even in remission, creates stress (Kangas, Henry, & Bryant, 2002). The resulting fear increases risk of PTSD (Cordova et al., 2007) and can produce what is known as the "Damocles Syndrome," a fear of recurrence, like a sword hanging over their heads (Wells & Turney, 2001). This contributes to intrusive thoughts being mainly future- rather than past-oriented (Sumalla, Ochoa, & Blanco, 2009). Survivors of traumatic illness do have flashbacks and intrusive thoughts of past events such as their diagnosis, but tend to dwell more on fears about the future. Because diagnosis of life-threatening illness has, seemingly, no beginning or end (Sumalla, Ochoa, & Blanco, 2009), patients can become preoccupied with it and tend toward: (1) continual study about the illness; (2) fixation on symptoms and treatments and (3) intensified self-care. On the other hand, these aspects of avoidance of the illness can also exist and even lead to fatality if they prevent treatment: (1) denial of the illness or its potential to harm; (2) lack of interest in self-care or (3) fear, lack of trust and/or numbness related to medical treatment, healthcare practitioners or information on illness and care.

Definitions

•   *Flashback* – Intrusive and involuntary re-experiencing of traumatic events through images, emotions or physical sensations

---

The ongoing nature of traumatic illness contributes to survivors feeling out of control, as do the ups and downs and varying symptoms and treatments along the disease trajectory. Illness proceeds in a direction and at a pace that is, for the most part, out of survivors' control (Levine & Karger, 2004). Knowledge of the illness process can help reduce stress and increase a sense of control (Cordova et al., 2007), but maintaining equilibrium presents a challenge. Ongoing signs of illness, such as blood tests, medication and pain, make it impossible to avoid stressful reminders of its progress (Kangas, Henry, & Bryant, 2002). Since these components of illness can also traumatize, survivors often cannot identify one cause of a trauma response (Sumalla, Ochoa, & Blanco, 2009), making it difficult to prepare themselves for stressors. Tests that appear innocuous, for instance, may have unexpected results, as with John, a cancer survivor in remission, who went for a routine bone marrow test result. Neither he nor his doctor expected to learn that cancer had entered his bone marrow and could spread to other parts of his body.

The internal source of the trauma – survivors' own bodies – exacerbates their feeling of being out of control. They cannot get away from the trauma or avoid reminders (Sumalla, Ochoa, & Blanco, 2009). It can even seem their bodies have betrayed them, with some blaming themselves for the illness or having other negative beliefs that create stress: That they deserve their disease as punishment or that pain indicates their illness is progressing even when this is not the case (Altilio, 2004).

Despite the way life-threatening illness creates feelings of lost control, survivors can have more of a sense of control than with other traumas because death and illness are a normal part of life (Sumalla, Ochoa, & Blanco, 2009). We expect to get sick and eventually die, but do not anticipate being raped. This may be part of the reason there is a high incidence of PTG among survivors of illness. Two studies cited by Wells and Turney (2001) found more positive changes than negative ones after serious illness. A study found significantly more positive emotions in the dreams of illness survivors than those surviving other traumas (Goelitz, 2009) and another found that 53% to 95% of breast cancer patients experienced increased spirituality, improved relationships with family and friends, greater self-confidence and personal strength and revised priorities and goals, resulting in generally more satisfaction and perceived meaning in life (Cordova et al., 2007).

Another aspect of PTG unique to this population is that survivors of serious illness have been found to be more aware of their bodies as a result of their experience. They are more conscious of their health, practice better self-care, avoid risky behaviors and participate in more healthy activities. These benefits of illness may be why some can say that their illness was a gift (Hefferon, Grealy, & Mutrie, 2009).

Tips

- *Do not expect PTG* – Although PTG can occur for survivors of any trauma, not all experience it. Expecting it or telling survivors it may occur can create feelings of guilt or despair for those who do not experience it. If you see an aspect of their response that indicates PTG, point it out so that they are aware and can gain strength from it. Help them see that this strength was a direct result of their tragedy and demonstrates their resilience

---

Cassandra, a survivor of childhood sexual abuse who was diagnosed with cancer as an adult, exemplifies of the development of PTG. She reacted to the cancer diagnosis traumatically, experiencing flashbacks of the scan that showed possible cancer and of getting the news of her diagnosis. She had difficulty with radiation treatment as well, frequently asking her providers to come in when they were ready to start treatment because she was frightened. She had head and neck cancer so she needed to wear a mask that kept her head still by being fastened to the treatment table. When this was done, she felt as though her abuser had come to get her.

Determined to find ways to cope, she told her providers about her difficulties. They offered support, talking to her during treatment which decreased her sense of isolation and referring her to a nurse who taught her guided imagery. Cassandra spoke to her therapist and they came up with a plan to imagine pushing her abuser away when scared. As a result of this and other coping she used during treatment, she reported that her cancer experience had become a positive and valued growth experience. Symptoms of PTG replaced her former PTSD symptoms.

Definitions

* *Coping* – Process of dealing with difficulties, problem solving and adapting to the environment in order to manage stress and conflict effectively

---

Tips

* *Coping toolbox* – Survivors need a toolbox full of coping skills so that if one does not work, they have others to choose from. Help them identify what they do naturally and add new skills to this repertoire. This empowers survivors, lowering stress

---

SPECIAL CONSIDERATIONS

A number of issues bear consideration when assisting survivors of illness-related trauma. Many recover without assistance, but individuals with these characteristics are more vulnerable to adverse effects of trauma: (1) prior physical and mental health issues; (2) emotionally labile, anxious and depressed personality types; (3) current life stressors and (4) a history of stressful life events. Adults with cancer have also been found to be more susceptible to PTSD than children (Smith, Redd, Peyserb, & Vool, 1999).

Although life is already stressful for most diagnosed with life-threatening illness, the following factors seem to increase the risk of psychosocial distress and heighten vulnerability to PTSD: (1) disease-related symptoms, that often cause both physical and emotional suffering, such as pain, shortness of breath and fatigue; (2) financial issues; (3) limited or inadequate access to medical or psychosocial care; (4) family distress (Walsh-Burke, 2004) and (5) inadequate social supports (Taïeb, Moro, Baubet, Revah-Lévy, Flament, 2003).

Individuals without supportive people in their lives can feel alone and scared when sick. Even those with friends and family can have difficulty. This is particularly true for people who do not talk openly about their experience. Both unavailability of support and reluctance to discuss their illness can lead to avoidance of feelings and becoming socially constrained. Research indicates that social constraint inhibits processing of trauma, increasing distress and the risk of PTSD (Cordova et al., 2007). Some cultural groups are more prone to the impact of this issue. LGBTs may be socially ostracized, for example, experiencing shame and guilt if their illnesses are considered socially undesirable, as can be the case with hepatitis, HIV and HIV-related cancers (Thompson & Colon, 2004).

Those who have mental illness prior to diagnosis are also at risk for social isolation and PTSD (Lanche, 2008). Even with no pre-existing condition, some develop these issues after being diagnosed and experiencing illness-related losses. Survivors often lose their work, financial security, old way of life, independence and body image. Illness can also lead to disability and the possibility of death, making adjustment to these losses difficult.

Access to needed healthcare, including information about their medical condition, is an essential social support that is not always available. Knowledge of the illness trajectory can help prevent PTSD, as it prepares survivors for what comes next in the disease process (Cordova et al., 2007). However, patients and families may not ask about illness treatment or recommended tests because their cultures discourage the questioning of authority figures (Del Rio, 2004). Language can also become an issue. One patient with a language barrier even believed doctors had begun treating his cancer against his will, causing him to feel out of control and helpless, when he was actually getting an X-ray.

Phone interpreters and family who act as non-professional translators can help, but this entails clinical challenges. Culturally based non-verbal communication is often missed with phone interpreters and non-professionals can selectively interpret conversations. Some people also fear lack of confidentiality when communicating with professional interpreters, refusing to use them or not sharing honestly with them present (Del Rio, 2004).

These access barriers can lead to marginalization and increase survivors' vulnerability to adverse trauma reactions. Other marginalization issues include: (1) disparities in healthcare available to minorities, including educational materials not being available in all languages; (2) significant barriers to care as indicated by most hospice patients being White middle class; (3) poverty that may mean transportation, housing and sufficient medication are difficult to obtain or non-existent (Otis-Green & Rutland, 2004) and finally (4) members of minority groups may have understandable trust issues with White middle-class practitioners. Those who are marginalized and whose healthcare is inadequate are more likely to be socially isolated and experience suffering related to untreated symptoms and lack of knowledge about their illness. These individuals are also less likely to be assessed and treated for trauma-related symptoms.

FAMILY MEMBERS AND CAREGIVERS

Since there is evidence that poor family functioning increases the risk of PTSD, it makes sense for social workers to work directly with family members and other caregivers when possible. Family distress tends to occur related to: (1) social isolation; (2) communication issues; (3) caregiver difficulties; (4) anger, abuse and violence; (5) substance abuse; (6) mental illness; (7) grief and (8) the inability to obtain illness-related resources or conflicts with resource providers (Walsh-Burke, 2004).

Demonstrating the incidence of family distress influencing trauma risk, one study that assessed family functioning in 144 adolescent cancer survivors and their parents found that (1) 47% of adolescents, 25% of mothers and 30% of fathers reported poor family functioning and 2) adolescents with PTSD were five times more likely to be members of low-functioning families (Alderfer, Navsaria, & Kazak, 2009). Family members can be at risk for PTSD as well. The incidence of PTSD in parents of pediatric patients is particularly high, with mothers most at risk (Pöder, Ljungman, & von Essen, 2008).

Another stressor, the burden on caregivers, increases family members' distress and vulnerability to traumatic reactions to their loved one's illness. Caring for the sick is financially, emotionally and physically taxing. Time constraints can also be an issue, particularly if caregivers work or care for other family members. Geographic proximity to patients is a factor as well, often requiring travel or causing concern because family members are too far away to see patients regularly. Healthcare professionals, including social workers, are not immune to stress associated with caring for those who are ill. See chapter 1 on secondary trauma for more information and be sure to discuss relevant concerns in supervision.

INTERACTIONS WITH OTHER FORMS OF TRAUMA

Another risk for PTSD with this population is a prior trauma history (Smith, Redd, Peyserb, & Vool, 1999). Past violent traumas are particularly problematic (Shelby, Golden-Kreutz, & Andersen, 2008). Holocaust survivors, for example, are vulnerable to adverse trauma reactions as a result of illness (Hantman & Solomon, 2007).

Current distress related to illness can interact with past trauma and loss by increasing survivors' feelings of vulnerability, triggering memories of past events so that survivors re-experience them through flashbacks and nightmares or have intense emotional reactions that may seem out of proportion to the situation at hand. Be on the lookout for this and for individuals who are sick and also living in stressful situations. Concurrently experiencing illness and another potentially traumatic circumstance may lead to severe trauma reactions. This includes individuals in abusive relationships or living in war zones. The impact of an abusive caregiver can be particularly devastating since caregivers should provide protection. Survivors sometimes even have trust issues with caregivers and healthcare providers who treat them well due to their trauma histories. These understandable trust issues often get in the way of effective care.

Those with serious illness can also encounter another trauma when sick and experience increased distress as a result. Denise, a lung cancer patient, was in the hospital during the September 11th disaster. She worked at the World Trade Center and had friends there. As a result, she was referred to a hospital social worker for support. The social worker helped allay the effects of the trauma by addressing Denise's feelings of guilt and reminding her of the importance of coping:

Denise:	I feel like if I hadn't gotten sick, I could have been there and helped them.
Social worker:	What do you think would have been different if you weren't sick?
Denise:	Well I'd have been there and we could've gotten away together.
Social worker:	You must have a lot of power. *Smiling gently.*
Denise:	Guess it wouldn't have been so easy, but maybe I'd have done something.
Social worker:	So let's talk about how you would have helped. It may help now.
Denise:	*Thinking.* Well, my office was full of angels – statues and pictures. I think they could have helped.
Social worker:	Were they still there when it happened?
Denise:	Yes, they were and I actually heard my colleague, Bernard, got out and was okay. He was in the office next to mine. *Pause.* Maybe my angels helped him.
Social worker:	Yes, and you can use the angels now, too. Call on them to help.

Tips

- *Build on past history with coping* – Discover how survivors have coped with difficult situations in the past and encourage them to use these methods with current stressors. This empowers them and increases their feelings of safety

---

Definitions

- *Safety* – State essential to trauma recovery and unique to each individual, in which: (1) risky behaviors, unhealthy relationships and negative emotions are reduced and (2) a sense of well-being, trust, calm and positive coping are increased

PRACTICE CONSIDERATIONS

Social workers are in a unique position to provide a range of services to individuals and families facing life-threatening illness. Research shows that these services can help with depression, sleep patterns, mood, emotional well-being and, in particular, quality of life (QOL) (Greer, 2002). What is more, social workers can help by assessing for and treating traumatic reactions to illness that can result in depression, anxiety and PTSD. Knowledge of PTSD is crucial because in our experience, healthcare practitioners tend to notice depression and anxiety, often missing PTSD.

Social workers need to learn about clients' illnesses and communicate with healthcare providers during assessment, since symptoms may interrelate with medical conditions. Metabolic imbalances and shortness of breath can cause anxiety, and fatigue can mimic depression (Walsh-Burke, 2004). In addition, somatic symptoms can be mistaken for PTSD symptoms. For example, what looks like dissociation may be fatigue or treatment side-effects. Also, arousal symptoms such as disturbed sleep, irritability and poor concentration may stem from illness or treatment (Kangas, Henry, & Bryant, 2002).

Tips

- *Be like Columbo* – When Peter Falk played the detective, Columbo, in an American TV series, he always asked many questions, learning from those he worked with. We can do the same in order to learn from survivors what they know about their illness. They are often good sources, but we can also do research or ask colleagues what they know. The more we learn, the more we can help coordinate survivors' care and support their effective coping

---

Definitions

- *Dissociation* – Disconnection from thoughts, memories or emotions that provides internal distance from reminders of traumatic events but also prevents integration of trauma material and disrupts normal psychological functioning

---

Multidisciplinary care – including practitioners communicating as they assess symptoms of shared patients, coordinating treatment and collaborating on how each practitioner can best help – provides a web of healing for those who are ill. Continuity of care is also important, enabling practitioners to follow patients during the course of their illness or to maintain communication as patients make the transition between different types of care, such as from hospital to home. This can ensure that identified traumatic reactions are followed and treated. Treating the whole person – spiritually and psychosocially, rather than just physically – also known as holistic care, is another component of care that tends to be practiced. Finally, integrative medicine and complementary and alternative medicine (CAM) are often components of care as well. These methodologies provide alternatives to traditional Western medical care and include: (1) yoga, acupuncture and other bodywork; (2) alternative medicine such as herbs and (3) relaxation techniques. Learn more about the use of these treatments in chapter 17 on other trauma interventions.

Since social workers are trained in an ecological approach that looks at all parts of clients' lives, working with these components of care makes sense and comes naturally, but social workers can help in other areas too. Crisis intervention is an important social work function because so many crisis periods occur in the disease trajectory – diagnosis, onset of disease symptoms and news of recurrence – when extra support can avert calamity and help prevent the onset of trauma reactions.

During times of crisis, social workers can advocate for survivors, helping them obtain services and information. Patients need someone to coordinate assistance with finances, housing, other concrete services or discharge planning (when social workers or other professionals ensure that patients have the equipment and care they need as they leave the hospital) (Blum, Clark, & Marcusen, 2001). Not only are these important services that help reduce survivors' stress and thus prevent traumatic reactions, but they also provide an avenue to connect with survivors who might not be open to talking to a social worker. Once the opening has been provided, many are willing to receive other psychosocial services as well.

Illustrating how concrete services can support survivors and potentially provide openings for other psychosocial services, a social worker was referred to a hospital patient who needed assistance with health insurance. The social worker gave her information and referrals and they then talked of other matters. The patient, Susan, had just had her leg amputated because of diabetes and was devastated. She said she had been terrified at night since she awoke from anesthesia unable to move. As they talked, she was reminded of when she was hospitalized as a child:

Denise:	I get so scared. It makes sense that it's similar to how I felt when I was in the hospital as a child because the feelings are so big. I can't stand it when it happens.
Social worker:	What would make it easier for you? Is there something you can hold or have with you like your bear? *Pointing to a stuffed bear on her bed.*
Denise:	I would be embarrassed if someone came in and saw me holding my bear.

Social worker:	You'd be surprised how many people do it. They see it all the time here. What else would help?
Denise:	Really? *Taking the bear and holding it in her arms.* Well it would help if my partner was here. He stayed one night and it was better, but he left and I was scared.
Social worker:	Can he stay again? If not, can you call him when you get scared?
Denise:	I think so. I'll ask him.
Social worker:	What else would help? *Pause.* What if you remind yourself that you're not that little girl, but actually an adult who can take care of herself?
Denise:	I like that and it's true isn't it?
Social worker:	*Nodding.* So we have a plan. If you get scared, you can hold your bear, call or talk to your partner and tell your little girl you are there and she is okay.

Tips

- *Safety plan* – Help survivors develop a plan that will empower and sustain them during an anticipated stressor. You can include ways to cope to reduce stress before and after; and resources to utilize during the challenging event, meeting with a difficult person or a stressful period of time

---

EVIDENCE-BASED PRACTICE

Careful assessment of survivor issues and needs is crucial when selecting appropriate psychosocial interventions. What some need most is assistance getting services or support during a crisis. For others, more robust interventions are called for. According to the literature, the following interventions are often used with this population: (1) psychoeducation, (2) emotional support and (3) cognitive behavioral therapy (CBT) to improve coping skills, challenge unhelpful thoughts and relax (Stanton, 2006).

Definitions

- *Psychoeducation* – Process of teaching about the nature and incidence of physical and mental illness, its impact, consequences and approaches to healing

---

CBT techniques, in particular, have a long history of use among practitioners caring for the seriously ill. Many social workers and nurses have training in relaxation techniques such as guided imagery and healing touch. Research shows that these practices improve emotional adjustment for cancer patients, not only lowering stress and positively affecting mood, but also significantly reducing anxiety and depression (Luebbert, Dahme, & Hasenbring, 2001). These and other CBT techniques have a positive impact on patients' quality of life as well (Osborn, Demoncada, & Feuerstein, 2006). A lower risk of PTSD after MI has even been found for those with effective coping and emotion regulation skills (Chung, Berger, Jones, & Rudd, 2008).

Both CBT and psychoeducation, another research-based practice that promotes adjustment to breast cancer (Zimmermann, Heinrichs, & Baucom, 2007), benefit survivors. In addition, authors reviewing the literature reported that the most effective intervention they found for adolescent cancer patients was psychoeducational. This intervention, which was geared toward improving psychosexual development, reduced illness-related distress and anxiety, potentially lowering the risk of adverse trauma reactions (Seitz, Besier, & Goldbeck, 2009).

Support groups also help the seriously ill with trauma reactions. Symptoms of PTSD were assessed for 181 women in unstructured psychoeducation support groups and in CAM groups that used yoga, meditation and imagery, movement and psychoeducation. Symptoms decreased by 91% in the support groups and by 80% in the CAM groups (Levine, Eckhardt, & Targ, 2005).

Addressing the need for effective coping, the Surviving Cancer Competently Intervention Program (SCCIP), a four-session, one-day group-based intervention geared toward reducing PTSD symptoms, integrates CBT and family therapy approaches and focuses on these topics: (1) cancer effects on patient and family; (2) coping skills; (3) how to get on with life and (4) consolidating what has been learned as the patient looks toward the future. Further research is required, but initial results indicate efficacy (Kazak et al., 2004).

Another group-based intervention, the Strength-focused and Meaning-oriented Approach to Resilience and Transformation (SMART), is a holistic approach to trauma that practitioners found effective with those suffering the impact of the Severe Acute Respiratory Syndrome (SARS) epidemic in Hong Kong. The intervention components include Eastern spiritual teachings, physical techniques such as yoga and meditation and psychoeducation that promotes meaning making (Chan, C., Chan, T., & Ng, 2006).

Narrative therapy helps clients challenge unhelpful thoughts by discovering new positive stories about their lives and dispelling negative ones. Replacing problem-based stories with more hopeful ones can provide meaning related to the illness experience and assist with integrating it. In particular, Narrative-Expressive Therapy is an intervention that was designed to address stress among the seriously ill and prevent PTSD. This is a three-session group intervention in which members tell their stories, engage in personally meaningful creative projects, and share the projects with group members (Petersen, Bull, Propst, Dettinger, & Detwiler, 2005).

Finally, social support seems to improve adjustment to illness, as seen with the Social Cognitive Processing (SCP) model. The model's primary tenet is that social support improves functioning and psychological response after trauma (Devine, Parker, Fouladi, & Cohen, 2003; Harper et al., 2007). Negative responses to disclosure of disease concerns can cause social constraint. Since constraint may interfere with processing the illness experience, lead to avoidance and prolong distress, interventions such as supportive counseling can be efficacious when they promote communication, validation, processing and reappraisal of the traumatic illness experience (Cordova et al., 2007). Further research is required in order to determine the efficacy of SCP, Narrative-Expressive Therapy and SMART.

Case Study

Mr. K was a 49-year-old freedom fighter brought to the United States by Amnesty International from the Czech Republic. He was admitted to the hospital for bleeding, pain, fatigue, excessive saliva and difficulty eating, related to head and neck cancer. Requesting pain medication, he refused all other treatment.

Socially isolated, with no family supports, he was suspicious of medical practitioners and refused to engage with hospital staff. He admitted to using cocaine and drinking alcohol daily and his living situation was tenuous. He lived in the unfinished attic of a friend's house where there was no running water or telephone and illegal activities precluded acceptance of home or hospice care.

On his hospital discharge date he was referred to the pain and palliative care team for consultation. He was motivated to communicate with them because he needed pain management and assistance with finances and insurance. The social worker coordinated obtaining an emergency two-week supply of medication and set an appointment for outpatient follow-up.

This man had experienced multiple traumas as a freedom fighter, had found his previous roommate shot in the head and now had cancer. He continued to live a precarious existence that increased his level of stress and added to the barriers preventing appropriate care. His PTSD symptoms made trusting healthcare practitioners and receiving treatment difficult. He was fearful of authorities and believed healthcare providers were "out to get him," exhibiting PTSD symptoms of hypervigilance and avoidance. He was vulnerable because he lacked financial resources and a stable home environment. Cultural and linguistic estrangement from providers increased his marginalization even more: He spoke English, but not well; had cancer-related sores in his mouth that added to communication difficulties and lived in a subculture that further alienated him.

The social worker engaged with Mr. K by providing the concrete services he sought – pain management and financial resources. Because of this, he was able to connect with and obtain support from pain management and hospice staff until he made the decision to come to the inpatient hospice unit to die. He died as he wanted, on his own terms, but also with support that made the process as comfortable as possible.

Tips

- *Lower stress and increase safety* – Interventions that lower stress and increase safety also help to prevent PTSD. Go where clients are and provide what they need. Concrete services like financial support can help some survivors more than therapy

RESOURCES TO HELP TUNE IN TO THE EXPERIENCE OF LIVING WITH LIFE-THREATENING ILLNESS

Albom, M. (1997). *Tuesdays with Morrie*. New York: Doubleday.
Wilber, K. (2000). *Grace and grit* (2nd ed.). Boston: Shambhala.

OTHER RESOURCES

Berzoff, J., & Silverman, P. (Eds.). (2004). *Living with dying: A handbook for end-of-life healthcare practitioners*. New York: Columbia University Press.
Lauria, M.M., Clark, E.J., Hermann, J.F., & Stearns, N.M. (Eds.). (2001). *Social work in oncology: Supporting survivors, families and caregivers*. Atlanta, GA: American Cancer Society.
Naparstek, Belleruth has produced guided imageries for the medically ill and traumatized. Search on YouTube or purchase copies for use with patients.

ONLINE RESOURCES

Association of Oncology Social Work (AOSW) including standards of care: http://www.aosw.org/
Association of Pediatric Oncology Social Workers (APOSW) including standards of care: http://www.aposw.org/
Online discussion group (listserv) for social workers working with the seriously ill: http://www.stoppain.org/for_professionals/content/information/listserv.asp

Practice Exercises and Questions

- Role-play meeting with a newly diagnosed breast cancer patient after tuning into your own fears of developing breast cancer. See chapter 1 for applicable information on secondary trauma
- Discuss how to communicate with and support a patient who does not speak English and was just diagnosed with HIV
- Provide examples of ways to connect with and support hospital patients. Consider concrete services as well illness related emotional support. Be specific
- Consider ways you could advocate for a medically ill patient. Keep in mind all areas of care and use the social work principle of going where the patient is
- Plan how to approach and work with a patient's family members, keeping in mind needs of both the patient and family

Life-threatening Illness Summary

Unique Signs of Trauma as a Result of Illness

- High rate of intrusion mostly due to anticipated danger
- High rate of avoidance, but difficult to avoid reminders
- Multiple traumatic stressors: diagnosis, symptoms, treatment
- Most sources of trauma are internal rather than external
- Duration of the trauma can be long, extending until death
- High rate of post traumatic growth, finding benefit in illness

Special Considerations for the Medically Ill

- High levels of psychological distress increase risk of PTSD
- Marginalized individuals can be even more vulnerable

Standards of Care After Diagnosis of Acute Illness

- Ongoing multidisciplinary coordination of treatment
- Holistic care of the whole person – mind, body and soul
- Integrative methods – yoga, herbs and other alternative care

Interventions That are Effective with This Population

- Crisis intervention, advocacy and psychoeducation
- CBT, including relaxation and coping skills
- Individual, group and family supportive care and counseling

Chapter 7

Witnessing Trauma

Just as experiencing trauma can be harmful, so can witnessing it. Not only are witnesses traumatized by their encounters, but they also blame themselves for not protecting victims or feel guilty that they were not personally harmed. These factors complicate both the effects of trauma and the recovery process.

Witnessing takes many forms. Children witness spousal abuse through direct observation and hearing it happen, seeing the aftermath (blood, bruises, broken items and tears), or feeling tension in the house – for example, from a parent's fear when the perpetrator returns home (Purvin, 1996). Even hearing neighbors arguing aggressively can be hard.

Witnessing can come from a distance. Family members who have never been exposed themselves can inadvertently absorb relatives' trauma-related distress (Motta, Joseph, Rose, Suozzi, & Liederman, 1997). Media reports often become traumatic and frightening, as does community violence. Natural disasters and serious accidents can also upset witnesses.

TUNE IN TO WITNESSING TRAUMA

Tune in to your own experiences with trauma. These can include witnessing difficult situations directly or in the media, and hearing stories related by loved ones of their traumatic experiences. Before tuning in to the witnessed trauma, make sure you feel safe and have the support you need to do so. If the memory you have chosen feels too anxiety-provoking, choose another less intense one.

Witnessing an adult aggressively chastising a child is an example of this type of experience. Even watching staff or customers admonish a store clerk is not pleasant. Most people have observed situations like these and felt helpless and stressed as a result.

When you have found a way to remember an experience safely, tune in with all your senses, noticing emotional and physical consequences of witnessing trauma. Keep the memory in mind as you read the following sections on types of witnessing, common responses and specific methodologies utilized when working with witnesses.

BACKGROUND INFORMATION

Those affected by witnessing trauma include professionals such as doctors, psychotherapists, nurses, social workers, social service workers, Peace Corps volunteers, hospice workers, battered women's and homeless shelter staff, sexual assault workers, suicide hotline staff, AIDS volunteers, foster parents, prison personnel, combat veterans, emergency medical staff, firefighters and police, criminal defense lawyers and prosecutors, judges, victim advocates (Saakvitne & Pearlman, 1996), journalists and others in the media (Weingarten, 2004), early responders and pastors (Naparstek, 2005). Even a university oral historian collecting stories from those affected by military combat, the September 11th disaster, and the Holocaust had to learn to counter the effects of exposure to trauma in order to do her work effectively. She regained a sense of well-being by praying for the survivors she interviewed and using images of her father hiking with her as a child to relax herself prior to sleep after she began waking with trauma flashbacks, having difficulty falling back asleep and feeling nervous and hypervigilant during the day (Naparstek, 2005). See chapter 1 on secondary trauma for more information on professionals who witness trauma.

Weingarten (2004) refers to the prevalence of trauma witnessing even outside the professional realm as "common shock." Common shock, as she describes it, is a widespread, collective disturbance caused by exposure to violence. Global media coverage of disturbing events magnifies this phenomenon (Weingarten, 2004).

We cannot predict, when witnessing events, which will have a traumatic impact. How individuals react in the moment varies, as does the trajectory of their responses over time. Some recover with no issues and others develop symptoms of post-traumatic stress disorder (PTSD). However, many people do not realize how events affect them and inadvertently accrue stress as a result. The cumulative impact can do harm, with individuals becoming inured to the effects of traumatic events even while "aroused and distressed" (Weingarten, 2004, p. 40) from witnessing them. Frequent exposure to atrocities through media reports contributes to these numbing influences of common shock (Weingarten, 2004).

Definitions

- *Common shock* – Widespread/collective physiological and psychosocial disturbance caused by exposure to traumatic events
- *Post-traumatic stress disorder (PTSD)* – A disorder resulting from exposure to traumatic events that causes symptoms lasting at least a month that include emotional responses of fear, horror or helplessness; flashbacks and/or nightmares of events; avoidance of reminders of the event and increased arousal

The global prevalence of witnessing is difficult to quantify because much is unconscious and thus under the radar. However, studies of 5th graders (10–11 years old) found that 91% of those in New Orleans and 72% of those in Washington, DC had witnessed violence such as shooting, stabbing or mugging (Weingarten, 2004). Other studies found 3–4 million children aged 3–17 at risk of exposure to domestic violence (Purvin, 1996).

Incidence of harm caused by witnessing war crimes has been documented as well. In a multi-stage, stratified, random cluster survey of 2,585 adults, conducted in villages and camps for displaced persons in Uganda, about 70% had PTSD symptoms after witnessing sexual abuse, family members and friends killed or abduction of children (Vinck, Pham, Stover, & Weinstein, 2007). In another study of evacuees with homes destroyed or damaged during the Gulf War, 80% had symptoms that qualified for diagnosis of PTSD if they had had them for at least a month; and a year later, 60% were diagnosed with PTSD (Solomon, Laor, McFarlane, 1996).

We also know that survivors of past trauma and other vulnerable individuals who witness current trauma have higher susceptibility to trauma symptoms. Children who survived trauma and later witnessed the September 11th disaster, for instance, had significantly more behavioral issues related to anxiety, depression, emotional dysregulation, aggression and sleep disturbances than those with no history of trauma (Chemtob, Nomura, & Abramovitz, 2008).

TYPES OF WITNESSING

Witnesses tend to have a hard time coping with traumatic events experienced by close family members and friends, even when witnessed indirectly. It has been found that the effects of trauma can pass on in an inter-generational manner to family members even though they were never exposed themselves, leading to emotional issues that are often undetected or attributed to other stressors (Motta et al., 1997). The physiological signs of stress from trauma, for example, have shown up in survivors and in their children born after the trauma occurred (Sternberg, 2000). There is even evidence that alterations to DNA caused by trauma can be passed transgenerationally to offspring (Youssef, Lockwood, Su, Hao, & Rutten, 2018).

Couples' relationships have been adversely affected by sexual or physical abuse experienced by their partners, adding credence to the idea that exposure to another's trauma creates distress (Nelson & Wampler, 2000). In support groups, parents of sexual abuse survivors expressed feelings of secrecy, shame and guilt; and parents of cancer patients expressed fear, anger, sadness and guilt (Jones, 1994; Schaefer & Pozzaglia, 1994), showing signs of common shock. A poignant example of parents' distress as they witness their children's traumatic experiences is a mother, Sarah, who was nursing her baby shortly after his birth when she saw he was turning blue. She called for a nurse who pulled him off her breast and took him for treatment and tests. Sarah never forgot the anxiety she felt until she found out her baby was fine. The anxiety was powered by the pain, love, terror, disbelief and helplessness she experienced until he was returned to her (Weingarten, 2004).

Children are witnesses too. The threat of danger as well as what they witness directly or through the media – including destruction of the environment, evacuation and harm to animals and humans – can traumatize them even when they are shielded from traumatic events and safe. Families, schools, law enforcement and even mental health practitioners often do not adequately consider the effect of witnessing. The ease of childhood can disappear as the traumatized suffer and sometimes lose hope for the future and trust in people (Ayalon, 1998). Traumatic events can confuse children. An example of this is children questioning why it was a good thing that Osama bin Laden was killed in 2011.

Children and adults are also affected by violence in their communities. This seems clear in the midst of war, but also holds true for those who live in neighborhoods where violence is considered the norm. A 6-year-old girl interviewed by a researcher reported that it was her job to protect her 2-year-old sister when there were gunshots. She felt the most secure in the bathtub (Weingarten, 2004). She may not have been physically hurt, but the experience must have traumatized her.

Media coverage can minimize disasters and paint them as a normal part of life. The reports do not depict the real suffering, including long-term trauma effects. Some media accounts even present events in ways that sensationalize them (McFarlane & Yehuda, 1996). When a 2-year-old Romanian girl fell into a well, millions watched the television coverage of her rescue. The collapse of the World Trade Center towers during the September 11th disaster was watched countless times by viewers, as were President Kennedy's assassination and the Rodney King beating. Some viewers experienced common shock as a result, but many watched the reports as though they were dramatic movie episodes (Weingarten, 2004).

Violent images that contribute to traumatic impact occur in television/movies, comics, song lyrics and video games (Weingarten, 2004). A 6-year-old boy recently showed me a cartoon video on his iPad that was violent and contained sexual innuendo and swearing. His mother sat beside us in the dentist's waiting room as he shared this. I commented on the violence and he had no idea what I meant. His mother said nothing.

COMMON RESPONSES

Common responses in witnesses include isolation/disconnection from others; despair, hopelessness and other emotions that can feel unmanageable; nightmares/flashbacks; sensitivity or cynicism, particularly regarding violence and disrupted feelings of safety (Saakvitne & Pearlman, 1996; Elklit & Kurdahl, 2013). Demonstrating this, many romantic partners in therapy after the September 11th disaster reported exaggerated neediness that generated fury if it was not responded to, coupled with numbness to the other partner's needs (Weingarten, 2004).

Children tend to react with fear, guilt, sleep disturbances, sadness, depression, anger, stomach/headaches, bedwetting, difficulty concentrating, resisting going to bed or school, hiding or running away, increased aggression, becoming withdrawn, self-injuring and delayed development of speech, motor and/or cognitive skills. Children often respond to the constant threat of danger from trauma such as domestic violence by worrying excessively about the victim and fearing or resisting separation from them. Studies have also found that child witnesses of domestic violence run a greater risk of abusing their partners (Purvin, 1996).

WITNESSES VULNERABLE TO HARM

Witnesses most vulnerable to harm include (1) socially, financially and culturally marginalized individuals; (2) helping professionals and (3) children. People with trauma histories are also more vulnerable as are those who have had intense exposure to trauma. In addition, exposure to human-made traumas such as terrorism and war creates more vulnerability than exposure to natural disasters (Weingarten, 2004).

Professional caregivers witness trauma both personally and professionally, increasing their exposure (Weingarten, 2004). With the September 11th disaster, for instance, social workers helped those affected and at the same time coped with their own reactions to the disaster. Professionals often feel the emotions of those they help, increasing their exposure (Rothschild, 2006). Finally, empathetic professionals and those exposed for long periods of time are more vulnerable. Symptoms of PTSD, for instance, were more prevalent among long-term human rights workers in Kosovo (Weingarten, 2004).

Witnessing becomes more difficult when there are multiple problems and limited resources. These stressors, which include emotional responses, current dangers and future prospects, increase vulnerability (Saakvitne & Pearlman, 1996). If survivors do not get organizational, political or societal support, the distress of witnessing can increase. Seeing that survivors are not getting proper care, as in New Orleans after Hurricane Katrina, can evoke helplessness in witnesses.

Children run even more of a risk of harm than adults, particularly young children. Factors that increase their vulnerability include intensity of exposure to violence (proximity, frequency, etc.), their relationship to victims and the vailability of adults or coping skills to assist with mediating the experience (Weinstein, 2002).

Marginalization increases vulnerability. Marginalization occurs for a number of reasons, including both issues that predate or directly relate to traumatic events. Separation from extended family, friends and community causes stress and cuts individuals off from supportive relationships that help them cope. Financial issues and discrimination also marginalize witnesses and increase vulnerability (Schaefer & Pozzaglia, 1994). "Linguistic and cultural isolation" (Schaefer & Pozzaglia, 1994, p. 335) also has an effect. Those who cannot speak the language or relate to the customs of those around them feel even more alone and unable to cope. See chapter 8 on vulnerable populations for more information on this topic.

SPECIFIC METHODOLOGIES

Testimonial psychotherapy, a form of narrative therapy, has helped witnesses of genocide and other traumatic events integrate, understand and find meaning in their experiences. With this intervention, which also decreases symptoms of PTSD and depression, mental health providers work with witnesses on compiling and, when appropriate, publicly sharing stories of their experiences. Having the stories witnessed by providers heals as it ensures that others remember and learn from them (Weine, Kulenovic, Dzubur, Pavkovic, & Gibbons, 1998).

Documentation of witnessed events can help create distance from their traumatic aspects. It can also be a political statement that empowers witnesses and allows those who would not normally do psychotherapy, for cultural and other reasons, an avenue for recovery (Lustig, Weine, Saxe, & Beardslee, 2004).

Weingarten (2004) has delineated other ways to decrease potential harm from witnessing traumatic events. She talks about the importance of consciously witnessing with kindness and respect. Compassionate awareness that something terrible has happened often forms witnesses' experiences, particularly when witnessing takes place through routine media coverage. Awareness includes: (1) satisfying resulting needs, obtaining support, talking about the traumatic event with others in order to support each other and utilizing coping/stress-management techniques; (2) institutions facilitating these functions for staff and constituents and (3) mourning the tragedy and teaching children to consciously witness, learn from and honor it. These processes can help to prevent current effects of witnessing trauma as well as future inter-generational effects (Weingarten, 2004).

Case Study

Roger was a firefighter who felt guilty that he did not personally respond to the September 11th disaster. He witnessed the reactions of colleagues who were there, supported families of firefighters who died, and went to the site to assist with the clean-up. He was also in the middle of a contentious divorce and had financial problems. He became tense, angry and unable to cope, spending his free time alone ruminating. He also developed a drinking problem. When support was offered through an organization that supports firefighters, Roger asked for help. At the third therapy session, he shared as follows:

Roger:	I just can't relax. I'm always tense and unhappy, even home alone.
Social worker:	Do you feel the tension in your body? Or is it more in your mind?
Roger:	My mind? I do feel it in my body, especially my shoulders and neck.
Social worker:	It can be in your mind too. Do you worry or think about that day?
Roger:	I do find myself imagining what it was like for my buddies who died and thinking I could have saved them if I'd been there. I worry a lot too about their families and about what's going to happen to me. My life is a mess. *He looks distraught.*
Social worker:	Do you want to try something to relax your mind and body? *Addressing his stated concerns rather than trying to analyze what he was feeling.*
Roger:	I'll try anything at this point. I don't know what to do. *He shakes his head.*
Social worker:	Guided imagery can help you relax and move your mind from disturbing thoughts. It may seem strange at first, but it can help. Will you give it a try?

Roger was surprisingly open to trying new things. He did quite well with guided imagery, a method found beneficial for trauma survivors (Naparstek, 2005). Feeling safer and less anxious as a result of the imagery, he drank less and could talk about and address the issues in his personal life. As his sense of safety increased, he could talk about the guilt and horror he felt related to the disaster. His trauma responses gradually decreased and his coping increased. See chapter 10 on the importance of safety for more information on why we need to address safety concerns first when working with those affected by trauma.

RESOURCES

Lustig, S.L., Weine, S.M., Saxe, G.N., & Beardslee, W.R. (2004). Testimonial psychotherapy for adolescent refugees: A case series. *Transcultural Psychiatry, 41*(1), 31–45.

Vinck, P., Pham, P.N., Stover, E., & Weinstein, H.M. (2007). Exposure to war crimes and implications for peace building in northern Uganda. *JAMA: Journal of the American Medical Association, 298*(5), 543–554.

Weingarten, K. (2004). *Common shock: Witnessing violence every day: How we are harmed, how we can heal*. New York: New American Library.

ONLINE RESOURCES

Child Witness to Violence Project: http://www.childwitnesstoviolence.org/

Practice Exercises and Questions

- Tune in to yourself, noting how you feel emotionally and physically and what your thoughts are. Go to a safe place inside yourself (a happy memory; what your feel during prayer or other spiritual practices, after exercise, or in nature; etc.). Watch a news report, really listening and watching. Tune into yourself again, noting how you feel has changed. This will give you insight into witnessing
- Role-play helping a trauma witness document and tell his/her story
- Find a news report describing a crime witness's experience. As you read it, look for possible trauma responses in the past, present or future
- Describe how you would explain the effects of witnessing trauma to a witness or their loved one
- Consider macro-level ways to work with witnesses including advocating and community organizing. See chapters 19 and 20 for more information

---

Witnessing Trauma Summary

Tune in to Witnessing Trauma

- *Awareness of prevalence in communities and the media*
- *Helplessness and stress felt as a result of exposure*

Types of Witnessing

- *Within intimate relationships such as family and friends*
- *In communities which suffer experiences such as war and natural disaster*
- *Accessed through the media including global news reports*

Factors to Consider

- *Effects of witnessing are magnified by global media coverage*
- *Previous trauma survivors are more susceptible to harm*
- *Those who have had long-term and/or intense exposure are also vulnerable*
- *Available support and coping reduce vulnerability*

Common Responses

- *Experiencing intense and at times unmanageable emotions*
- *Symptoms of PTSD such as nightmares and hypervigilance*
- *Becoming numb or inured to atrocities witnessed*

Treatment Methodologies

- *Testimonial psychotherapy promotes healing by documenting*
- *Consciously witnessing with respect, sadness and kindness*
- *Acknowledging potential for harm and practicing self-care*
- *Sharing experiences with others for mutual support*

Chapter 8

Vulnerable Populations

Vulnerable populations, including children, the elderly and mentally ill, immigrants, previous trauma survivors and those with substance abuse issues, are at risk of adverse effects from trauma. Experiencing trauma also creates vulnerabilities for survivors that increase their risk of complex reactions to trauma or further traumatization. Some develop substance abuse or mental health issues, while others manifest difficulties with relationships and work that can lead to marginalization. This chapter focuses on how trauma and vulnerability interact and highlights specific issues for social workers to consider.

TUNE IN TO VULNERABLE POPULATIONS

In preparation for reading this chapter and understanding survivors' vulnerability, tune in to their unique backgrounds. You can get a sense of this without having experienced trauma yourself. Imagine their situations by remembering moments of vulnerability when you experienced a crisis. For example, bring to mind a time when you were sick or not doing well financially. Then think about the problems you had at that time. Maybe your boss criticized your work and threatened to take action, your child had serious problems at school or close friends told you they would soon divorce. You would have had difficulty with these circumstances at any time, but sickness or worry about money magnified them. This is a classic situation for survivors. Life stressors lessen resiliency, increasing the impact of traumatic events. Keep this in mind as you read the chapter and work with vulnerable survivors.

FACTORS CONTRIBUTING TO VULNERABILITY

Vulnerabilities to harm from trauma (Briere & Scott, 2006) include: (1) gender, with women more at risk; (2) age, with the young and elderly more at risk; (3) race – for instance, with African-Americans and Hispanics more at risk as compared to Caucasians; (4) lower socio-economic status; (5) pre-existing psychological issues; (6) family problems and (7) prior trauma history.

Those with life stress or trauma occurring soon after the traumatic event, past histories or family histories of psychiatric issues and the inability to cope with their post-trauma reactions are also at risk. Although these vulnerabilities do not necessarily lead to post-traumatic stress disorder (PTSD) and can also lead to post-traumatic growth (PTG), they are red flags and bear monitoring (McFarlane & Yehuda, 1996).

Definitions

- *Post-traumatic stress disorder (PTSD)* – A disorder resulting from exposure to traumatic events that causes symptoms lasting at least a month that include emotional responses of fear, horror or helplessness; flashbacks and/or nightmares of events; avoidance of reminders of the event; and increased arousal
- *Post-traumatic growth (PTG)* – Condition resulting from exposure to traumatic events that causes symptoms that include the ability to see trauma from positive perspectives, to find benefit in it, to attach meaning to it that makes sense and inspires and to make constructive and helpful behavioral changes as a result

---

Prior trauma history increases the risk of harm from trauma. Therefore survivors are a vulnerable population. It has been documented, for example, that trauma survivors are more likely to experience depression, medical issues, relationship problems, substance abuse and self-injury, among other issues. One study even found that (1) most psychiatric issues for children related to trauma and (2) adult survivors had more psychiatric hospitalizations and cost more to treat than individuals without trauma histories (van der Kolk, 2009). Specific vulnerability factors and tips for working with them are explored in the following sections.

SOCIO-ECONOMIC STATUS AND CULTURE

Since life stress following a traumatic event is a risk factor, people who are marginalized in any way have a greater vulnerability to harm. This includes those living in poverty, with less education and opportunity for work or those dealing with cultural issues such as prejudice, immigration or the inability to speak the primary language of the community. Not only do these individuals have a greater risk, they also tend to have more difficulty obtaining assistance from professionals.

Immigrants often have complex trauma histories. Their trauma experiences may include events, prior to immigrating, that forced them to leave their country of origin (Perez Foster, 2001). Seventeen-year-old Maria, for example, left Ecuador because a man made her his girlfriend and she did not want him. He tried to force himself on her sexually and she saw no way to stop him except to leave. Others encounter trauma as they immigrate (Perez Foster, 2001). This includes dangers involved in illegally entering countries and traveling with few resources or protection. Settling in temporary locations such as detention centers and in new host countries are stressful transitions that create vulnerability from lack of resources, loss of social networks, poor living conditions and the inability to find work. These conditions are particularly difficult for those traumatized en route who have not yet recovered (Perez Foster, 2001).

Nina, an immigrant from Central America where her parents were murdered, illustrates how language can create vulnerability as well. Nina suffered from chronic mental illness after she settled in the United States, and practitioners always assessed her in English, which she spoke fluently. Forty years later, when she was assessed in both English and Spanish, it became clear that the trauma of her parents' deaths remained unresolved. Nina thought that people from her country still sought her to kill her. This did not come out during the English assessments because she apparently expressed her deepest fears only in her native language (Perez Foster, 2001). This case highlights the importance of keeping in mind survivors' vulnerabilities when working with them. Not only did Nina fail to deal with her trauma experience adequately because no one assessed her in Spanish, but the isolation of facing her trauma memories alone in the ensuing years probably traumatized her even further.

AGE AND GENDER

As discussed in chapter 9 on culture, gender poses a risk factor for trauma, with women more at risk than men. Children and the elderly also risk harm from trauma. In fact, studies show that many survivors function well posttrauma until they encounter aging-related losses that include retirement, a partner's death and illness. The elderly are also vulnerable to abuse and neglect which can be both detrimental emotionally and also trigger past trauma memories (Graziano, 2003).

Aging involves individuals grieving their losses, accepting and finding meaning in life experiences and re-establishing balance as they create identities as older adults. Traumatic events sometimes resurface during this process and can lead to PTSD and other trauma reactions. Older adults are therefore developmentally more vulnerable to risk from trauma (Aarts & Op den Velde, 1996).

Children are even more vulnerable to trauma than their adult counterparts. Homeless youth, for example, suffer more than adults, exhibiting health and mental health issues and developing learning and behavioral disabilities at rates twice those of children with homes. They are also more at risk for traumatic events such as experiencing or witnessing violence and many are traumatized, for instance, by witnessing intimate partner violence (IPV), prior to becoming homeless (National Child Traumatic Stress Network, 2005).

Compounding their vulnerability, less than one-third of homeless children with serious emotional issues, such as from trauma, receive treatment. Homeless children also live with more stress which makes coping with trauma difficult (National Child Traumatic Stress Network, 2005). Moreover, traumatic reactions in both children and older adults often go undetected because they exhibit behavioral and health issues rather than PTSD symptoms. This is discussed in more detail in the section on interventions for vulnerable populations below.

EMOTIONAL AND PSYCHOLOGICAL ISSUES

Besides being at risk for trauma reactions such as PTSD, those who experience trauma are vulnerable to other psychiatric issues, such as panic disorder, phobias and depression, that can manifest later in life as a result of life stressors (McFarlane & Yehuda, 1996). Anxiety, somatic disorders, antisocial or aggressive behaviors and dissociative identity disorder can become factors as well (McCann & Pearlman, 1990a). Personality and eating disorders are also not unusual. Illustrating this, Sandra, a 32-year-old survivor of abuse as a child and rape as an adult, developed anorexia and was also diagnosed with borderline personality disorder. She used the Dialectical Behavioral Therapy (DBT) skills she learned to manage her symptoms so that she could function in life. See chapter 17 for more information on DBT.

The nature of survivors' trauma experiences can also increase their risk for harm. This includes individuals who experience retraumatization, which often occurs among those abused as children (McCann & Pearlman, 1990a); and those who experience traumas of long duration, such as war or IPV (Naparstek, 2005). These individuals could have more severe symptomatology as a result of the severity of their traumas. In addition, grief plays a role and awareness of this aids recovery from traumatic experiences. Survivors experience many losses (McCann & Pearlman, 1990a). They lose their sense of well-being and safety, their trust, their childhood if traumatized as children or even their homes and loved ones.

As explored in the next section of the chapter, survivors are not only vulnerable to mental health issues, but also to substance abuse. In fact, Newmann and Sallmann (2004) found that 95% of the women they studied who had both mental illness and substance abuse issues, also had trauma histories. This draws attention to the need to assess for both mental illness and substance abuse when working with survivors. It also means that we must gear interventions to both of these issues when treating those with co-occurring disorders (Newmann & Sallmann, 2004).

SUBSTANCE ABUSE

Substance abusers – women in particular – have a high incidence of trauma (Najavits, 2002). Many use substances because of difficulties in coping with trauma experiences and symptoms, reporting that substances allow them to express feelings such as anger or stop memories and "numb them out." Some even learn to depend on substances to "cope" and take care of themselves, as illustrated in this survivor's comment: "I developed a love/trust relationship with drugs that I never had with people. I knew they would never fail me the way people had" (Courtois, 2010, p. 312).

It can be difficult to work with this population because attempts to stop using often worsen trauma symptoms, leading to relapse (Najavits, 2002). Quite simply, substances help relieve trauma symptoms and withdrawal symptoms exacerbate them. Agitating substance withdrawal symptoms, for instance, often increase hyperarousal (Jacobsen, Southwick, & Kosten, 2001). To offset the propensity to relapse when trauma and substance abuse co-occur, interventions need to address both issues (Newmann & Sallmann, 2004). This is discussed in more detail in the section on interventions for vulnerable populations below.

Definitions

- *Hyperarousal* – Heightened emotionality that can lead to agitation, anger, difficulty sleeping and/or hypervigilance
- *Hypervigilance* – State of increased attention to the environment, in order to detect threat and prevent harm, that can increase anxiety, prevent sleep and cause fatigue

---

Substance abuse and the way of life that accompanies it also increase the risk of trauma (Najavits, 2002). Substance abusers often find themselves in unsafe situations where they are more likely to experience trauma (Jacobsen, Southwick, & Kosten, 2001). In fact, many substance abusers share about rape, robbery or assault that occurred while under the influence. This vulnerability can create a detrimental cycle that counters recovery.

DISABILITY

People with disabilities experience all kinds of trauma, but are particularly at risk – more so than the general population – for abuse, neglect, assault and other crimes. Compounding this, they also have more difficulty accessing trauma services (Charlton, Kiliethermes, Tallant, Taverne, & Tishelman, 2004). Survivors of IPV, for example, report difficulty in finding services due to inaccessibility issues such as stairs, hallways with obstructions, healthcare aides not being allowed in IPV shelters, transportation, forms such as restraining orders not being written for those with limited language abilities and lack of interpreters for people who are deaf. Staff with prejudiced and negative attitudes toward disabled survivors also limit accessibility and discourage use of services (Lightfoot & Williams, 2009).

The culture of specific disability groups can also affect accessibility. In the deaf community, for instance, community members often connect so well that they know each other's issues. This leads to survivors of IPV not seeking help because others in their community will quickly find out about the abuse, creating distress and shame that they do not want to contend with (Lightfoot & Williams, 2009).

The nature of abuse can differ for people with disabilities as well. Isolated and alone (Charlton, Kiliethermes, Tallant, Taverne, & Tishelman, 2004), they are more vulnerable to caregivers who can abuse them by not providing assistive devices, medications, special meals and aid in getting out of bed (Baladerian, 2009; Lightfoot & Williams, 2009). People with disabilities are also abused at their most vulnerable moments such as being dressed or bathed. Some disabled people do not even know they are being abused because (1) they do not understand what is happening or (2) it has become the norm and they have learned to expect it (Charlton et al., 2004; Lightfoot & Williams, 2009).

Experiencing trauma can also lead to disability, increasing survivors' vulnerability. Examples include physical injuries such as blindness, hearing loss and cognitive issues resulting from traumatic injuries (Baladerian, 2009); and other physical ailments such as cardiovascular, neurological, gastrointestinal and pain issues that seem to be more prevalent with survivors. In addition, survivors often have occupational or relational issues (McFarlane & Yehuda, 1996).

INTERVENTIONS FOR VULNERABLE POPULATIONS

Since vulnerable populations have more of a risk of harm from trauma, it is important to work closely with them and to monitor for signs of PTSD and other trauma-related disorders. Vulnerability decreases safety, so we must diligently work to increase survivors' safety, making it the number one concern (Herman, 1992; Najavits, 2010). Adequate coping is also important and social workers can help to build survivors' repertoire of skills in this area. See chapters 10 and 11 on safety/safe relationships and chapter 12 on coping skills for more information.

Safety is particularly important in treatment environments. These trauma-informed care approaches have been found beneficial for vulnerable individuals: (1) helping them maintain as much autonomy and control as possible; (2) showing respect and acceptance and (3) relating in a conciliatory way that promotes trust and goodwill (Levenson, 2017; National Child Traumatic Stress Network, 2005). Trust is essential when assessing individuals for trauma histories and symptoms.

Vulnerable individuals' trauma symptoms can be hard to identify. Cognitive impairment, for instance, can cause problems because questions in trauma screening tools may be too intellectually challenging (Mitchell, Clegg, & Furniss, 2006). Deficient language, intellectual, communication or social skills can also be barriers to assessment. Open-ended and somewhat focused questions tend to work best. Obtaining collateral information from caregivers can also help (Newman, Christopher, & Berry, 2000).

Recognizing non-standard trauma symptoms facilitates assessment. For children, the aging and people with intellectual disabilities, for instance, physical ailments can indicate trauma (Graziano, 2003; Mitchell, Clegg, & Furniss, 2006). As survivors age, they may have more chronic pain, cognitive issues, difficulty sleeping, sexual problems and poor health-related self-care than those with no adverse trauma reactions (Graziano, 2003). Abused/neglected older adults may also exhibit disorganization, agitation, memory issues and poor self-care (Graziano, 2003). Children may have developmental delays (National Child Traumatic Stress Network, 2005).

Training professionals to identify these symptoms is important. This includes shelter, healthcare and mental healthcare staff (National Child Traumatic Stress Network, 2005). Educating other caregivers in the community also makes sense (Graziano, 2003). This includes emergency and law enforcement workers, staff in the judicial system and teachers.

Educating vulnerable populations can help as well. For instance, sex education geared toward the disabled can help to prevent sexual abuse (Baladerian, 2009). Seeking Safety, a treatment model designed to treat both substance abuse and trauma, incorporates psycho-education and focuses on safety first, then on mourning what was lost as a result of the trauma and finally on reconnecting with the world and others. It is a manualized evidence-based treatment with topics that include safety, learning about PTSD and substance abuse, coping, setting boundaries and developing healthy relationships. Addressing both substance abuse and trauma simultaneously, it has helped many survivors stay clean and sober who had previously relapsed because of their trauma symptoms (Najavits, 2002). See the Resources section at the end of the chapter for more information.

Case Study

Nadine, a 45-year-old married woman, was being seen in a trauma clinic that utilized Seeking Safety, a protocol specifically designed for those with co-occurring trauma symptoms and substance abuse issues. Nadine was referred to a Seeking Safety group. She participated in the group, but insisted that she did not have a substance abuse problem, although some of what she shared in the group indicated otherwise. Then, in about the tenth session she was in the group, she arrived in crisis:

Nadine:	I can't believe what happened. My husband's been arrested. *Out of breath.*
Social worker:	Sit down and tell us about it.
Nadine:	*Proceeded to tell how her husband got caught with drugs in their car. Finishing dramatically with:* I told him! He wouldn't listen to me.
Marge:	But why were there drugs in his car?
Nadine:	*Looking down.* We make extra money that way sometimes.
Sue:	*Incredulously.* I thought you didn't have a problem with drugs!
Social worker:	You have been saying that for weeks, Nadine. And getting arrested does fall into the category of having a problem.
Nadine:	Well I wasn't arrested and I don't use like he does. I just smoke sometimes to relax. There's a lot of stress in my life.
Social worker:	I think that's why a lot of women with trauma histories use drugs and alcohol. *She looks around the room and several members nod.* Learning the coping skills we talk about here helps. You can use them instead of smoking.

Nadine became more involved in the group after this and began to use coping instead of drugs. Her trauma symptoms decreased and she had less stress as a result. She was subsequently able to work on her substance abuse issue safely and without worsening her stress which would not have been possible without adequate coping skills.

RESOURCES

Briere, J., & Scott, C. (2006). *Principles of trauma therapy: A guide to symptoms, evaluation, and treatment.* Thousand Oaks, CA: Sage Publications.

Courtois, C.A., Ford, J.D., van der Kolk, B.A., & Herman, J.L. (Eds.). (2009). *Treating complex traumatic stress disorders: An evidence-based guide.* New York: Guilford Press.

Najavits, L. (2002). *Seeking safety: A treatment manual for PTSD and substance abuse.* New York: Guilford Press.

ONLINE RESOURCES

Najavits, L. (2010). Seeking Safety: http://www.seekingsafety.org/

Practice Exercises and Questions

- Think about vulnerable individuals you have worked with and delineate ways in which they could be affected by trauma
- List reasons vulnerable populations are more at risk of adverse effects of trauma
- How can vulnerable individuals react differently to traumatic events?
- What are some of the conditions that cause individuals to be vulnerable?

Vulnerable Populations Summary

Tune in to Vulnerable Populations

- *Think about times you have felt vulnerable such as when you are sick*
- *Imagine a calamity occurring while you are sick, increasing your vulnerability*

Culture and Socio-Economic Status

- *Marginalization increases vulnerability and risk of harm from trauma*
- *Includes poverty, lack of education and work, prejudice and immigration*

Age and Gender

- *Women, children and the elderly are vulnerable and at risk*
- *Age increases vulnerability to abuse or neglect and to experiencing loss*

Emotional and Psychological Issues

- *Survivors are vulnerable to loss or stress that leads to psychiatric issues*
- *There is risk of anxiety disorders, depression and personality disorders*

Substance Abuse

- *(1) Increases trauma risk; and (2) Survivors use substances to ease trauma symptoms*
- *It is important to treat substance abuse and trauma concurrently*

Disability

- *People with disabilities are at risk for abuse, neglect and crimes like assault*
- *As with many who are vulnerable, accessibility of treatment is an issue*

Interventions for Vulnerable Populations

- *Assessment can be challenging with vulnerable individuals*
- *Recognizing non-standard trauma symptoms is essential*

Chapter 9

Cultural Considerations

Survivors' backgrounds determine their experience of trauma and healing. Cultural influences help prevent harmful psychological side effects by "furnishing social support, providing identities in terms of norms and values, and supplying a shared vision of the future" (de Vries, 1996, p. 400). Cultural groups also help as they support their members and encourage responsibility among them. In addition, culture can provide healing rituals and belief systems that promote recovery and finding meaning related to trauma (de Vries, 1996; Bryant-Davis & Wong, 2013).

Correspondingly, lack of cultural supports impedes healing from trauma. When trauma disrupts culture, individuals often become further traumatized by the loss of its protective influence. Soldiers, for instance, killed a young girl's father and brother, kidnapping her from her village in Uganda. When she was freed two years later, life had no meaning for her without her family/village culture. She walked the countryside trying to recapture it, becoming more and more hopeless and depressed (de Vries, 1996).

In order to help survivors heal from traumatic events such as this, social workers need to comprehend how culture affects their experience and recovery process, always keeping in mind survivors' individual nuances in order to avoid stereotyping them. This chapter explores the place where trauma and culture intersect. It defines and contextualizes culture as it relates to trauma and discusses ways to become competent in this area.

TUNE IN TO CULTURAL CONSIDERATIONS

Prepare yourself to read this chapter and work effectively with survivors from a variety of backgrounds, by tuning in to the impact of cultural factors on trauma experiences. Learn from survivors about their cultural contexts and attempt to enter them so that you can understand their meanings when trauma occurs.

> **Tips**
>
> - *Be like Columbo* – When Peter Falk played the detective, Columbo, in an American TV series, he always asked many questions, learning from those he worked with. We can do the same in order to learn about cultural aspects of coping, letting survivors and their families teach us their traditions. We can also do research or ask colleagues what they know. The more we learn, the more we can help survivors incorporate culture into their coping

Think of your own cultural backdrop and how it influenced difficult experiences you have had. Ask yourself questions to clarify how culture operated in your life. Did it help you or get in the way of your recovery from difficulty, and how would you use it in the future to make the most of its healing aspects? What was it like when people expected you to react in ways that did not fit your culture's norm? Use the information you garner from this process as you work with survivors.

BACKGROUND INFORMATION

Society is a blend of "various racial, religious, and ethnic groups, as well as other distinct groups, each of which has different values and lifestyles" (Barker, 1999, p. 113). Other distinct groups in society include those based on class, sexual orientation, education level and socio-economic status (Lantz & Harper-Dorton, 2007). Historically, members of cultural groups like these have banded together for support, safety and survival, creating niches of security, protecting each other from external forces and providing nurturance.

Membership in cultural groups, however, has hazards as well as benefits. Trauma affects some cultural groups more than others. According to one study, Latinos/Hispanics, the most prevalent and quickest growing minority in the United States, have a higher incidence of domestic and community violence than Caucasians, with Latinos/Hispanics experiencing almost three times more community violence. Compounding this, Latinos/Hispanics, like most minorities, have more poverty, another risk factor for trauma (Conradi, Hendricks, & Merino, 2007).

Other trauma risk factors that many minorities confront include inadequate housing, single-parent families, substance abuse, stress related to discrimination and acculturation, lack of education and history of cultural oppression (Conradi, Hendricks, & Merino, 2007). Minorities also tend to have less access to healthcare, including mental healthcare (Bernal & Saez-Santiago, 2006). Therefore, the onset of post-traumatic stress disorder (PTSD) symptoms after trauma can be as much a product of culture as of individual pathology (Bracken, 2002).

Definitions

- *Post-traumatic stress disorder (PTSD)* – A disorder resulting from exposure to traumatic events that causes symptoms lasting at least a month that include emotional responses of fear, horror or helplessness; flashbacks and/or nightmares of events; avoidance of reminders of the event; and increased arousal

---

Besides the risk factors discussed above, society has marginalized cultural groups in myriad ways that include genocide, slavery, exclusion and bigotry. This generally occurs with minority groups and can encompass not only current issues, but also historical traumas such as the Nazi Holocaust and slavery of African Americans in the United States (Tummala-Narra, 2007).

THE IMPACT OF CULTURE

Culture has an impact on individuals' vulnerability to trauma. In addition to the trauma risk factors previously mentioned, cultural beliefs promote vulnerability that, for example, discourages women from reporting intimate partner violence (IPV). Migration creates an environment for trauma, particularly for cultural groups forced to migrate or who became minorities after migration. And minority-related stress increases the risk of PTSD (Tummala-Narra, 2007).

Cultural racism – with their language, art, way of life and beliefs considered substandard – can mark these individuals, increasing stress and vulnerability. Survivors can also be culturally disadvantaged; i.e., unable to take full advantage of what their societies have to offer, due to cultural marginalization, geographic isolation and strife (Barker, 1999).

Cultural groups and related beliefs can also foster resilience in the face of trauma. Religious groups provide spiritual support and a sense of connection. Support received from family and groups of individuals, such as artists, who share similar beliefs and backgrounds, is important as well. Ideals of individualism and/or collectivism can also be supportive, but must be matched to cultural beliefs. Many middle-class Westerners need to maintain strong personal boundaries and feel safe within themselves after trauma, whereas Easterners with a collectivist focus may have more of a need for community and sharing (Tummala-Narra, 2007). We must therefore take care to promote coping that fits with survivors' backgrounds.

Finally, culture affects how individuals respond to trauma. Differing responses range from cultural avoidance of displaying emotion or of dealing directly with what occurred (Turner, McFarlane & van der Kolk, 1996) to variations in endorsed PTSD symptoms. In fact, non-Anglo Saxons are less likely to be diagnosed with PTSD because they have fewer avoidance and numbing symptoms, and some non-Western cultures experience more somatic and dissociative symptoms (Briere & Scott, 2006).

Definitions

- *Avoidance* – Individuals staying away from people, places or activities, even when not dangerous, because they are reminders of trauma
- *Dissociation* – Disconnection from thoughts, memories or emotions that provides internal distance from reminders of traumatic events but also prevents integration of trauma material and disrupts normal psychological functioning

---

This differentiation in response to trauma can lead to misdiagnosis of trauma symptoms. Because of the way they depict their symptoms, African Americans (AAs) are often diagnosed with psychotic disorders when they have anxiety disorders such as PTSD. In a study of combat veterans with PTSD, for instance, AAs endorsed more symptoms that could be linked to psychosis. They also reported more dissociation than Caucasian Americans, which researchers surmised may have been mistaken for symptoms of psychosis (Tummala-Narra, 2007).

ETHNICITY

As noted above, ethnicity can increase trauma risk. Non-Caucasians are more likely to experience trauma in the United States. Hispanic and AA Vietnam veterans studied had higher rates of PTSD and were exposed to more severe combat stress (Briere & Scott, 2006). We do not know if the incidence of sexual abuse is higher for particular ethnic groups, but the impact does seem to differ by ethnicity, with Hispanics affected the most, followed by AAs and then other ethnic groups (Courtois, 2010).

Social workers need to pay close attention to risk factors and other issues related to ethnicity when working with survivors. Louisa, for instance, came to the attention of Child Protective Services when, after a school janitor molested her, it was found that her father had been sexually abusing her as well. Her mother became distraught, saying that others knowing what had occurred would disgrace the family. Her Central American culture considered these private matters, not to be shared with others, particularly if denigrating to men (Courtois, 2010). Culturally sensitive care of Louisa and her family needs to be considered in cases like this.

Studies show that many IPV interventions lack ethnic sensitivity, and consequently, a large number of AA women in the United States do not seek help (Gillum, 2009). Most IPV interventions, for instance, incorporate individualist Western values, rather than the collectivist focus of AA cultures (Gillum, 2008). Demonstrating how culture can be incorporated in trauma interventions, increasing their ethnic accessibility, Trauma-focused Cognitive Behavioral Therapy has been modified to fit American Indian and Alaskan native cultures, adding traditional healing techniques such as sweat lodge, drumming, smudging and vision seeking (Wilmon-Haque & BigFoot, 2008).

RELIGION

Generally considered to be a key coping method, religion and spirituality can offer a form of protection for those who are traumatized. Survivors of IPV, for example, with committed faith, had fewer PTSD symptoms. Spiritual leaders, such as clergy and chaplains, can also be a source of support for individuals after trauma. In studies, Armenian survivors of genocide reported that prayer and faith inspired them and helped them cope, and Holocaust survivors exhibited greater faith and hope than control groups, demonstrating religion's contribution to resilience (Weaver, Flannelly, Garbarino, Figley, & Flannelly, 2003).

Religion and spirituality engender support and healing, increasing resilience, but can also cause trauma; this occurred with children sexually abused by priests, who were invalidated by family and church when they shared what happened. These sexual abuse survivors often could not practice religion as adults and were therefore cut off from a source of support that could have aided their trauma recovery (Tummala-Narra, 2007; Farrell, 2009). Betrayed by their intended spiritual guides, many have lost not only their feelings of connection to the church, but also their trust in all authorities (Horst, 2000). This can be amplified by media attention to sexual abuse in the Catholic Church around the world.

Those sexually abused by clergy are not the only survivors who feel they lose religion as a result of trauma. Many feel abandoned by spiritual forces posttrauma, even when their experiences do not relate to religion. Social workers can offer vital assistance by helping them to come to terms with this, discover a new form of spirituality or find other ways to cope.

SEXUAL ORIENTATION

The stressors of prejudice and stigmatization can cause PTSD symptoms for sexual minorities. Events such as witnessing discrimination and violence, either in person or through the media, compound the daily stressors of: (1) wondering if they will also become victims; (2) hiding their sexual identities and relationships; (3) deciding what to reveal and to whom and (4) working out legal and financial issues in relationships often not acknowledged by workplaces, family and the legal system (Kaplan, 2007).

Social workers need to give careful consideration when working with lesbian, gay, bisexual and transgender survivors. Surmising, for example, that a survivor of sexual abuse became gay because of the abuse would hinder the therapeutic process. When leading groups, practitioners would do well to watch for group members making similar assumptions. Generally a sensitive topic, sexuality merits cautious exploration because shame and hopelessness related to trauma are easily triggered in survivors (Courtois, 2010). Finally, social workers should respect survivors' preferences for groups and therapists of the same sexual orientation (Courtois, 2010).

Gender can also factor into the mix. Women have higher rates of PTSD than men because they have more exposure to trauma (Briere & Scott, 2006) and men react differently to trauma than women. Male survivors of sexual abuse, for example, have many of the same reactions as women, but may also try to regain control and their manhood through forceful behavior that can lead them to become perpetrators themselves. Men are also less likely to tell others, including therapists, about their sexual abuse. Once they have been told, therapists need to sensitively: (1) explore survivors' fear that they caused the abuse since it may have involved their own arousal and (2) find out if they molested others (Courtois, 2010).

OTHER CULTURAL GROUPS

The young and the elderly have a higher vulnerability to trauma and a greater likelihood of developing PTSD (Briere & Scott, 2006). Their developmental life stages affect their responses to trauma and have an impact on future growth. Adolescents, for instance, who go to war, may have difficulty developing healthy egos as adults because of the violence they encountered (McCann & Pearlman, 1990a).

The culture of the military and foreign service can complicate experiences of trauma in other ways. Survivors of sexual abuse may have less stability and more isolation from community supports as a result of frequent moves. This culture tends to have a more traditional family structure, with the father as the authority on whom others depend; this can influence recovery, particularly if he is frequently away from home. Finally, medical and mental healthcare practitioners in these communities often lack sensitivity to sexual abuse issues (Courtois, 2010).

Another cultural group with vulnerability to trauma, those with physical and emotional disabilities, are: (1) more likely to suffer sexual abuse; (2) less able to stop the abuse; (3) have a more difficult time getting treatment and (4) may need treatment with special skills such as sign language. Their disabilities may require other adjustments to treatment as well. Those with cognitive issues, for example, may benefit from concrete treatment geared toward protection from further abuse because they do not respond to traditional therapeutic methods (Courtois, 2010).

CULTURALLY COMPETENT TRAUMA CARE

Survivors often look for trauma care in agencies that incorporate their cultures. When African American (AA) women, for example, seek help for IPV, they usually go to agencies in AA neighborhoods with AA staff (Gillum, 2009), because they fear others will not be sensitive to their AA experience. They also look for facilities with family-centered holistic care, a spiritual focus, outreach, support for incarcerated women, substance abuse treatment, transportation and help with safely retrieving belongings. A reflection of their culture in agencies' curricula and environments is also important. This includes featuring AA language, art, photographs, posters, magazines and books (Gillum, 2008).

Illustrating the need for culturally focused trauma care, The National Child Traumatic Stress Network made these recommendations (Conradi et al., 2007) for treatment of Latino/Hispanic survivors: (1) note how survivors perceive agencies, focusing on being friendly, human and accessible and on providing an environment that welcomes through cultural touches; (2) assess survivors from a cultural perspective that takes into account level and process of acculturation, cultural identity, values, beliefs and attitudes, as well as culturally related stressors and traumas and (3) emphasize cultural values during treatment, exploring their impact on understanding the meaning of traumatic events. Examples of important Latino/Hispanic cultural values include: (a) *personalismo*, the ability to connect and build trust, which is imperative in treatment; (b) *simpatia*, avoiding conflict to smooth over relations; (c) *respeto*, respect for boundaries and social hierarchies and (d) *fatalismo*, the idea that God determines destiny – this is key in terms of how individuals interpret the meaning of traumatic events and also bears exploration.

Other recommendations include: (1) engage families; (2) provide survivors with adequate resources and (3) ensure that bicultural trauma clinicians receive training/support (Conradi et al., 2007). These recommendations reflect the need for cultural literacy or "information and knowledge that members of a culture must have to function effectively in that community" and for culturally sensitive practice or being "knowledgeable, perceptive, empathetic, and skillful about the unique as well as common characteristics of clients who possess" cultural differences (Barker, 1999, p. 113). Becoming culturally competent requires incorporating these recommendations and engaging in ongoing education, training, consultation and supervision, continually honing these skills and remaining open to new ideas (Brown, 2009b).

Case Study

Mr. Hussani was from Afghanistan and of Hazara ethnicity. He was traumatized prior to seeking refuge in Australia where he lived a life of poverty and had no permanent visa. He was treated in Australia by a female therapist from Afghanistan, of Pashtun ethnicity, the cultural group that had murdered his brothers in his country. She was also different from him because she was a woman and had more money and education. Further complicating the cultural backdrop of Mr. Hussani's therapy, she was supervised by a Christian Anglo-Saxon woman (Bowles & Mehraby, 2007).

His therapist had the advantage of knowing something of his life in Afghanistan. She respected him as a member of an ethnic group that was hardworking and had experienced much hardship. The difference in their socio-economic and educational status also challenged her at times. She tried to show him deference, at times ignoring the differences neither could forget, but he said she knew more, so he should do what she told him to do (Bowles & Mehraby, 2007).

Although the supervisor and the therapist came from very different backgrounds, they had worked together for many years and built a relationship based on trust. Mr. Hussani and his therapist proceeded similarly to establish a safe connection. He did not come to therapy to discuss his trauma issues or their cultural differences, but the work they did together and the relationship they built established trust and he began to heal (Bowles & Mehraby, 2007).

The main fracture Mr. Hussani suffered due to trauma was to his relationships with others. He had lost not only many family members, but also his home and community in Afghanistan. As a result of learning to trust his therapist, he began to trust others as well and to form a new community in Australia. Even though they never discussed the cultural diversity within their relationship in depth, it became a route for his overall healing (Bowles & Mehraby, 2007). This could not have happened without his therapist and her supervisor consistently working with their own countertransference and with Mr. Hussani's cultural values and trauma issues.

RESOURCES

Bracken, P. (2002). *Trauma: Culture, meaning and philosophy*. London and Philadelphia, PA: Wiley.

Drozdek, B., & Wilson, J.P. (Eds.). (2007). *Voices of trauma: Treating psychological trauma across cultures*. International and Cultural Psychology series. New York: Springer.

Weiss, T., & Berge, R. (Eds.). (2010). *Posttraumatic growth and culturally competent practice: Lessons learned from around the globe*. Hoboken, NJ: Wiley.

ONLINE RESOURCES

The National Child Traumatic Stress Network recommendations: http://www.nctsn.org/nctsn_assets/pdfs/culture_and_trauma_brief_v2n3_LatinoHispanicChildren.pdf

---

Practice Exercises and Questions

- Role-play a session with Mr. Hussani from the case study in this chapter exploring some of the issues described
- Role-play a session between Mr. Hussani's therapist and her supervisor exploring some of the issues described
- Talk about why safety is even more important when there is marginalization of survivors due to cultural issues
- List some of the approaches you would use with the marginalizing cultural issues and with maximizing safety

---

Cultural Considerations Summary

Tune in to Cultural Considerations

- *Think about how culture has affected you in times of crisis*
- *Enter clients' cultural contexts, imagining trauma impacts*

Culture Defined

- *Discrete societal groups with unique ideals and ways of life*
- *Includes race, ethnicity, religion, class and education level*

Background Information

- *Cultural groups can be: safe/supportive and promote survival*
- *Marginalized by genocide, slavery, exclusion and bigotry*
- *At risk for trauma and unable to access trauma treatment*

The Impact of Culture

- *Contributes to vulnerability to trauma and PTSD*
- *Promotes resilience, protecting from trauma and PTSD*
- *Causes variations in trauma responses and symptoms*
- *Influences the recovery process post-trauma*

Culturally Competent Trauma Treatment

- *Be friendly, human and accessible to all cultures*
- *Conduct initial and ongoing cultural assessments*
- *Emphasize cultural values during treatment*
- *Develop cultural literacy and competency*
- *Maintain cultural competency with education/supervision*

Part III

Coping with Trauma

Chapter 10

The Importance of Safety

Social workers need to understand the safety issues trauma survivors confront. Trauma overrides survivors' inherent adaptive functions, leaving them helpless in a world that feels out of control and unsafe. Trauma experiences so sharply affect their physiological arousal, emotions and memory that at times they have no memory of the traumatic event, but experience intense emotion; or have clear recall with no emotion. Because the emotions generated by the ordeal fall so far out of the scope of human understanding and coping, survivors tend to avoid them, thus cutting themselves off from current experiences as they build a protective shell. This dissociation can be both conscious, as individuals avoid memories of the incident; and unconscious, as they shy away from emotional experiences that triggers unwanted memories.

Trauma recovery requires integration of distressing events and reconnection with daily life. In order to heal, survivors must also learn to manage symptoms and tolerate feelings associated with trauma (Herman, 1992). Although many integrate their experiences and recover on their own with no intervention necessary, the intense emotions endured as a result of trauma can make integration difficult. Often survivors fluctuate between re-experiencing the trauma via flashbacks and feeling numb as they deny and repress their emotions.

Definitions

- *Coping* – Process of dealing with difficulties, problem solving and adapting to the environment in order to manage stress and conflict effectively
- *Dissociation* – Disconnection from thoughts, memories or emotions that provides internal distance from reminders of traumatic events but also prevents integration of trauma material and disrupts normal psychological functioning

---

Instinctual reactions related to the freeze, flight, fight, fright, faint emergency response can also become habitual and maladaptive after distressing events if survivors do not restore their sense of safety. This habitual response causes stress, impeding recovery and contributing to trauma's erosion of survivors' sense of safety. Healing requires creating a new safety (Rothschild, 2000). The healing process includes attaining physical, emotional, social and financial stability.

Definitions

- *Flashback* – Intrusive and involuntary re-experiencing of traumatic events through images, emotions or physical sensations
- *Freeze, flight, fight, fright, faint emergency response* – Physical reaction to perceived threat or danger that leads to discharge of hormones such as adrenalin and cortisol, increased heart rate, shallow breathing and slowdown of non-essential activities such as digestion so that the body can mobilize to protect itself

---

TUNE IN TO SAFETY

When reading about survivors and hearing their stories in person, some of us may not connect with their loss of safety because we unconsciously distance ourselves from their suffering. Although this is not a healthy approach, it is natural to try to protect ourselves in this way. We need to create a safe space when we work with trauma survivors and it is difficult to do so without first opening ourselves to their emotional experience (Bromberg, 2006). A safe workspace requires witnessing how unsafe they feel, but doing so while grounded in our own internal safe place. This protects us from secondary trauma and allows us to connect with survivors as we help them.

Definitions

- *Safety* – State essential to trauma recovery and unique to each individual, in which: (1) risky behaviors, unhealthy relationships and negative emotions are reduced and (2) a sense of well-being, trust, calm and positive coping are increased

---

The stories of survivors may seem foreign to social workers who have not experienced trauma. If so, think of your own losses and hardships and the associated feelings. Often we find it easier to relate to the emotions than to the actual events a survivor has endured. For me, September 11th is such a touchstone. I worked at a hospital not far from the disaster and met with the survivors who came in. I also talked with many more family members in search of their loved ones and with hospital staff and Emergency Medical Services (EMS) workers who helped survivors and family members. I lived in Manhattan, so I experienced the trauma too and had feelings of fright and vulnerability. I dealt with the traumas of the survivors, the families and the practitioners along with my own feelings about the event. I remember going home after long days at work with tears in my eyes. I had difficulty taking good care of myself and wanted to watch the replays on television instead.

The pain of this experience and my own loss of safety help connect me with survivors and their horrific stories. The coping I managed to do to take care of myself at the time and my constant awareness of the need for self-care keep me grounded as I work with survivors. To tune in, connecting with any kind of loss will work. The loss of a loved one, being diagnosed with a serious illness or witnessing an accident can bring up feelings similar to those of survivors. Try to imagine any time you felt vulnerable and then join it with a familiar feeling of comfort. Together, these emotions allow us to be close to survivors, understanding how unstable they feel, without losing ourselves in the process. This chapter discusses how survivors lose their sense of safety when trauma occurs and explores the need to re-create it in order for survivors to cope with the stress generated by traumatic events. For more information on coping and self-care, see chapter 12.

Tips

- *Tune in to personal loss or trauma* – Remember a trauma or loss you experienced or witnessed. Do not pick a raw or unprocessed incident. As you think of it, become aware of your physical, emotional and cognitive sensations, telling yourself that these are the kinds of feelings survivors encounter. Then think of something safe to balance the loss. Breathe into the safe feeling or use other means to relax and nurture yourself

---

THE STRESS OF TRAUMA

Intense trauma emotions can cause physiological stress. Research has found that emotions affect the body. If repressed during upsetting times, they can become physically trapped, causing individuals to lose contact with both the painful feelings and the body parts holding them. The intestines, for instance, contain an abundance of emotion-regulating neuropeptides and receptors (Pert, 1999). This may explain experiences such as butterflies in the stomach and emotional difficulties that lead to indigestion and ulcers.

Similarly, the immune system operates more efficiently when individuals express, rather than repress, their feelings. Studies have noted better recovery rates in cancer for those who expressed anger. Tumors were also found to grow more quickly when transplanted into rats that were under stress (Pert, 1999). Not only does repressing emotions create stress, but life without access to safe feelings can also relegate trauma survivors to a life of disconnection and isolation. Recovery will not occur until survivors resolve trauma emotions, and integration of emotions must take place in order to heal wounds caused by traumatic experiences.

Emotions can be either biologically adaptive instinctual reactions, such as warnings of danger, or learned reactions that are not necessarily adaptive. Reactions to shocking occurrences are maladaptive when they warn of danger that no longer exists or lead to numbing of feelings that are painful to bear. Maladaptive responses include: (1) avoidance where survivors stay away from people, places or activities with no danger because they are reminders of their ordeal and (2) hyperarousal or arousal of the autonomic nervous system, causing tension, an exaggerated startle response, insomnia and fatigue. These two features of survivors' responses to trauma particularly influence their abilities to experience and express emotion (Litz, Orsillo, Kaloupek, & Weathers, 2000). Usually difficult to unlearn even with professional help and medication, these reactions make regulation of affect a feat for survivors (Greenberg & Paivio, 1998).

Definitions

- *Avoidance* – Individuals staying away from people, places or activities even when these are not dangerous because they are reminders of trauma
- *Hyperarousal* – Heightened emotionality that can lead to agitation, anger, difficulty sleeping and/or hypervigilance
- *Hypervigilance* – State of increased attention to the environment, in order to detect threat and prevent harm, that can increase anxiety, prevent sleep and cause fatigue

---

Signs of stress and stress adaptation also present physiologically in survivors' brains. These include heightened amygdala activity, causing a fear response and neurochemical, neuropeptide and hormonal changes, induced by stress and prevented by adaptation (Charney, 2004; Vermetten & Bremner, 2002). The inability to heal, integrate trauma material and regulate trauma emotions have been linked to continuation of trauma symptoms. This may be related to the cortical processes in the brain. These processes normally store memories in permanent memory as narrative. When the cortical processes break down during distressing events, the brain stores memories as sensory fragments, causing nightmares and flashbacks to persist (Siegel, 2001). The resulting stress erodes trauma survivors' basic sense of well-being.

THE FREEZE, FLIGHT, FIGHT, FRIGHT, FAINT EMERGENCY RESPONSE

The freeze, flight, fight, fright, faint emergency response triggered by traumatic events can also contribute to survivors not feeling safe. Emotions generated by trauma often deter the recovery process, but can be protective as the trauma occurs, activating the emergency response and causing survivors to act quickly to protect themselves and others (Goleman, 1995). Goleman explains these functions of emotions from the viewpoint of the brain (see Figure 10.1). The amygdala monitors affect and connects it to emotional memories. It also controls the emergency response, taking over during danger and using feelings such as fear to encourage quick reactions to threats.

This process differs from that of the neocortex, another part of the brain that works actively with emotions. Its response is slower and more methodical. The neocortex essentially "thinks" about how to respond, utilizing cognitive

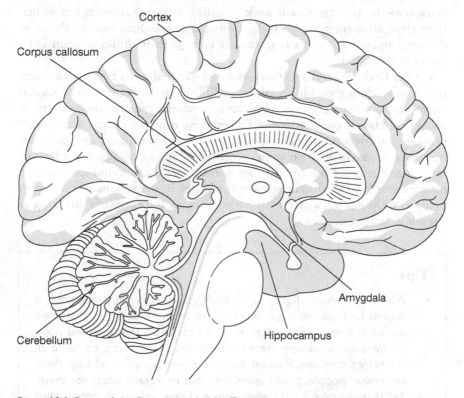

Figure 10.1 Parts of the Brain Impacted by Trauma.

Source: "Alcohol and the adolescent brain: Human studies" by S.F. Tapert, L. Caldwell and C. Burke, 2004/2005, *Alcohol Research & Health, 28*(4), p. 207. Copyright S.F. Tapert. Reprinted with permission.

functions such as comparison, analysis and contemplation, whereas the amygdala acts quickly, without thinking. Both functions are important when processing affect.

On the one hand, without the amygdala, memories would not be associated with feelings. Response to danger would also happen slowly. On the other hand, without the neocortex, all responses would be impulsive and lack cognitive control. We could not make decisions without the neocortex's ability to problem solve and reason. The amygdala's ability to safeguard us by sensing danger and prompting protective action also plays a role in decision making, contributing to making choices that increase safety during crises. The amygdala uses fear to rush us out of the path of an oncoming vehicle. If we waited for the neocortex's slower cognitive process, we could get hurt (Goleman, 1995; Greenberg & Bolger, 2001).

With trauma, the emergency response dominates while the "thinking" part of the brain takes a back seat. This keeps survivors in the emergency mode the distressing event set off. As a result, survivors can seem to stay always in crisis. Some come for treatment each week reporting very real stressors but identifying them all as emergencies. If this occurs, they may have lost the ability to differentiate everyday stress from danger because their thinking brain is no longer in command.

van der Kolk (2014) likens this process of habitual crisis to a smoke alarm that goes off during cooking, making it difficult to distinguish an accidental alarm from a real emergency. As he says, we need a reliable smoke alarm to protect us. Having one that goes off when there is no fire creates unnecessary physiological stress. Our bodies release stress hormones, blood pressure rises, muscles tense and digestion stops, potentially causing an upset stomach or other health issues. Not only this but scientists have also found a connection between this kind of chronic stress and changes in the volume of the brain's gray and white matter, with both the hippocampus and amygdala shrinking as a result (Chetty et al., 2014).

Tips

- *When the freeze, flight, fight, fright, faint emergency response is activated* – If possible, get survivors to sit or lie down so that their bodies can relax. Encourage them to focus on the here and now; for instance, by having them count things in the room or name all the colors they see. Remind them that they are safe and help them remember people, places and things that represent safety for them. Tell them to take it easy when they go home, talking to people they trust, getting a lot of rest, drinking water and eating things that are not hard to digest

If this defensive process becomes chronic, as with many survivors, it no longer fulfills its mobilizing function, but instead begins to weaken the sympathetic nervous system. This can lead to suppression of the immune system, headaches, indigestion, hypertension, backaches, sleep disorders, anxiety and depression. It can also suppress reproductive hormones (Kabat-Zinn, 1991; Sternberg, 2000). These symptoms increase survivors' stress levels and decrease their sense of security.

An example of how the emergency response can affect survivors physically is an 8-year-old boy named Chris who witnessed his father beating his mother. After four sessions of counseling, this boy's mother reported he was complaining of feeling too sick "in the tummy" to go to school. She took him to his pediatrician who knew Chris had witnessed intimate partner violence and determined he had indigestion, probably caused by stress. He encouraged the family to stay in counseling.

At the next counseling session, Chris's therapist learned that he was protective of his mother and did not want to leave her to go to school. School was stressful because he worried about her. He began to learn coping skills and the complaints lessened. His therapy remained mostly non-directive until he felt comfortable. Then, Chris blew bubbles with his therapist. He learned to breathe properly in the process since bubbles require blowing slowly and deeply, promoting relaxation. Music also helped Chris to cope. His therapist played drumming games with him to release stress and taught his mother so she could encourage it at home. The two of them drummed on their laps as they traveled to school, helping him feel safe and lowering his anxiety as he approached his most stressful time of the day.

THE SAFE PLACE SHATTERED

The real world is never completely secure or in control. Catastrophes can occur at any time. Despite this, parents encourage children to believe that they live in a safe place. This learned safe place grows out of familial love and getting needs met. When trauma at an early age prevents development of a safe place, or trauma later in life crushes the sense of safety, creating a new refuge is essential. One of the most important aspects of this process is connection with safe people (Herman, 1992). Self-care, coping skills and learning to tolerate what seem like intolerable emotions are also key (Najavits, 2002).

Living without a sense of well-being in the aftermath of trauma, survivors become vulnerable. There is a loss of coping as well because feeling safe is essential to coping. This loss creates a void that something must fill. Some survivors learn good coping skills, such as meditating and talking to safe people, and use these techniques to fill the void which contributes to safety. Those with less access to coping or with unstable lives that make creating a new safe place more difficult may turn to less effective means of "coping" which include substance abuse or other activities that numb the pain and help them forget the trauma.

Overstimulation can be an ineffective means of "coping" as well. Survivors may work themselves up into intense emotional states that overwhelm them in order to escape the pain of losing a sense of basic security. The intense emotions are powerful and decrease feelings of vulnerability. Although survivors may still feel that they are in pain, it is a frenzied display of emotion rather than a soft and open suffering that accesses deep feelings. Some survivors even become aggressive. Getting into a physical fight can offer relief. This type of aggression distracts, helping survivors forget trauma emotions.

In an anger group for survivors of trauma, one member, Juanita, became increasingly distraught over several sessions. She had resisted joining the group, but when she did participate, she related to and liked the other women immediately. She became very protective of them and had difficulty when they expressed emotions such as sadness or fear. She demonstrated her protectiveness by giving advice, was frustrated when members did not do as she said, and then became silent. This came to a head in this session where she was able to talk about how hard it was to communicate without anger:

Juanita:	I don't understand what's the matter with you women. Can't you stand up for yourselves? *Speaking loudly and looking each member in the eye as though trying to stare them down. There is an uncomfortable silence.*
Group facilitator:	What's going on, Juanita? We know you worry about the women in the group. Is there something you are afraid of now?
Juanita:	*Scornfully.* I'm not afraid of anything. I can take care of myself and do. It's these women who are like bumps on logs. *Pounding her fists on the table.*
Group facilitator:	I know you want to help, but right now you are making the group unsafe. You know the rules about no yelling or being aggressive. Let's talk about this safely.
Juanita:	You're as bad as them. All you want to do is teach them to be doormats.
Group facilitator:	I don't want to have to do this, but if you continue to yell, I'll have to ask you to leave. Can't you just talk about how much you care about everyone here? We can all feel it can't we? *Looks around and several members nod.*
Jan:	You know me, Juanita. I get mad too. That's why I'm here. It's gotten me in some real trouble. We don't want you to get in trouble over us. We care about you too.
Juanita:	*Putting her head down and speaking softly.* I just don't know how to do it. I try not being mad and my family doesn't

understand it. They take advantage of me too. And it hurts. It's hard to hear all you've been through. I can't do it …

Group facilitator: You are doing it, but it's not easy. The anger had a use. It makes us feel strong and invulnerable so it seems like it will keep us safe. Unfortunately it doesn't always work so well. Am I right? *Several members laugh and others nod.*

HYPERVIGILANCE

As the stress of trauma continues and subsequently triggers the emergency response, many survivors become hypervigilant to perceived threats and have exaggerated startle responses. When they experience flashbacks and otherwise remember the traumatic event, these symptoms can recur (Bromberg, 2006). The strong smell of sweat reminded one rape survivor of her rapist. Another always got scared when she was in the neighborhood where she was attacked. Seeing or hearing airplanes often triggered survivors of September 11th. One reporter found himself ducking each time he heard an airplane for weeks after the attack.

This experience of hypervigilance led to the hypothesis that the amygdala, the portion of the brain responsible for monitoring threat, becomes overly responsive after upsetting ordeals (Shin, Rauch, & Pitman, 2006). The prefrontal cortex is also involved in the fear response. A role of this portion of the brain is to notify the amygdala when the fear response is no longer needed. One theory suggests that trauma damages this portion of the brain so that it does not signal the amygdala, and the fear response continues to trigger when a threat no longer exists (Shin, Rauch, & Pitman, 2006). This is probably what happened to the reporter who kept ducking each time he heard planes after September 11th.

Tips

- *Coping with hypervigilance* – Remind survivors that this is a symptom caused by trauma, not a response to actual danger. If it began unexpectedly, try to determine what set it off – knowing this can make survivors feel less out of control. Help them to feel grounded in the moment, moving away from thoughts of trauma. Do relaxation techniques with them and discuss safe references, telling them that they are safe now

---

These theories regarding the effects of trauma on the brain may explain why even trauma events unrelated to the original incident can be triggering.

Survivors are often more on edge than most individuals. A sudden loud noise during a trauma support group generally startles group members in an exaggerated way. This hypervigilance can also present when an abused child in day care jumps because another child taps her to invite her to join in a game. These stressful reactions take their toll on survivors, who are always on alert for a possible threat. Hypervigilance is also the antithesis of a sense of security. The constant search for danger not only causes stress, but provokes anxiety as well.

LIVING IN FEAR

Survivors often live in some form of fear after the event. Many fluctuate between emotion overload and dissociation. Hiding emotionally charged memories in the unconscious, removing feelings from factual details of the traumatic event or essentially erasing particularly salient memories all cause dissociation. The split-off parts of the self live on, with the affect stored within the survivor's physical body and memories filed in an unconscious part of the mind. Like forgotten landmines, until they are integrated, these memories can inadvertently trigger flashbacks of the traumatic event or associated emotions and dissociation (Kalsched, 1996; Rothschild, 2000). Nightmares can be a form of flashback as well, so that survivors cannot escape, even during sleep, from the feelings evoked by trauma. These symptoms and the defense mechanisms required to cope with them take tremendous energy that survivors can use for more productive purposes when recovering and healing.

The film *In the Valley of Elah* (Haggis, 2007), based on real-life events, depicts the horrific effects of combat-induced dissociation that result in murder. In combat, circumstances force a soldier to run over a child in the road. He never recovers from this or from subsequent shocking war events that he experiences with his buddies, who are also traumatized. They lose the ability to regulate their emotions and control their aggressive impulses, resulting in a sad ending that impacted them all. The soldiers who confess to the murder do so in a detached and unemotional way, exhibiting profound dissociation.

Flashbacks are particularly prevalent for survivors with post-traumatic stress disorder (PTSD). One study examined the brain processes of 24 survivors (11 with PTSD and 13 without) and found that those with PTSD experienced traumatic recall as flashbacks, whereas those without it experienced it as narrative memory. Unlike narrative memory, flashbacks are disconnected fragments of sensory experiences. Based on magnetic resonance imaging (MRI) analysis, investigators determined that the brain retrieves flashbacks differently from narrative memories, possibly revealing a neural basis for this PTSD symptom (Lanius et al., 2004).

Other studies have focused on how the brain processes survivors' emotions. One study with survivors (10 with PTSD and 10 without) found through MRI that certain parts of the brains of survivors with PTSD (areas of the limbic system and the thalamus, a part of the brain integral to emotion regulation) were less stimulated than expected by attempts to activate sadness, anxiety and traumatic memories. These portions of the brain monitor sensory input and attempt to identify it as related memories are compared. The investigators postulated that this finding could reflect dysfunction in these brain areas and with the emotion and arousal functions they monitor (Lanius et al., 2003).

Definitions

- *Post-traumatic stress disorder (PTSD)* – A disorder resulting from exposure to traumatic events that causes symptoms lasting at least a month that include emotional responses of fear, horror or helplessness; flashbacks and/or nightmares of events; avoidance of reminders of the event and increased arousal

---

Because these areas of the brain regulate affect, dysregulation of emotion may be another cause of at least some PTSD symptoms such as hyperarousal, flashbacks and numbness (Lanius et al., 2003). Affect arousal is stressful and flashbacks can be terrifying, feeling so real that survivors can hardly function when experiencing them. One therapist described a sexual abuse survivor's experience this way:

> She couldn't leave the house and called saying that parts of her genitals were hurting or that there was pressure on her chest and she had to keep her hand there pressing on it. It turned out that her grandfather had probably penetrated her and pushed down on her chest as he did.

Dreams can also be reminiscent of the trauma event, replaying it over and over as survivors sleep. They can seem as real and scary as daytime flashbacks. This one comes from a survivor of sexual abuse:

> I dreamt that I was a witness to terrible gangland violence. A vicious guy had another guy and was holding a large pair of industrial scissors up to him, like Edward Scissorhands. He was backing away from the bad guy. (Well, they were both bad guys.) And saying no, no, no. The vicious guy takes the scissors and puts one part inside his mouth and one outside and cuts back from the mouth to the jaw hinge. I watch and can't do anything.

These examples demonstrate the emotions such as vulnerability and helplessness that nightmares and flashbacks can invoke, making it difficult for survivors to experience the sense of well-being needed for recovery and healing.

Tips

- *Coping with flashbacks* – Remind survivors that they are safe now and that the trauma is no longer occurring. For those still living in traumatic environments, tell them that even in the midst of this, they can find a safe place inside themselves. Help them to feel grounded in the moment, moving away from thoughts of the trauma and/or flashbacks. Try to determine what triggered them – knowing this can help survivors to feel less out of control

---

DISPLACING FEAR

In addition to feeling fright about traumatic events, survivors can become fearful in other areas of their lives. Sometimes these fears directly relate to the incident, as was the case with those who avoided the subway after September 11th out of fear that something else might occur. Survivors of attacks by other humans often emotionally react to people who resemble their attacker so that women who are raped may worry about men in general. There is also a pervasive loss of trust among survivors who may become overly attentive to how people treat them and easily feel abandoned, attacked or disrespected (Turner, McFarlane & van der Kolk, 1996). These reactions reflect the lack of safety felt by survivors after traumatic occurrences.

Fear can extend to other areas of life such as finances, work or home. The fear of losing all three can become exaggerated, creating even more stress. Some survivors worry when they hear noises, afraid of being attacked even in their homes. Others have difficulty with anyone who tries to control them, including doctors and bosses, because they had such a loss of control and personal power during traumatic events. The presence of someone in control or powerful, such as an authority figure, can feel unsafe and intimidating. This affects personal relationships as well. Survivors can be sensitive to changes in the balance of power in relationships and become defensive if they feel a partner or friend wants to control them or tell them what to do (Graber, 1991).

Tips

- *Safe relationships* – Encourage survivors to engage with safe people. If they need to encounter those who do not feel safe, recommend using coping skills before to prepare and after to relax and feel safe. This includes encounters with friends, family, work colleagues and bosses, doctors and other authorities. Talk about ways to increase safety in relationships. This can include ending unhealthy friendships and finding trustworthy healthcare providers

---

Despite sometimes having difficulty with the authority aspect of doctors, survivors tend to have more medical issues than most because of the physical effect of trauma-related stress (McCann & Pearlman, 1990a). This can also create a feeling of not being safe, as if even their bodies have betrayed them. Compounding this sense of betrayal, sickness naturally creates vulnerability.

In addition, survivors overprotect themselves in response to their fear. This can include staying in relationships that do not work because being alone feels unsafe and the partner seems to offer some kind of protection. Parents can also become overprotective of their children in an attempt to respond to the fears they harbor that their children will never be secure and will be traumatized as well.

Demonstrating the vulnerability and fear that survivors experience, this excerpt comes from a session with an adult survivor of child abuse who often felt scared in his apartment at night and whose fear had recently increased:

Joel:	It's terrible. I can't even sleep without the light on. Even then I don't really sleep. I lock all the locks and then when the phone rings, I feel like they will get in.
Social worker:	Who do you think will get in?
Joel:	Whoever's calling.
Social worker:	Who is calling?
Joel:	Afraid it's my uncle. He's been calling lately. Even came over once.
Social worker:	What's he like?
Joel:	Pushy, loud. Keeps saying I should be more of a man. Don't like him.
Social worker:	Sounds kind of like how your father (*the abuser*) was.
Joel:	*Surprised.* You're right, he is a lot like him. Reminds me of him.
Social worker:	Doesn't it make sense you're scared lately?

RE-CREATING TRAUMA

When survivors inadvertently re-create trauma in their daily lives, it has an impact on their safety. Some attempt to re-create the trauma in order to understand and reach for mastery of the situation. Survivors can choose relationships where they become victims. This includes overbearing or abusive bosses, partners with histories of intimate partner violence and aggressive friends. At times survivors are victimized again or become perpetrators of violence themselves (van der Kolk, 1996). This happens for a number of reasons.

Individuals who have lived with trauma and crisis can also become habituated it, so much so that it feels familiar and strangely safe. Re-creating the trauma can feel safe in other ways. It offers an escape from day-to-day fears as the survivor is flooded with feelings and detaches from reality as a result. One survivor became an EMS worker. She said she did it to help people, but as we explored further, she admitted that the crises she encountered also gave her a "rush" and helped her to forget about her own problems. The habit of crisis can also cause the emergency response, further upping the ante and re-creating the stress of the trauma.

Survivors can trigger memories of the traumatic event as another means of re-creating trauma (McCann & Pearlman, 1990a). They often want to talk about the occurrence, going over minute and often painful details with no emotion expressed. They can also seek out other survivors' stories, wanting details of these as well. Survivors can be drawn to violence as in the case of a man who survived September 11th and could not stop watching coverage of the war in Iraq. Others are drawn to movies about trauma or that contain other types of violence including horror films or to violence on the street, such as car accidents or physical fights.

Tips

- *Healthy avoidance of trauma reminders* – Encourage survivors not to dwell on their trauma experiences or participate in activities that could be reminders. When they need to talk about the event, such as in court, recommend using coping skills before to prepare and after to relax and feel safe. Discourage them from watching traumatic or scary movies if these trigger thoughts of trauma. Even watching war footage or violence on the news can be upsetting and may need to be avoided. If reminders need to be encountered, encourage use of coping skills

---

Individuals who talk about trauma without the skills to cope with underlying feelings or who repeat trauma in other ways are like people who pick at scabs on their wounds. They never allow the wounds to heal properly and this can cause problems as a result. For survivors, one result of this process is further erosion of security in their lives.

TOLERATING EMOTIONS

Learning to tolerate and modulate emotion is essential to trauma recovery. Even when survivors know that their reactions to feelings are not helpful, many do not know how else to cope. Expressing and processing emotion is an integral part of life and one of the primary ways to connect with others (Goleman, 1995). The effects of trauma can cause survivors to lose their awareness of emotion. Consequently, many lose the ability to talk about feelings and make informed decisions based on them. This may have adverse effects on relationships, impulse control and self-care (van der Kolk, 1996).

As we process emotions, we learn adaptive behavior that helps us live more effectively (Greenberg, 2004). Positive emotions provide feedback that encourages certain behaviors while negative emotions discourage others. Through this feedback loop, we learn to avoid situations that engender fear and anger and to move toward those that generate joy and happiness (Carver, 2001). Harnessing this process, so that it becomes conscious rather than mechanical, is "emotional intelligence." Goleman (1995) describes it as individuals learning to identify and name feelings and to recognize how the feelings connect to ideas and behaviors so that the results of decisions become clear. By utilizing emotional intelligence techniques, survivors can become aware of their emotional responses, self-soothe when needed and replace trauma-related emotions with adaptive ones such as compassion for self (Greenberg & Bolger, 2001).

Reappraisal and self-awareness are components of emotional intelligence (EI) that are beneficial for survivors. EI: (1) reduces impulsivity, as situations and the emotional responses they engender are reappraised before reacting to them (Gross & John, 2003; Ochsner, Bunge, Gross, & Gabrieli, 2002) and (2) increases regulation of emotions as distinguishing them increases (Feldman Barrett, Gross, Conner, & Benvenuto, 2001). These attributes contribute to survivors' sense of safety.

CREATING A NEW SAFE PLACE

Since trauma destroys safety, creating a new safe place is essential to the healing process (McCann & Pearlman, 1990a). This includes finding physical, emotional and financial stability. Healthcare is also important. Although survivors can be somatically focused and have many health issues, they are often not good at regular self-care (Najavits, 2002). The somatic or bodily focus tends to take the form of obsessive examinations of physical changes and fears of severe illness rather than healthy habits. Creating new healthy habits to add to the ones they already have is crucial, so that survivors will have a toolbox to turn to in times of stress. Healthy habits will contribute to coping and support the process of learning how to tolerate and regulate the intense emotions brought on by the traumatic event.

In addition to developing healthy habits, survivors may also need help finding safety in their relationships. Trauma-related loss of trust and protective habits that isolate survivors can make relationships difficult. Many have difficulty choosing positive healthy people to relate to. Where there has been family violence, familial relationships can be troubled and potentially triggering.

Despite this, establishing safe relationships heals more than anything (Herman, 1992). Learning good boundaries can help make this possible and contribute to creating a new safe place.

These steps toward creating safety will be discussed more in chapters 11 and 12. They include developing effective coping skills and building safe relationships. These positive actions help create well-being for survivors.

Safe place is unique to each individual's personal preferences, history and culture. The documentary *War Dance* (Nix & Fine, 2007) depicts an interesting example of safe place. This movie shares stories of African refugees of genocide including children with horrific pasts who were living in a refugee camp without their families, often not knowing if their families were alive or having witnessed their deaths. Other children were forced to kill and torture as child soldiers.

This traumatized community created a tenuous safe place as they danced and made music together. Then, they had the opportunity to participate in a countrywide music and dance competition and all became involved as they prepared. Even inadequate food did not dispel the intense security and feeling of empowerment and joy generated by this process.

As social workers, we need to work with survivors to find "their" own new refuge. We must also keep in mind that this safe place can change. Survivors need to learn how to add to their safe place when it comes time for it to change. Social workers can be guides and companions in this process, as the following extract shows.

Social worker:	Seems like the things that normally keep you safe aren't working.
Steve:	I just keep remembering his face as he died. Nothing feels safe.
Social worker:	Can you think of a place you like, maybe where you went as a kid?
Steve:	That picture kind of reminds me of where I went fishing with my dad.
Social worker:	*Getting picture from desk.* This one?
Steve:	Yeah. That path in the woods goes to a stream. I really liked it there.
Social worker:	So that's your safe place. Try to remember everything about it and use it when you think of him dying. Can you tell me more about this place?

The details of this safe place alleviated Steve's flashbacks and increased safety.

Case Study

Susan was a 49-year-old woman in therapy for marital issues. In therapy for years, she had worked in the past on issues related to surviving child abuse. She had not been herself lately and it had affected her relationship with her husband. Always a strong woman, she had become quite dependent on her husband. She could not make household decisions on her own and he even took over the cooking, something they had always done together.

Her husband complained that she did not hear what he said when he talked to her, and she often seemed "spaced out" in therapy, needing help to refocus. Her husband was also concerned that she might lose her job because she had missed a lot of work. He worried about finances since she was contributing less than usual. Susan's health was poor because she had two major surgeries that year. The recovery from the second surgery was slow. She missed work because of the surgeries and her poor health.

Not only was Susan's safety affected by her health and resulting financial issues, she also moved to a new home shortly before the injury that required the first surgery. Her husband was out of town on a job so she had to face this event on her own with no one in the vicinity to lean on. Because of the move and her husband's absence, she lost some sense of her safety even before the injury. And she had no time to find safety in her new home before the accident occurred.

Susan made the connection between her loss of safety and the way it triggered her past trauma when she talked about this recurring nightmare:

> I'm in a big cavernous building with high walls and I am running. Running from someone – monsters or something else very scary. Every time I go down a hall I think, "This is the one," and then when I get closer, I see it is the same as the others, with still no way out.

She had this recurring dream when she was a child as well, a dream she realized reminded her of her abuse. Once she understood that she was having the dream because she was feeling traumatized, Susan became more conscious and much improved. The awareness made her feel safer and reminded her to take care of herself and focus on the present. Given this sense of security, she began to heal.

RESOURCES

Herman, J.L. (1992). *Trauma and recovery*. New York: Basic Books.

Najavits, L. (2002). *Seeking safety: A treatment manual for PTSD and substance abuse*. New York: Guilford Press. See also http://www.seekingsafety.org/

Rothschild, B. (2000). *The body remembers: The psychophysiology of trauma and trauma treatment*. New York and London: WW Norton & Company.

van der Kolk, B.A. (2014). *The body keeps the score: Brain, mind, and body in the healing of trauma*. New York, NY, US: Viking.

Practice Exercises and Questions

- Role-play tuning into yourself as you prepare to work with a trauma survivor
- Pick a traumatic event such as a mugging from the newspaper and imagine what the survivor must be experiencing. Come up with ways to work with him/her and suggestions for coping
- Explain why safe relationships and safety in general are so important to survivors
- List some of the ways the brain operates post-trauma and talk about how this makes life difficult for survivors
- Describe the smoke alarm example of how survivors get stuck in emergency mode

The Importance of Safety Summary

Tune in to Safety

- *Be aware of survivors' sense of safety*
- *Remember past losses in order to relate to survivors*
- *Focus on your own safe place*

Use Coping to Stay with Survivors

- *Check in with self regularly*
- *Notice your reactions to survivors*
- *Stay present with breathing, touch and other coping strategies*

Assess Stress of Trauma

- *Disconnected from or overwhelmed by emotions*
- *Hypervigilance, flashbacks and nightmares*
- *Avoidance of or attraction to things related to trauma*
- *Difficulty with relationships*
- *Insufficient or inconsistent self-care*

Assess Survivors' Sense of Safety

- *Effective coping skills*
- *Network of supportive relationships*
- *Financial, physical, social and emotional stability*

Help Survivors Create a New Safe Place

- *Discuss survivors' ideas relative to safety*
- *Identify safe things to add to their coping repertoire*
- *Help survivors reintroduce safety into their lives*

Chapter 11

Building Safe Relationships

Healing from trauma begins with building safe reliable relationships. Survivors' recuperation process may even be hindered if they are unable to bond with people (Herman, 1992). Rapport with trustworthy individuals is crucial to trauma recovery and provides a healing environment within which to strive for understanding of what occurred. This chapter focuses on rebuilding current relationships and finding new healing connections. Developing healthy boundaries and avoiding or leaving unsafe relationships are also explored.

TUNE IN TO RELATIONSHIPS DURING AND AFTER TRAUMA

Think about your most comfortable relationships. Remember how accepted and appreciated they make you feel. Disagreements in these relationships may not have even posed a problem because you maintained your connection with the individuals even when your views differed. Or you may have always known that you could go to them for kind words, supportive hugs or nurturing meals.

Tips

- *Accessing safety of relationships* – Safe relationships are low-stress and positive, but also challenging because people who are close and care often help us see ways to eliminate obstacles and grow. In safe relationships, it is alright to say no and set appropriate boundaries. It is also important to share concerns and fears because this helps create the strong bonds that promote safety. Finally, the ability to laugh together even when facing difficulty is essential to safe relationships

---

Picture life without those relationships or with relationships that feel unsafe, making it difficult or impossible to talk about how you really are or to relax and have fun, both of which are important to effective and satisfying relationships. Sense how alone and disconnected you would be.

Imagine how it would be to have safe relationships, but not know how to talk about your fear after experiencing a trauma. Instead of feeling surrounded by people who care, as you did before the traumatic event, you feel alone with the fear and do not know how to reach out and get the support you need. Perhaps you feel even more alone and misunderstood when people minimize the trauma in an attempt to help you forget (McCann & Pearlman, 1990a). You may struggle to believe you can have safe relationships after a distressing event hurts you and others in ways you never anticipated.

This exercise can give practitioners a glimpse of survivors' difficulties relating to others during and after traumatic events. It can help to use the exercise prior to meeting with a survivor or when learning about trauma. Relationship issues often encountered by survivors are outlined further in the sections that follow.

TRAUMA CREATES ISOLATION

Symptoms of post-traumatic stress disorder (PTSD) often impede relations with others and lead to isolation. Hypervigilance or poor sleep caused by nightmares of the event can make survivors jumpy, nervous and hard to approach and connect with. Intrusive memories of what occurred can get in the way. Friends and family may have difficulty hearing about the trauma or tolerating survivors "spacing out" as they focus on intrusive thoughts. Survivors also frequently have trouble feeling emotions such as affection and lose interest in social interaction (American Psychiatric Association, 2013); this contributes to survivors feeling disconnected and isolated. These reactions, which often occur after trauma even without a PTSD diagnosis, can be particularly prevalent for individuals experiencing ongoing trauma such as those involved in abusive relationships or living in war zones.

Definitions

- *Post-traumatic stress disorder (PTSD)* – A disorder resulting from exposure to traumatic events that causes symptoms lasting at least a month that include emotional responses of fear, horror or helplessness; flashbacks and/or nightmares of events; avoidance of reminders of the event; and increased arousal
- *Hypervigilance* – A state of increased attention to the environment, in order to detect threat and prevent harm, that can increase anxiety, prevent sleep and cause fatigue

Illustrating trauma's influence on relationships, research indicates that veterans have more work, family, social and sexual issues after exposure to combat. Their children can also become withdrawn or aggressive and often have difficulty playing (Nader, 2004; Solomon, Labor, & McFarlane, 1996). Experiencing interpersonal trauma can even have an impact on pregnant women's ability to attach with their unborn children (Schwerdtfeger & Nelson Goff, 2007).

Part of the difficulty with relationships revolves around damage to survivors' feelings of competency, ability to trust and sense of self – all essential to intimacy (Herman, 1992). Suspicion of others who may seem unsafe because of past trauma (Bromberg, 2006) and fears related to relationships – that include fear of hurting others, abandonment, attack, rejection or vulnerability and loss of control – abound as survivors open up to others. These fears can cause survivors to avoid connection, instigate arguments, cut off relationships, abuse substances, work excessively or use other means to create distance (Schiraldi, 2009).

CONNECTION HEALS

Research shows that just as trauma can lead to isolation, connection can heal and aid recovery. Holocaust survivors, for example, who spent time with groups of peers had less trauma-related psychological impairment (Schiraldi, 2009). Studies also show that lack of bonding after traumatic events promotes development of PTSD (van der Kolk, 1989). This impact is seen in female rape victims who, in one study, had more severe trauma symptoms if they had controlling fathers who did not express affection (Hauck, Schestatsky, Terra, Kruel, & Ceitlin, 2007).

Herman (1992) goes so far as to say that survivors cannot heal from trauma if they are isolated from others, stressing the importance of empowering by helping them regain a sense that they control their lives so that they feel safe enough to take a chance on interacting with others. Social workers can help by encouraging survivors to ask for and accept help from dependable individuals who may or may not include mental health professionals. This can take some effort since survivors often find it difficult to reach out in this way (Herman, 1992). It is important that they limit these post-trauma relationships to supportive individuals who help survivors feel good about themselves, increasing their sense of competency and of integration in their world (McCann & Pearlman, 1990a).

Social workers can also help by creating a safe enough environment for survivors to open up and be themselves. This is crucial, since the effects of trauma can cause survivors to pretend everything is fine in order to make those who care about them feel better (McCann & Pearlman, 1990a). Working with survivors in this way allows them to grow and develop as their feelings of being protected and safe increase, enabling attachment rather than isolation (Pearlman & Courtois, 2005).

RELATIONSHIPS TIPS FOR SURVIVORS

Social workers help survivors feel attached rather than isolated by guiding and educating them as they negotiate relationship issues. The tips outlined below aid this process. The following sections also address ways in which practitioners can facilitate survivors' relationship skill building. These skills include:

1. tolerating, working with and safely expressing emotion
2. setting appropriate boundaries with others and
3. identifying safe and unsafe relationships

Tip 1: Pay Attention to Signs of Potential Relationship Issues

Since survivors can have an almost desperate need for nurturance, they can tend to ignore the inappropriate behavior of people in their inner circles. Some even turn to their abusers for support (van der Kolk, 1989). Help survivors watch for subtle and overt signs of abuse as well as a lack of balance in their relationships; e.g., caring for others rather than themselves or hiding feelings upsetting to loved ones.

Tip 2: Ask Trusted Individuals When Unsure About How to Proceed

Survivors can have a hard time seeing relationships clearly when they are involved in them. Encourage them to ask others and to listen to their viewpoints when what they say makes sense, or when they hear the same message in a variety of ways from different sources (Najavits, 2002). Remind them to stay open to other perspectives, realizing that theirs may be skewed by proximity and a need for support. They need to ask for help, carefully choosing individuals whom they respect and learning to trust their own instincts when getting help, remembering that if what they hear does not seem to fit, they can let it go. Being specific about what they need from others is also important, asking for support, ideas, viewpoints and/or resources, depending on their needs (Najavits, 2002).

Tip 3: Talk Appropriately About Thoughts and Feelings

Sharing beliefs and emotions honestly and sincerely strengthens intimacy if done safely (Schiraldi, 2009). Particularly with couples, withdrawal after trauma can become an issue, weakening relationship ties and creating loneliness and vulnerability (Johnson & Williams-Keeler, 1998). Help survivors find ways to share openly with safe individuals.

Tip 4: Try to Understand and Accept What Cannot Be Changed

Remember that many people cannot comprehend trauma's impact. When survivors try to communicate about it and ask for support, it may be best for them to desist if recipients seem unable to hear. They may need to find understanding elsewhere and to communicate at a level that fits the unique personality of each individual. Emphasize that this reflects relationship capacities and is not the fault of survivors (Najavits, 2002).

Tip 5: Focus on Changing What Can Be Controlled

Coach survivors to consider relationships carefully, weighing their pros and cons. Encourage working on what they can change such as their own behavior, being careful not to add to the self-blame and guilt with which survivors often grapple. Remind them that some relationships with negative aspects are worth maintaining because they nonetheless offer significant benefits (Graber, 1991). These relationship decisions often require distance, perspective, input from others and even temporary separation (Graber, 1991).

Tip 6: Remember That Relationships Require Attention and Effort

Assure survivors that everyone needs to work on their relationships, normalizing the process (Najavits, 2002). Help them by providing support and pointing it out when you see them encountering obstacles or experiencing abuse.

Tip 7: Know That Unsafe Relationships Are Not Acceptable

Watch for signs of inappropriate or abusive behavior in survivors' relationships and do not hesitate to discuss this. Help survivors to see that they should never accept aggressive behavior and that being alone, although it may seem impossible and frightening, is actually safer and more conducive to growth than remaining in a relationship where someone hurts or takes advantage of them (Najavits, 2002). Provide resources such as intimate partner violence shelters and hotlines for those currently experiencing abuse.

THE ROLE OF EMOTION

Because trauma emotion can impede relations, skill building in this area also helps. Survivors may use dissociation and numbing to protect themselves from the intensity of emotion (Pearlman & Courtois, 2005). This process cuts them off not only from the feelings, but also from loved ones because individuals of all cultures bond by sharing what they feel. Keep in mind that everyone expresses emotion, but how it is expressed it can vary. Unlike Westerners, for instance, non-Westernized Asians express less positive emotion about themselves, tending toward self-effacement (Goleman, 2004).

Trauma survivors often have difficulty expressing intense emotion. This can cause children who have experienced trauma to disconnect from the environment (van der Kolk, McFarlane, & van der Hart, 1996). It can also disrupt their attachment to adults, a potentially serious problem depending on their stage of development and the severity of the rift. Since children learn to regulate and tolerate emotion through secure attachments (Pearlman & Courtois, 2005), failing to attach impedes learning these skills and can consequently stunt emotional development.

Survivors who lack emotion-regulation skills may have relationships plagued with fear and lack of trust. Others may use substance abuse and other ineffective means of "coping" (Najavits, 2002). These ineffective "coping" skills also get in the way of relationship intimacy and the ability to connect, increasing isolation.

One couple's experience shows how trauma emotion affects relationships. The wife, Julie, survived incest and had a history of flashbacks and self-harm. The couple undertook emotion-focused couples counseling (EFT) to help them cope with her trauma reactions. Emotion-focused therapy (EFT) is a short-term (12–20 sessions) methodology that facilitates processing emotional responses in order to create secure attachment. In the twelfth session of treatment, Julie talked about cutting herself when distressed at night and feeling she could not wake her husband, Larry, because he would get angry and lecture her. The therapist helped them to access underlying emotions, including (1) Julie's fear that asking for help would bring abuse, as it did during her childhood; and (2) Larry's fear and sadness about what she had experienced. This work enabled Larry to support Julie in ways he could not previously and she began to use their relationship, instead of self-harm, as a means to cope (Johnson & Williams-Keeler, 1998).

BOUNDARIES THAT WORK

Setting appropriate boundaries, where survivors do not feel too close to or far away from others, helps establish secure attachment after traumatic events. Without knowledge about how to accomplish this, tolerating and regulating proximity in relationships can become troublesome. Children who may not have learned these skills or who regress after experiencing trauma can have a particularly hard time. As a result, survivors can become confused as they try to ascertain who they are as individuals and how to separate from others (McCann & Pearlman, 1990a).

Trauma interrupts the individuation process through which children learn to see themselves as discrete entities. Even adults can have difficulty in this area because trauma disrupts safe attachments (Pearlman & Courtois, 2005). Parents teach children the intricacies of establishing boundaries in order to form safe attachments. Unfortunately, many do not have effective skills to teach their children (Davis, 1991). Trauma complicates this, particularly when both parents and children are survivors. Many survivors react to trauma by clinging to loved ones or pushing them away out of fear. Combat veterans, for instance, can develop hypervigilance about their personal space, setting firm and excessive boundaries because physical closeness feels threatening (McCann & Pearlman, 1990a).

As social workers, we can assist survivors by helping them learn these skills, pointing out areas where they can make boundaries more secure or open, enabling safe attachment to others. Types of boundaries requiring attention include physical space, eye contact, interpersonal boundaries and touch. It is important for us to remember to honor and work with survivors' difficulty with emotional and physical proximity, touch and eye contact (Rothschild, 2000). By doing so, we can help them discover their own personal space limitations and how to avoid uncomfortable contact with others.

Tips

• *Making comfortable eye contact* – If direct eye contact is uncomfortable, suggest that survivors look at the side of the face or the forehead instead of the eyes and, if appropriate, ask others to do the same. This tactic mimics direct eye contact

---

Examples of ways you can coach survivors regarding boundaries include:

1. being aware of autonomy
2. learning to say "yes" and "no" and
3. the need for balance

Both autonomy and the ability to care for themselves are essential to survivors who may have been out of control and/or dominated by others or circumstances during the trauma. Saying "yes" lets others in and allows closeness, and "no" provides distance when needed. These boundaries require balance. Saying either "yes" or "no" all the time is not healthy. Nor is spending too much or too little time alone, focusing too much on selves or others, or moving too fast or too slow in relationships – for example, by revealing intimate details immediately or sharing almost nothing about themselves within clearly safe interactions (Najavits, 2002). Remember to explain that developing good boundaries is a trial-and-error process and that it improves with practice over time (Davis, 1991).

Survivors need boundaries because they usually find it easier to accept themselves and others when they know that separateness and autonomy mean less confusion about which needs and feelings belong to survivors and which belong to others. When they know how to set appropriate boundaries, they also have less need to control or depend on others to feel safe (Davis, 1991).

The experience of 3-year-old Lane, who was traumatized by medical issues, illustrates how boundaries can help. As a result of her trauma background, she became overstimulated and fearful with groups of people. When distraught at a family gathering, gently rubbing her back and telling her that this was Lane who was here and being touched, calmed her. Having felt physically invaded by her medical issues, she needed to be reminded of her body and its separateness from others (Rothschild, 2000).

POTENTIALLY SAFE RELATIONSHIPS

Potentially safe relationships can come in many forms, with the most important ingredients being (1) connection; and (2) support for survivors and their recovery (Najavits, 2002). Banding together rather than going it alone evolved historically because humans could hunt, gather food, stay safe from predators, and reproduce more effectively as part of a community (Harvey & Miller, 2000). This safe, protective quality of community is paramount for survivors who often feel isolated and alone after traumatic events. Safe relationships vary and can come through family, pets, spiritual entities and others, as is discussed in this section. Even memories of past supportive relationships can help survivors feel secure (Rothschild, 2000).

INTIMATE RELATIONSHIPS

In intimate partner relationships, safety and support for recovery from trauma become most crucial. Trusting partners enough allows survivors to share their helplessness and pain related to the traumatic event (Turner, McFarlane, & van der Kolk, 1996). This can be difficult, since many survivors withdraw from their partners and do not talk about feelings (Johnson & Williams-Keeler, 1998).

Tips

- *See selves as safe houses* – Help survivors to understand boundaries by comparing themselves to safe houses with doors, gates and windows that they can open and close as needed for fresh air and to let others in, but can securely close for safety (Schiraldi, 2009).

As documented with survivors of sexual abuse, combat and intimate partner violence, survivors of trauma commonly struggle with both marital and sexual issues (McCann & Pearlman, 1990a). Discussing these issues honestly, which can be particularly difficult with sexual issues, is essential (Graber, 1991). Social workers can help by teaching communication skills and rehearsing or role-playing the skills with survivors.

Family and Friends

Relationships with family and friends have a healing influence on recovery. When social workers encourage survivors to reach out appropriately, share their needs and wants and ask to for help when necessary, they can act as watch-dogs in the process, pointing out signs of unsafe relationships. At times, coaching survivors to ask for what they need may help the situation. In other cases, practitioners may need to intervene more directly.

Pay particular attention to bonds formed between the abuser and the abused during traumatic events. This usually leads to damaging relationships with bonds formed, for example, between those involved in intimate partner abuse and between children and their adult abusers (James, 1994). Even if these relationships cease to be abusive, it takes time and effort to create safe connections. See the Resources section at the end of the chapter for more information on this topic.

Community Ties

Community – a supportive feeling of connectedness that includes shared culture, history, ideas, goals, activities and the ability to communicate and identify – can heal trauma survivors and go a long way toward dispelling the isolation they so often endure (Ayalon, 1998; Farwell & Cole, 2001–2002). Community includes friendships and familial/intimate relationships. Geographic areas; groups of those with similar racial or ethnic backgrounds; schools and workplaces; spiritual networks; and connection to animals, nature and even with the deceased or imaginary friends can also form community, potentially providing support and a sense of being cared for.

Illustrating how the imagination can provide connective community, a mother found her husband dead in his study after sending her 6- or 7-year-old daughter to get him. The girl returned saying an angel stopped her going in the door, protecting her from finding him herself. Another severely neglected 9-year-old girl, Lenore, had a fairy godmother who protected her by preventing her suicide (Kalsched, 1996).

Animals also protect and help survivors. Research shows that riding and relationships with horses contribute to healing from a variety of traumas (Yorke, Adams, & Coady, 2008). Sexual assault survivors benefit from animal-assisted therapy (Lefkowitz, Paharia, Prout, Debiak, & Bleiberg, 2005). And a combination of animals and storytelling can help sexually abused children talk about their experience and associated feelings (Reichert, 1998).

Empowering and supportive resource providers, including peers who are also survivors, can be an important component of community for those who have experienced trauma (Najavits, 2002). Addressing survivors' needs for resources in the aftermath of trauma, specific community interventions have been developed including the Community Oriented Preventive Education (COPE) project for Israelis affected by war; the Belief, Affect, Social interaction, Imagination, Cognition and Physiology (BASIC-Ph) model that stresses coping resources; and the Graça Machel project which works toward involving children in creating peace and stopping violent altercations and traumatization (Ayalon, 1998).

Bosses, Doctors and Other Authorities

Survivors can have difficulty and even re-enact trauma with social services professionals as well as with bosses, doctors, priests and other authorities. Some may encounter people in authority who are abusive, resemble abusers, or bring up feelings related to traumatic events (Naparstek, 2005). When this occurs, social workers can help survivors work with their feelings and establish safety. This includes helping them leave unsafe relationships and enter healing connections. Therapeutic relationships with mental health professionals can also create community. For more information, see chapter 15 on individual, couples and family therapy.

Case Study

Joan was in her sixties when her husband, George, became sick suddenly and almost died. She spent months by his bedside in the hospital. In the beginning he was in a coma and unresponsive, but even as he slowly recovered, she did not. She had lost hope and caring for him wore her out. A nurse told her about the hospital's caregiver center which in turn referred her to a social worker. She shared the following during a therapy session:

Joan:	I don't feel like myself.
Social worker:	How so?
Joan:	I feel damaged, like I won't get better even if he does and he won't.
Social worker:	Isn't he getting better? *Joan nods.* Have you felt this before?
Joan:	*Looking thoughtful.* I felt damaged as a kid.
Social worker:	This illness has been quite a shock. Could it remind you of difficult times when you were a child?
Joan:	Those were hard times for me till I met my husband.

The social worker learned that Joan had been neglected by her mother because she was unable to deal with the grief of losing her husband. Busy working to support the family, she hardly talked, expressed no affection, nor did she attend to Joan's needs for proper food, clothing and healthcare. Fortunately, her grandmother took care of Joan's basic needs, but she was a lonely and unhappy child.

In 7th and 8th grades at school, fellow students repeatedly beat her up because she was quiet and dressed shabbily. She said that she felt like something was wrong with her until she met her husband. They fell in love and she adopted his more "normal" family. Her life changed. The healing power of the familial community and of her safe relationship with her husband gave her confidence and she became happy. After establishing a healing relationship with the social worker and realizing in therapy that her husband's illness had reminded her of the difficulties with her family of origin and triggered unhappy feelings, she began to regain her self-confidence.

RESOURCES

Davis, L. (1991). *Allies in healing: When the person you love was sexually abused as a child.* New York: Harper Perennial.

James, B. (1994). *Handbook for treatment of attachment-trauma problems in children.* New York: The Free Press.

Johnson, S.M., & Williams-Keeler, L. (1998). Creating healing relationships for couples dealing with trauma: The use of emotionally focused marital therapy. *Journal of Marital and Family Therapy, 24(1)*, 25–40.

Pearlman, L.A., & Courtois, C.A. (2005). Clinical applications of the attachment formula: Relational treatment of complex trauma. *Journal of Traumatic Stress, 18(5)*, 449–459.

Rothschild, B. (2000). *The body remembers: The psychophysiology of trauma and trauma treatment.* New York and London: W. W. Norton & Company.

Practice Exercises and Questions

- Review and discuss the seven relationship tips
- List the three ways you can coach survivors regarding boundaries
- Role-play a session with a survivor who has become quite isolated and is resisting connecting with others. Keep in mind the relationship tips and ways to coach regarding boundaries
- Tune in to yourself as you think about meeting with a trauma survivor whose friends and family have become distant probably because they are unsure what to say. Think of what it would be like to be in that position and the kind of support that would help

Building Safe Relationships Summary

Tune in to Safe and Unsafe Relationships

- Safe relationships are healing and there is a feeling of ease
- Trauma isolates survivors and decreases relationship safety

Relationship Tips for Survivors

- Pay attention to signs of potential relationship issues
- Ask trusted individuals when unsure about how to proceed
- Talk appropriately about thoughts and feelings
- Try to understand and accept what cannot be changed
- Focus on changing what can be controlled
- Remember that relationships require attention and effort
- Know that unsafe relationships are not acceptable

The Role of Emotion

- Intense trauma-related emotion can be difficult to express
- Learning to express emotion facilitates bonding with others

Boundaries That Work

- Survivors ascertaining when and how to say "yes" and "no"
- Awareness of own autonomy; taking responsibility for self

Potentially Safe Relationships

- Intimate relationships, family, friends, peers, colleagues
- Community including resources, spirituality, nature, animals
- Bosses, doctors, therapeutic relationships, other authorities

Chapter 12

Coping Skills and Self-Care

Coping is not a new concept. All beings, including animals, adapt to their environments by making adjustments so that they fit in. Depending on their adaptive abilities, everyone reacts differently to stress and crisis (Vattano, 1978). Some panic, while others take it in their stride. When the adaptation process falls short, stress occurs and can even trigger the freeze, flight, fight, fright, faint emergency response in a crisis. Coping is integral to minimizing these responses since it encourages adaptation (Lazarus, 2006). As Lazarus says, coping is "concerned with our efforts to manage adaptional demands and the emotions they generate" (2006, p. 10).

Definitions

- *Coping* – Process of dealing with difficulties, problem solving and adapting to the environment in order to manage stress and conflict effectively
- *Freeze, flight, fight, fright, faint emergency response* – Physical reaction to perceived threat or danger that leads to discharge of hormones such as adrenalin and cortisol, increased heart rate, shallow breathing and slowdown of non-essential activities such as digestion so that the body can mobilize to protect itself

---

Because stress is a part of life, coping is too, not just for crises, but also for the day-to-day strain of interpersonal conflict, frustration and disappointment. Therefore, everyone needs to cope to maintain balance and adapt (Lazarus & Folkman, 1987). This includes methodologies such as meditation and yoga and eating, hygiene and other basic self-care. Examples of coping are: Music for relaxation, reading for distraction and a new perspective, physical exercise for the positive effects of endorphins and discharge of negative emotions, talking to friends for connection and support, spiritual activities for support and motivation, spending time in nature for relaxation and rejuvenation and using humor to change perspective and relax.

Trauma survivors often experience high levels of stress, so familiarity with coping is crucial to their healing. Evidence-based treatment approaches, such as Trauma-focused Cognitive Behavioral Therapy for children and Seeking Safety for adults, benefit survivors as they provide much-needed coping skills and stress management. Both models encourage increasing survivors' expertise in these areas before embarking on in-depth psychotherapy. Even without therapy, daily functioning and well-being improve and trauma symptoms reduce with this skill-building process (Cohen & Mannarino, 2008; Najavits, 2002).

TUNE IN TO COPING

In order to work with survivors regarding their coping, we need to pay attention to our own. Since we normally cope through unconscious processes, with skills utilized automatically without thinking, this requires work. For instance, we do not generally think about our morning showers and getting a restful night's sleep as examples of good coping, but they are. We do not often realize that a cup of tea or a greeting from a colleague as we start the workday also help us cope. Becoming aware of these actions helps us to assist survivors with becoming aware of their own. As an added benefit, the awareness helps improve our own coping as survivors improve theirs.

An exercise that can help with awareness of coping is to draw a circle and put ourselves in the center. Think about the people and things most important to you and put them in the inner circle. This will usually include our closest friends and family; beloved pets; homes or favorite rooms; important music, books or artwork and nature or spirituality. Only include the things that are most special in this inner circle. Keep drawing consecutive circles until the outer circle lists those things most removed from you, but that offer support of some kind. Figure 12.1 is an example of how this exercise works (much more coping can be listed).

Once we become aware of our own coping, we can think about how well it works. Perhaps one of the ways we cope is to get quiet when we are upset. However, this prevents us from talking about what bothers us so that it does not always end up working effectively. This does not mean we should never be silent, but it does mean we should think about the costs when we are and we may ultimately decide to incorporate a better solution. Thinking this way will help us to work with survivors on finding their ways to cope effectively.

To help survivors with coping, pay attention to what they say and do. A survivor who liked the actress and singer, Jennifer Lopez (J.Lo), and saw her as strong and confident, came for treatment one day, triggered by walking through the neighborhood where she had been seriously hurt when hit by a car. We talked about ways to feel safer, both at that moment and any time she had to be somewhere she felt scared. I brought up J.Lo and she smiled. "Yes,"

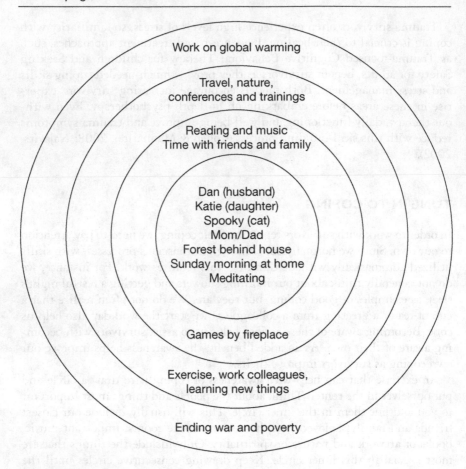

Work on global warming

Travel, nature,
conferences and trainings

Reading and music
Time with friends and family

Dan (husband)
Katie (daughter)
Spooky (cat)
Mom/Dad
Forest behind house
Sunday morning at home
Meditating

Games by fireplace

Exercise, work colleagues,
learning new things

Ending war and poverty

Figure 12.1 Circle of Coping

she said, "I'll be J.Lo and that will keep me safe." Her whole demeanor changed as she said this. She clearly felt stronger and more confident with this image in her mind.

As we pay attention, we will notice things that we can point out as components of survivors' automatic and unconscious coping, including what they do naturally, but do not think of as coping – such as cooking traditional foods, respecting family and ethnic customs and caring for loved ones. Identifying these actions as coping supports survivors' understanding that they can take steps to feel better on their own and alleviates their fear that a feeling of safety is unattainable after trauma. The following sections elaborate on coping benefits and on how we, as social workers, can help survivors develop these skills. Doing this in a way that helps them re-establish safety in their lives is crucial to recovery and healing.

THE BENEFITS OF COPING

According to the literature, coping skills benefit diverse populations including individuals with life-threatening illness, combat veterans and those affected by serious accidents, terrorism and the Holocaust (Boothby, Crawford, & Halperin, 2006; Desai, Harpaz-Rotem, Najavits, & Rosenheck, 2008; Krysińska & Lester, 2006; Najavits, 2002; Owen et al., 2005; Schnyder, Moergeli, Klaghofer, & Buddeberg, 2001; Silver, Holman, McIntosh, Poulin, & Gil-Rivas, 2002; Tarakeshwar, Pearce, & Sikkema, 2005; C. Telch & M. Telch, 1986). Research indicates that post-traumatic stress disorder (PTSD) symptoms and the ability to cope interrelate. This relationship includes decreased PTSD symptoms in survivors with effective coping skills and increased symptoms among older adults, as stress increases and coping wanes (Aarts & Op den Velde, 1996), and with those who stop their coping efforts after exposure to trauma (Silver et al., 2002; Desai et al., 2008; Schnyder et al., 2001).

Definitions

* *Post-traumatic stress disorder (PTSD)* – A disorder resulting from exposure to traumatic events that causes symptoms lasting at least a month that include emotional responses of fear, horror or helplessness; flashbacks and/or nightmares of events; avoidance of reminders of the event; and increased arousal

---

Research also indicates that coping groups where trauma survivors actively learn and support each other's development of coping skills are efficacious. Symptoms of PTSD were decreased for group members studied, including some who found it difficult to engage, such as prison inmates (Najavits, 2002). A coping skills phone group for HIV/AIDS patients was also evaluated in a controlled study that compared symptoms of group participants with those of individuals on the waiting list. Stress and psychological symptoms diminished for patients who participated in the group. Not only did their symptoms lessen, but they did so with the obstacles of a membership who were at least 50 years old, with more medical problems than younger adults, and general resistance to discussing issues and asking for help (Heckman et al., 2006).

In addition to reducing psychological symptoms, coping also improves survivors' welfare as it reduces stress (Kabat-Zinn, 1991) and contributes to physical well-being since stress can have a negative impact on health. Illustrating this, a member of an anger-management coping group began with dangerously high blood pressure with onset after she was sexually molested at work. When she left the group to return to work a few months later, her blood pressure and health had normalized. She attributed this to awareness and expertise with coping skills.

Here is another example of how coping helped a survivor of sexual abuse. Sharice, a young African American woman, went for trauma treatment at the advice of her residential care service providers. She came to the first session wearing a baseball cap with the brim pulled low so that when she looked down, her face was not visible. She looked down for the entire first session and talked little, responding in monosyllables to questions asked and expressing no emotion throughout the process. After several sessions, she slowly began to talk about herself:

Sharice:	I'm scared a lot. Can't even take my clothes off to shower. Too scared someone'll get me. I was in the [psychiatric] hospital for years. Don't even remember how long. Nothing seems to help. *She looks down even more and her body tenses up.*
Social worker:	That must be hard for you. Are you scared now? You look anxious. *Sharice continues looking down and does not answer.* Let's do some coping to help the anxiety. Can you look around and tell me the colors you see?
Sharice:	*Looking at the lower part of the room and speaking softly.* Green, brown, white.
Social worker:	Can you look up and say the other colors in the room?
Sharice:	*Looking up slowly and speaking a little louder.* Red, blue, purple, yellow … *Tears begin to fall down her cheeks as she recites. This was the first emotion she had expressed since beginning treatment.*
Social worker:	Sharice, it makes sense that you're sad. You've had a hard life and lost much of your childhood because of it. I'm glad you can let yourself feel that. And you don't have to be alone with it anymore. I'm here with you.

Tips

- *Focus on the here and now* – Helping survivors focus on their immediate physical environment encourages coping as it moves them away from often scary memories of the past or worries about the future. Examples include counting chairs in the room, identifying colors around them, describing a picture in great detail or touching objects and noticing their texture and weight. This is also beneficial when survivors dissociate

---

After this session, where coping helped her get in touch with loss and sadness, Sharice slowly began to open up, both in one-to-one sessions and groups. Her coping and PTSD symptoms improved so much that she was able to get married a few years later to someone she met at her residence. Not only was she more comfortable with emotion, but she also felt much happier with her life.

COPING IS LEARNED

Sharice's case demonstrates one way we can help survivors learn to cope. This process of learning coping is manifold. It begins at birth and continues as we progress through life and is related to the adjustments we make to fit into our surroundings. As humans, we have choices about how we adapt, and can either modify how we respond to our environment or learn to make it work for us (Hartmann, 1958).

Unfortunately, not all our learning about coping occurs with consciousness and volition, so choice is not always involved. We absorb coping methods without realizing it and those we learn from often do not know what they have passed on, particularly in families where children learn to cope by copying their parents. In homes with alcoholism, for instance, children may learn to drink as a way to cope. Parents also teach self-soothing. When told that we did a wonderful job and tried the best we could, we learn to tell ourselves this as well.

Survivors learn coping from family, friends and through their own experience. Some coping does not relate to the trauma and some develops as a direct result of what occurred. Survivors have a variety of skills that may or may not work well, and then acquire new ones in the aftermath of trauma. They often forget to use their repertoire of skills after what occurred, but with support can regain lost skills, develop new ones to manage their experience, and thus learn to adapt.

Those who have experienced a trauma tend to develop "survival skills" such as dissociation and hypervigilance (Dinsmore, 1991). When used excessively, these can get in the way of functioning, but their intent is to protect. Dissociation can be helpful for survivors (Raphael, Wilson, Meldrum, & McFarlane, 1996) as it lessons pain and allows them to move away from frightening memories or circumstances.

Definitions

- *Dissociation* – Disconnection from thoughts, memories or emotions that provides internal distance from reminders of traumatic events, but also prevents integration of trauma material and disrupts normal psychological functioning
- *Hypervigilance* – State of increased attention to the environment, in order to detect threat and prevent harm, that can increase anxiety, prevent sleep and cause fatigue

---

Adjusting to trauma can also promote positive coping. In concentration camps during the Holocaust, activities such as smuggling and stealing food to help orphaned children, joining illegal study groups, keeping a diary, spreading good news and positive rumors, telling jokes, praying and sharing stories all helped to act as antidotes to the trauma (Krysińska & Lester, 2006). Part of the process of healing from trauma involves attempting to understand why it occurred in order to make sense of it. Positive coping can ameliorate the hopelessness often experienced as a part of this reflective process.

CULTURAL ASPECTS OF COPING

As survivors consciously and unconsciously learn coping, the process is affected by personal tastes, upbringing and cultural background. Because of this, social workers are uniquely qualified to help them ascertain effective ways to cope. Our background and training focus on the ecological perspective, orienting us to where survivors fit in the socio-economic, family and other systems intersecting their lives. We are also trained to follow the social work principle of going where the client is. Both skills play an essential role in investigating the cultural roots of survivors' coping.

In the spirit of going where the survivor is, the best way to learn what type of coping best fits their cultural patterns is to ask survivors about what helps them when they have difficulties, and to observe how they respond to stress (Najavits, 2002). This matters when working with those at the end of life, for instance. It is crucial to die at home for some cultures. Others have special meanings associated with medications that require sensitivity and education prior to treating pain. Spiritual beliefs also hold significance when facing the possibility of death. Learning about these cultural aspects of dying can help us to optimize the dying person's coping process.

Tips

- *Be like Columbo* – When Peter Falk played the detective, Columbo, in a American TV series, he always asked many questions, learning from those he worked with. We can do the same in order to learn about cultural aspects of coping, letting survivors and their families teach us their traditions. We can also do research or ask colleagues what they know. The more we learn, the more we can help survivors incorporate culture into their coping

---

Examples of cultural coping methods include religious beliefs, rituals, traditions, food preparation, dance, music, art, clothing and costumes and ideologies. Traditional belief systems can have a great deal of power. It has been found, for example, among African Americans, that individuals who believe they have a purpose, and have mastered aspects of life that allow them to work toward this purpose, have greater resilience from trauma (Alim et al., 2008). This holds true for survivor Indigenous women as well. Enculturation, or becoming aware of and believing in native culture, including traditional spiritual and health practices such as sweat lodges, can enhance coping processes after a traumatic event (Walters & Simoni, 2002).

Having a history of trauma and of discrimination can complicate the coping process. Because of this, we need to be aware of survivors' cultural beliefs and issues they may encounter as members of certain cultural groups. This includes considering the impact of racism when working with survivors of combat. Racism can be both emotionally painful and have socio-economic consequences that affect coping (Jones, Brazel, Peskind, Morelli, & Raskind, 2000).

Tips

• *Coping that fits* – When practicing coping with survivors, choose methods that fit them. Children and those with impaired functioning need uncomplicated methods such as counting. Count with them slowly and feel their stress reduce as you proceed. Another simple way to cope is to have survivors use a self-administered eye movement desensitization and reprocessing (EMDR) technique, the "Butterfly Hug" (for more on EMDR, see chapter 15 on other trauma interventions). Cross the arms over the chest so the fingers touch the shoulders. Alternately tap just below the left and right shoulders while focusing on something positive. The tapping reinforces and strengthens the positive focus

---

Coping also depends on factors such as survivors' ages, levels of functioning and cognitive developmental states. Higher functioning adults, who have insight and the ability to analyze, can utilize more sophisticated coping methods; whereas those with lower functioning need concrete and uncomplicated skills. This includes those with lower cognitive abilities such as children, people with disabilities, the elderly and those with high stress or debilitating symptoms. Many survivors, for example, present as lower functioning when they begin treatment due to PTSD symptoms.

SELF-CARE AS COPING

Not everyone thinks of basic self-care as coping, but healthy habits have been tied to happiness (Schiraldi, 2009). For survivors, coping starts with the body. This includes eating, sleeping, bathing and having as safe a home as possible (Herman, 1992). Many survivors have difficulty sleeping due to nightmares and hypervigilance. Exercising, learning sleep hygiene techniques, like avoiding scary movies or heavy meals prior to going to bed can improve sleep and decrease nightmares. Pre-sleep coping and relaxation can also help to reduce stress and the chance of nightmares.

Tips

* *Dream incubation* – Survivors can utilize visualization to "ask" for the types of dreams they want, describing them on a piece of paper they put under their pillows or just imagining themselves waking up after no dreams or dreams that are not scary. They should imagine this frequently throughout the day. Survivors are often so scared of their nightmares that when given a choice, they "ask" for no dreams, rather than happy ones. This technique can not only reduce nightmares, but also increase empowerment

---

Feeling safe, secure and relaxed in their homes is complicated for survivors who (1) have PTSD symptoms that upset their equilibrium; (2) use "coping" methods that are harmful, such as substance abuse and cutting; (3) still experience trauma or (4) continue to be in the environment where trauma occurred, as with those living in the midst of war or staying with someone who abused them in the past (Herman, 1992).

Financial problems reduce safety in the home as well, particularly for those living on the streets or without enough to eat. Poor health also reduces safety, so medical attention is important for survivors (McCann & Pearlman, 1990a).

In general, improving the ability to function effectively on a daily basis helps trauma survivors (Rothschild, 2000). This includes feeling in control of their daily schedules, being organized, and having a plan for what they want to accomplish (Schiraldi, 2009). The positive effects of this kind of coping became clear when working with those affected by the September 11th disaster, many of whom worked in the area and were thus out of work. One survivor talked about how walking the neighbor's dog was healing for him. He said it helped him most because it gave structure to his day and made him feel he had something worthwhile to do. The canine company and unconditional love animals provide, although also beneficial, only motivated him secondarily.

INEFFECTIVE COPING

Despite the benefits of practicing coping skills, some attempts to cope do not work well and can even do harm. Examples include substance abuse, self-injurious behavior, gambling, aggression, excessive shopping and eating disorders. It is important to note that although these behaviors generally do not work as coping and can also do harm, they represent attempts to cope and stem from a healthy desire to adapt and establish equilibrium. For instance, self-injurious behavior has been studied and it was found that, at times, it is an attempt to avoid more serious responses such as suicide (Whitlock & Knox, 2007). Survivors who injure themselves often describe feeling temporary relief from psychic pain as a result of the injurious behavior.

Responses to trauma such as the symptoms of dissociation, numbing and avoiding can be ineffective coping as well. Although unconsciously meant to protect, these responses do not work as coping when they impede daily functioning and cause well-being to deteriorate (Raphael, Wilson, Meldrum, & McFarlane, 1996). Approaching reminders of trauma can overwhelm and stimulate survivors as when veterans of war watch war footage and become upset as a result. On the other hand, if a victim of rape by a man cannot associate with men after the event, work opportunities could be severely limited, making financial security tenuous and demonstrating how complete avoidance of trauma reminders can impede recovery. Coping will help reduce these adverse responses so that survivors who successfully cope in other areas of life, such as their general level of safety, will be less affected by trauma symptoms (McCann & Pearlman, 1990a). See the following section for ideas on how survivors can use their responses to trauma constructively.

Definitions

- *Avoidance* – Individuals staying away from people, places or activities, even when not dangerous, because they are reminders of trauma
- *Safety* – State essential to trauma recovery and unique to each individual, in which: (1) risky behaviors, unhealthy relationships and negative emotions are reduced and (2) a sense of well-being, trust, calm and positive coping are increased

---

Lack of balance can also get in the way of effective coping. Finding a comfortable balance between approaching and avoiding trauma material makes processing the material more manageable. Balance helps to prevent survivors' blocking out trauma material, overusing avoidance or being triggered by the material as they approach it repeatedly. Another aspect of balance is that even good coping can be overused, as is the case with survivors who exercise excessively and physically hurt themselves as a result. Social workers can help survivors incorporate balance into their coping plans.

Shame and self-blame can thwart effective coping too. Not only do survivors often feel guilt about their inability to prevent the trauma or help others enough when it occurred, but some also feel ashamed of their responses to trauma. Responses that can cause shame include PTSD symptoms and difficulty coping (Dinsmore, 1991). Self-blame is also common (Najavits, 2002) to the point that some survivors do not feel they deserve nurturing attention and thus neglect self-care (Herman, 1992). In order to cope effectively, survivors may need to learn compassion for and acceptance of themselves and what they have been through. We can encourage this by providing survivors with psychoeducation so that they can recognize that what they are experiencing is a normal response to an abnormal event (Dinsmore, 1991).

Coping helps trauma-associated shame and does not have the pathological stigma of some interventions. Survivors generally accept recommendations to adopt coping without the sense that it is needed because of their "craziness" or weakness. The attitudes of members learning coping in one trauma group reflected this. Many taught the skills they learned to their children, improving their families' coping as a result. The ordinariness of practicing coping also means that it is less likely to add to the shame many feel as a result of traumatic experiences, increasing the likelihood of effective coping.

HELPING SURVIVORS FIND NEW WAYS TO COPE

Optimizing coping includes replacing ineffective coping with coping that works. This means survivors need an arsenal of skills to choose from. Start the process of building that arsenal by helping them discover coping they do now that works. Also encourage borrowing ideas for coping from other survivors. This works particularly well in groups where survivors can share how they cope. Keep these points in mind while helping survivors optimize their coping (Table 12.1).

In addition to these points, to be effective, coping must fit survivors' resources and specific environmental situations (van der Kolk et al., 1996). Coping that costs money will not work for those without financial means, and a busy person will need help finding ways to cope that work while engaged with other activities, or that take little time. Helping survivors come up with a coping plan is also helpful (Schiraldi, 2009). This can be a general plan for any time that crisis or stress occurs, or a specific plan for before and after difficult events such as a gynecological appointment for a survivor of sexual abuse.

When helping survivors develop a coping plan, remind them that the goal is to "thrive," not just "survive." Some skills developed to survive the trauma may seem unnecessary after the trauma has ended, but still have worth and contribute to thriving. Hypervigilance, for instance, protects from danger (Dinsmore, 1991). It also heightens awareness so that survivors often have increased sensitivity to others' feelings and actions and are attentive to minute details in the environment. This skill can work constructively and become effective coping by translating the sensitivity to increased empathy toward others and the awareness of the environment to mindfulness or attention to the present moment.

Table 12.1 Coping Teaching Points

Coping	Teaching Point
Individual	Coping varies based on personal taste, upbringing and cultural background. Effective coping for one person may not work for another. No coping will work under all circumstances, even if it has in the past.
Automatic	Coping skills tend to be responses requiring little attention. This lack of consciousness means that many people are not aware of how they cope.
Learned	Skills are often acquired from others, who may be unaware of what they are teaching, or during the traumatic event experienced.
Efficacy	Attempts to cope can be both effective and helpful; or ineffective, and at times harmful.
Harmful	Harmful attempts to cope, such as substance abuse, overeating, aggression and self-injury, are prompted by the healthy desire to adapt.
Awareness	Improved coping requires not only utilizing effective coping skills, but also becoming conscious of automatic coping responses. Awareness makes it possible to ascertain when coping is effective. Individuals can work consciously to make new effective coping methods automatic.
Balance	Balance is an important aspect of coping. Even effective coping can be harmful if utilized excessively, as with overeating.
Toolbox	Everyone needs a large arsenal of coping skills to choose from.
Keep trying	If one coping skill does not work, others must continue to be tried until an effective solution is found.

Sometimes dissociation has positive aspects. With the guidance of a qualified instructor who is knowledgeable about trauma, meditation comes naturally to some survivors who are accustomed to shifting their consciousness while dissociating and can thus enter a meditative state easily. This skill can also help with consciously and purposely moving awareness away from uncomfortable thoughts, emotions or stimuli. Even flashbacks and nightmares can be beneficial, enabling reclamation of lost memories (Dinsmore, 1991). Survivors of child abuse, for instance, may lose childhood memories, many of which were pleasant, as they block out the abuse. Avoidance or running away can also be positive if it involves leaving a bad situation. As social workers, we can help survivors see the strengths behind their responses to trauma and how to use them productively.

Learning how to respond effectively to PTSD symptoms, such as nightmares, can also improve coping. A survivor of sexual abuse had terrifying nightmares like this:

> I am a mermaid in a pond, sitting on a rock. The rock is partly in the water so that my legs are in the water. There is music and a narrator is saying something like "Your Prince Charming is coming, sometimes it comes in the form of a big fish." Just then a big fish swims by me, brushing my leg. It has big teeth. As it comes by again, I see it is a fucking shark. I get scared. Then there is water all around and I want to leave …

The dream reflects how out of control the survivor, Jane, felt. She woke up regularly from dreams such as this and did not know what to do when awake and feeling the terror they engendered. Then she came up with a process that helped her cope. She got up, wrote down the dream to bring to her therapist and discuss. The process contained and held at bay the horror of the dream until it could be brought out in order to find some resolution in the safe place of therapy. Even without the outlet of therapy, this technique can help survivors because it provides a way to get dreams out and on paper where they can be looked at with some distance or disposed of.

IF COPING DOES NOT WORK

It is important that survivors find effective ways to cope as Jane did by writing down her nightmares. Social workers need to remind them not to give up, to keep trying to cope no matter what, to use baby steps as they proceed and to have a large toolbox of skills to choose from. Unfortunately, initial coping attempts do not always work. Since coping helps create a feeling of control and stability, it can be frustrating and scary for survivors when it does not work immediately, potentially increasing the loss of control they already feel as a result of their trauma experience.

This loss of control and frustration with coping results can particularly affect those who stop ineffective coping and do not replace it with sufficient skills. Survivors often use substances such as alcohol and drugs, for instance, in an attempt to block out what happened to them. When they become clean and sober, memories of the event, including emotions such as helplessness and fear, often come rushing back to them. They may make a few attempts at coping and then give up, feeling hopeless and perhaps falling back on their old habit of using substances to cope.

Encouragement to take baby steps can help survivors as they learn to eliminate unhealthy coping and incorporate effective coping methods. Harm reduction aids this process because it acknowledges and accepts without judgment that survivors are individuals who have suffered and need to find their own ways to change (Collins, et al., 2012). Harm-reduction involves engaging with survivors, helping them identify pros and cons of ineffective coping behavior, establishing goals toward change, creating a climate conducive to change and predicting and coping with crisis (Collins et al., 2012). Helping survivors develop workable coping plans is also a part of this process.

A COPING TOOLBOX

Survivors need to have a toolbox of coping methods so that if one style of coping does not work, there is always another to try. Coping methods fall into categories, including: (1) relaxation and soothing; (2) distraction; (3) changing perspective; (4) self-care; (5) emotion recognition and regulation, including positive thinking; (6) connectivity and support; (7) fun; (8) spirituality; (9) problem solving; (10) altruism; (11) creativity; (12) personal growth and learning, including psychoeducation; (13) awareness and orientation to the present, also known as mindfulness; (14) physical activity and (15) attention to thoughts, perceptions, ideas and beliefs.

Many types of coping fall into more than one category. For example, drawing a picture can be relaxing, creative, distracting and mindful. It can also change the survivor's perspective as they help others who get pleasure from the picture, or focus on drawing instead of negative thoughts.

Children can benefit from coping that include storytelling, imagining heroes and heroines and creativity such as drawing and expressing what they drew through music or movement (Kagan, Douglas, Hornik, & Kratz, 2008). Planning for safety, restructuring unhelpful thoughts and beliefs to be more helpful, learning how to measure stress levels, preparing for upcoming stressors, enhancing social supports and improving attachments to safe people, benefit both children and adults (Kagan et al., 2008; Najavits, 2002; van der Kolk, 1996).

Coping imagery can help as well. Survivors can, for example, picture being triggered by a distressing memory and then imagine feeling happy and relaxed, saying positive statements as they do (Schiraldi, 2009). (Survivors should be cautioned to focus on their reactions to the memory not its details. If they cannot do this, they should not use the exercise, because remembering details can be triggering.) Self-nurturance (including praise for coping efforts), animals, nature and any activities that enhance life are also healing for survivors (Dinsmore, 1991; Najavits, 2002). Life-enhancing activities include rituals and cleansing ceremonies that help them come to terms with what occurred (Boothby et al., 2006; Schiraldi, 2009). For examples of rituals, see the sample toolbox in Table 12.2.

Tips

- *Measuring stress level* – It can help survivors to put a number or name to their stress or level of arousal, because what can be measured often feels more manageable. It can be given a number from 0 to 10 with 10 being their highest level of stress and 0 none. Naming is easier for some. It can be labeled high, low or medium; or intense, relaxed or neutral

Table 12.2 Coping Toolbox

Coping Skill	Description	Which Survivors?
Blowing bubbles	Relaxes children because they need to be conscious of their breathing process and breathe deeply to make bubbles.	Children
Deep breathing	Involves breathing deeply and slowly into and out of the abdomen. The breathing should be as natural and unforced as possible. This can increase anxiety for those with breathing issues.	All but those with breathing issues
Music	Help survivors be cognizant of the effects of different kinds of music, using some to relax and others to invigorate or just for fun.	All
Story telling	Use stories that are appropriate to culture, circumstances and age, or help survivors create stories that support their recovery.	All
Creative arts	Utilize creative movement, music, art and writing to help survivors constructively express and expel difficult emotion.	All
Imagery	Suggest that survivors think of an imaginary or real place that engenders positive emotion. Have them focus on every detail, including smells and tastes and sounds.	All
Muscle relaxation	Guide survivors through progressively relaxing muscles, from head to toe. Or first have them tighten their muscles and then release them. Tell them to look for tense places in their body and breathe into them. They can also imagine light or water flowing through them. With children add a story about the sun making flowers grow, telling them to be a flower or suggest they stretch like a cat, raise their shoulders like a turtle or go stiff like a statue.	All
Problem solving	Puzzles, cross word puzzles and many games encourage problem solving, empowering and moving the mind away from negative or difficult thoughts.	Requires some cognitive ability
Physical activity	Exercise, walking and other physical activities are invigorating, fun and an outlet.	Dependent on physical ability

Table 12.2 **(Continued)**

Coping Skill	Description	Which Survivors?
Meditation	This can be as simple as looking at a candle or a sunset or even just sitting quietly. Meditation can increase confusion for those with thought disorders such as psychosis.	Not for those with thought disorders
Nature	Nature can be healing and relaxing. If survivors cannot be in it, suggest they enjoy it from a distance or look at pictures.	All
Rituals	Rituals can be healing if not associated with trauma memories. Examples include cultural foods, religious/spiritual rituals, holidays and traditions. Social workers can also help survivors come up with their own rituals such as a grief ceremony for all they lost as a result of the trauma.	All
Volunteer work	Helping others has been found to help survivors heal. Even the elderly, infirm and children can do little things to help such as drawing pictures or sending prayers.	According to abilities
Get support	Suggest that survivors spend time with a safe friend, family member or well-loved animal. They can also go somewhere people congregate such as a church, concert or the park. Making medical, dental or haircut appointments if needed, is supportive too.	All
Laugh	Help survivors incorporate humor and fun in their lives. They can watch a funny movie, play with a puppy or baby, think of something funny, tell a joke or see someone who makes them laugh.	All
Learn	Learning something new about topics they find interesting makes survivors feel like they are growing and promotes healing. This includes getting a degree or certification.	All
Notice thoughts	Social workers can help survivors notice thoughts, emotions, ideas and beliefs that create discomfort and then transform them in ways that support the healing process. At first this will seem impossible but little by little change will occur over time.	According to cognitive abilities

Case Study

Michael was a 45-year-old divorced African American man who was raised by and lived with his aunt. He witnessed community violence as a child, including his brother being fatally shot. He experienced violence in his home as well and his parents abandoned him when he was 12 years old, complicating his trauma.

As with many survivors, Michael was constantly in crisis. He had many health issues and required oxygen to breathe as a result. He thought of death and dying often, due to his experiences with violence and disease, and consequently felt scared and alone. Compounding his difficulties, Michael's trauma-induced fear made him resist medical care and distrust doctors, so that he did not always get the care he needed.

He would generally come to treatment in an anxious state. Here is an example:

Michael:	I just can't seem to get a breath today. *Breathing heavily and sitting tensely after sharing a litany of concerns.*
Social worker:	Seems like some coping might help. *Michael's face hardens, making him look angry, and he becomes very still.*
Social worker:	*Feeling Michael is angry and nervous that the coping she has suggested will not work.* Shall we try something together?
Michael:	I'm counting. *Eventually his face relaxes, he smiles, and looks up.*

The coping had worked, and Michael became very good at it to the point that he became much more self-sufficient, despite his poor health, and began to take steps toward getting his own apartment. The coping skills he learned also increased his confidence, helping him to stand up for himself with medical practitioners so that he no longer distrusted them and could get the care he needed.

RESOURCES

Cohen, J.A., & Mannarino, A.P. (2008). Trauma-focused cognitive behavioural therapy for children and parents. *Child and Adolescent Mental Health, 13*(4), 158–162.

Herman, J.L. (1992). *Trauma and recovery*. New York: Basic Books.

Kabat-Zinn, J. (1991). *Full catastrophic living: Using the wisdom of your body and mind to face stress, pain, and illness*. New York: Dell Publishing.

Najavits, L. (2002). *Seeking safety: A treatment manual for PTSD and substance abuse*. New York: Guilford Press.

Rothschild, B. (2000). *The body remembers: The psychophysiology of trauma and trauma treatment*. New York and London: WW Norton & Company.

Schiraldi, G.R. (2009). *The post-traumatic stress disorder sourcebook*. Los Angeles: Lowell House.

Practice Exercises and Questions

- Identify ways you cope and rate them according to effectiveness. Make adjustments to improve effectiveness if needed
- Do the exercise above with a client or friend, helping them to identify coping and effectiveness
- Consider why balance is important with coping and explain this to a client or friend, giving examples as you do
- Why is it important for coping and rituals to be culturally appropriate? Explain in a way your client would comprehend
- Role-play discussing how attempts to cope such as substance abuse are harmful and can be replaced with positive coping

Coping and Self-Care Summary

Tune in to Coping

- *Remember how you cope in order to support survivors*
- *Be aware of how survivors cope and how well it works*

Coping Skills are Learned

- *Coping tends to be automatic and unconscious*
- *It is learned during childhood and in response to trauma*
- *Some attempts to cope, such as yelling, can do harm*
- *New effective and conscious coping can become automatic*

Cultural Aspects of Coping

- *Coping methods vary among individual survivors*
- *Personal tastes, upbringing and culture affect coping*
- *Effective coping for one survivor may not work for another*

Shame and Blame Impede Coping

- *Some survivors may not think they deserve to be treated well*
- *Others may blame themselves for not coping effectively*
- *They may need help with self-compassion and acceptance*

Building a Toolbox of Coping Skills

- *Survivors need an arsenal of skills from which to choose*
- *Self-care is an essential form of coping*
- *Balance and awareness are important aspects of coping*
- *Encourage trying a variety of skills until coping works*

Part IV

Healing Trauma on a Micro Level

Chapter 13

Assessment

This chapter examines the ways in which social workers can aid trauma survivors by utilizing assessment techniques and referring those in need for further assistance. The topics covered include assessing for a trauma history, PTSD, lethality and other safety and risk factors. Specific screening tools and approaches will be discussed.

Definitions

- *Post-traumatic stress disorder (PTSD)* – A disorder resulting from exposure to traumatic events that causes symptoms lasting at least a month that include emotional responses of fear, horror or helplessness; flashbacks and/or nightmares of events; avoidance of reminders of the event; and increased arousal.
- *Safety* – State essential to trauma recovery and unique to each individual, in which: (1) risky behaviors, unhealthy relationships and negative emotions are reduced; and (2) a sense of well-being, trust, calm and positive coping are increased.

TUNE IN TO ASSESSMENT

Tune in, noticing how you are feeling as you read this. This will provide you with a benchmark that you can check in on as you read this book and work with survivors. If/when you veer from where you are now mood-wise, it will be a signal to take care of yourself so that you can maintain your equilibrium and be available for your clients. Also, note your feelings about assessment including any of your own past experiences being assessed or any concerns you have about assessing clients.

ASSESSMENT PROCESS

Assessment for trauma is important in all areas of social work where there is direct client care. This is true because trauma is prevalent. It has been reported, for instance, that more than half of survey respondents have experienced trauma

(Center for Substance Abuse Treatment (US), 2014) and it touches all of us at one time or another via: (1) direct experience, (2) witnessing directly or indirectly through the media and other means or (3) simply by absorbing it from loved ones who have experienced trauma themselves. Think of how you are effected by others' anger or joy. This same process can occur as we are exposed to trauma through others and often without our being aware of it. Therefore, trauma assessment is imperative.

Tip

- Always be aware of the possibility of survivors' trauma memories being triggered as you work with them. Ensure adequate coping skills are in place and prompt them to use the skills as needed during the assessment process. Watch for dissociation and help them to come back to the present moment if it occurs

---

The assessment process is hierarchically layered and begins with assessing for trauma and, if a history of trauma is found, then also for PTSD. Where PTSD is a possibility, assess (1) trauma based on DSM-5 criteria, (2) lethality, (3) functionality, (4) medical and treatment history and (5) family history (Department of Veterans Affairs & Department of Defense, 2017). Knowing whether survivors are safe and secure is also important and should be determined before going into any depth with their trauma experience so as not to trigger flashbacks. This is key because healing from trauma requires safety and self-care.

Assessments of individuals' strengths/resilience and social/coping skills gives us a picture of how they are set in this area and where they can use assistance. Assessing their stress is also important including their levels of distress, difficulty and need. Then comes attending to their vulnerabilities as these can negatively impact the effects of trauma. Finally, we need to watch out for risk factors such as substance abuse and lethality/suicidality (Center for Substance Abuse Treatment (US), 2014). Assessing these areas also provides a sense of their functionality.

While conducting assessments, be sure to keep in mind (1) explaining what the assessment process entails so there will be no surprises, (2) establishing an atmosphere that engenders trust and exudes positive regard and acceptance, (3) maintaining appropriate boundaries so that clients feel safe, (4) adjusting for culture and language, (5) providing clients with opportunities to control the process, increasing their feelings of safety, (6) helping them remain comfortable throughout the assessment, utilizing coping if needed and (7) considering mandated reporting and other legal issues related to the information gathered (Center for Substance Abuse Treatment (US), 2014).

Definitions

* *Coping* – Process of dealing with difficulties, problem solving and adapting to the environment in order to manage stress and conflict effectively
* *Dissociation* – Disconnection from thoughts, memories, or emotions that provides internal distance from reminders of traumatic events, but also prevents integration of trauma material and disrupts normal psychological functioning
* *Flashback* – Intrusive and involuntary re-experiencing of traumatic events through images, emotions or physical sensations

Practitioners conducting assessments must also keep their purpose in mind. Crisis assessments, for instance, differ from psychosocial assessments done at the start of mental health treatment when considering longer term care. Crisis situations call for sensitivity to both safety/risk factors and survivors' requests for immediate assistance. Time is of the essence in crises. Ultimately, we must assess the urgency of identified wants and needs (Wainrib & Bloch, 1998).

TRAUMA HISTORY AND PTSD

In addition to detective work uncovering aspects of our clients that require consideration, we also need to differentiate stressors from traumatic events and identify symptoms of PTSD and other mental health disorders such as anxiety, acute stress, complex PTSD, traumatic bereavement, depression, dissociative and psychosis.

The first order of business is assessing clients' history of stressful and potentially traumatic events. Screening tools that aid this process include: the Traumatic Stress Schedule (TSS), the Traumatic Events Questionnaire (TEQ), the Traumatic Life Events Questionnaire (TLEC) and the Stressful Life Events Screening Questionnaire (SLESQ). We can ask children simple questions to quickly screen for traumatic impacts as well, such as whether anything scared them recently or made them feel like crying, hiding or running away (Cohen, Kelleher, & Mannarino, 2008). See the resources section at the end of this chapter for links to information on these scales.

Some specialized tools uniquely fit particular populations when assessing trauma. These tools are useful when assessing those in crisis situations: (1) the Crisis State Assessment Scale (CSAS), which measures the magnitude of the crisis state (Lewis, 2005); (2) the Crisis Triage Rating Scale (CTRS) (Lewis & Roberts, 2001), which provides recommendations for inpatient or outpatient mental health treatment, if needed, based on the scoring; and (3) the Triage

Assessment Form: Crisis Intervention (TAF) (Lewis & Roberts, 2001), which assesses the severity and type of crisis.

Other examples of specialized tools include the Mississippi Scale for Combat-related PTSD (M-PTSD) and the Child Trauma Screening Questionnaire (CTSQ). The latter facilitates intervention with children post accidents. It does not take long to complete and is easy to comprehend (Kenardy, Spence, & Macleod, 2006).

In the United States, the Veterans Administration and the Department of Defense utilize these two instruments in particular to screen for PTSD – the Primary Care PTSD Screen (PC-PTSD) and the PTSD Checklist (PCL). Both have multiple versions some of which can be used for different purposes. The PC-PTSD was originally a 4-item DSM-IV based scale and has since been expanded to the 5-item DSM-5 version, the PC-PTSD-5. The PCL-5 is a 20-item DSM-5 based tool derived from the original DSM-IV based PCL measures. These DSM-IV measures include the PCL-C for civilians, the PCL-M for military, and the PCL-S for non-military, very stressful events. The PCL tools not only screen for PTSD but also for symptom intensity (Department of Veterans Affairs & Department of Defense, 2017).

The Clinician-Administered PTSD Scale (CAPS) is another reliable instrument for assessing trauma. There is a DSM-5 based version, CAPS-5, and a child and adolescent version, CAPS-CA-5 (Weiss, 2004). CAPS can also be used to assess for acute stress disorder. See the resources section at end of the chapter for links to these and other assessment instruments. Links to assessment tools for related psychiatric issues such as depression, anxiety and disassociation, are also included.

STRENGTHS AND COPING SKILLS

One of the goals of assessment is to identify those imminently at risk as a direct result of their traumatic experiences. Exploring this involves evaluating survivors' and family members' safety in the aftermath of distressing events. Assessing for resilience, coping/social skills and strengths aids this process. See Chapter 12 on coping for more information on this topic. As you will see, coping includes all the ways survivors obtain support and engage in self-care.

Coping is not necessarily an easy task. While conducting support groups for practitioners caring for survivors, I have seen that even professionals can have difficulty with coping and self-care. When asked to identify how they took care of themselves, many practitioners were at a loss. Some even shared activities such as having a glass of wine or eating sweets that are not necessarily healthy or nurturing. Others admitted they did not take good care of themselves, demonstrating how important it is to address this underutilized skill while conducting assessments.

Scales exist for measuring resilience, coping/social skills and strengths and can be useful in the assessment process. This is particularly true for trauma survivors since coping and safety are essential to recovery. Examples of such scales include The Resilience Scale (Wagnild & Young, 1993), The DBT-Ways of Coping Checklist (DBT-WCCL) (Neacsiu, Rizvi, Vitaliano, Lynch & Linehan, 2010) and The Strengths and Difficulties Questionnaire (SDQ) (Goodman, 2002). See the resource section at the end of this chapter for links to these scales.

LEVEL OF DISTRESS

Social workers work with survivors to identify needs and come up with plans that include referrals or recommendations that will work toward fulfilling them. Since unmet needs can create vulnerability and feelings of danger, potentially intensifying trauma symptoms and causing distress, this is a crucial step in the assessment process (Wainrib & Bloch, 1998).

Of paramount importance is considering survivors' basic needs are met such as for food, water, shelter, financial resources and safety. This includes resolving any areas of imminent danger. Toward this end, Roberts (2005a) outlines these questions which aid the stress assessment process: (1) Were survivors physically hurt during crisis events? Are they in need of medical attention? (2) Are they suicidal? If so, do they have a plan and is the plan for a certain time or place? (3) Are they in danger of hurting themselves including self-mutilation? (4) Were they victims of abuse or crime? If so, are they currently in danger? (5) Are there any children in danger? (6) Are there violent individuals in their homes? If so, have they been able to protect themselves and their children from them in the past? (7) What are the violent individuals' histories of violence, arrest, mental illness and substance abuse? (8) What are survivors' histories of physical harm/hospitalization, mental illness, suicidal/self-harm behavior and substance abuse? (9) Are there weapons in survivors' homes? What is the history of weapons usage? (10) Have survivors been threatened, including terrorist threats? (11) Are they under the influence of alcohol or drugs? (12) Is transport needed to a hospital or shelter? Many of these items will be covered in more detail in the following sections. All contribute to distress and assessing for distress is key.

Having multiple stressors, including past or present traumas, compounds the situation for survivors, as seen with the Hurricane Katrina disaster in New Orleans in 2005 (Jaycox et al., 2007). Survivors felt the effect of the hurricane from: (1) flooding; (2) loss of homes and the ability to financially support and feed themselves; (3) looting and assault including sexual assault; and (4) separation from and loss of family and friends. This interrelation of stressors and traumas devastated survivors of Katrina just as it can with any crisis.

During the assessment process, social workers act as detectives, unearthing other underlying issues that might contribute to survivors' current stress. For example, Dan was traumatized when beaten by a gang of men because he was gay. Sensitivity to the fact that he had not told his family he was gay was essential when conducting an assessment with Dan, because his parents' questions about what had occurred increased his anxiety about his "secret" and made re-establishing equilibrium after the attack difficult (Herman, 1992).

Fifteen-year-old Janet's experience after being raped also required attention to details not readily apparent. In the midst of family conflict about whether to forget about the rape or report it, nobody considered Janet's needs. During the crisis intervention conducted after she attempted suicide because of the rape, those helping her learned that she craved safety and privacy, but also needed to feel she had the power to make her own decisions, rather than let her family determine her legal processes related to the rape (Herman, 1992).

There are tools that can aid the assessment process by measuring distress. The Children's Hassles (CHS) and the Children Uplifts (CUS) scales, for instance, measure the ups and downs of children's lives. These can be used in tandem or separately and have been found to be among the most Well-Established instruments studied (Blount, Simons, Devine, Jaaniste, Cohen, Chambers, et al, 2008).

SPECIFIC VULNERABILITIES

Besides stressful factors directly related to trauma, many survivors also have general life conditions that create vulnerability. These areas of vulnerability include (Hillman, 2002): (1) histories of substance abuse; (2) physical or mental illness including being disabled or cognitively impaired; (3) being very young or elderly; (4) the presence of current stressors or traumas; (5) having experienced trauma in the past and (6) being members of underserved populations. Recent marital separation can be another area of vulnerability for many (Institute of Medicine, 2003).

It is crucial to know about survivors' substance abuse histories. Those who have a history of substance abuse but no longer use substances run the risk of relapse. Therefore, both those in recovery from substance abuse and those actively using may need help finding more effective coping strategies, particularly those at risk of hurting themselves or others, since substance use increases impulsivity and decreases inhibitions (Roberts & Yeager, 2005). See the resources section at the end of this chapter for links to substance abuse screening tools.

Stress can exacerbate physical and mental illness, so we also need to pay attention to survivors' psychiatric symptoms. Disabilities can make individuals more vulnerable to harm from others or create barriers to getting needs met. Focus on cognitive ability as well. For example, 3-year-olds need to be

approached differently from 16-year-olds because they have coping requirements unique to their cognitive abilities and associated age-appropriate methods of processing emotion (Sandoval, Scott, & Padilla, 2009). Children and
adolescents in general are also vulnerable as are females since this gender has
been found to be more at risk (Institute of Medicine, 2003).

Barriers to getting aid due to marginalization can also add to survivors'
vulnerability. Underserved populations who encounter poverty, lack of health
insurance and other factors, which include difficulty obtaining support from
mental and physical healthcare practitioners, often do not know how to take
care of themselves post-trauma. This includes minorities, refugees, immigrants
and those in underserved areas such as rural communities and makes the support of social workers via community outreach and other intervention methodologies essential (Institute of Medicine, 2003; O'Donnell, Joshi, & Lewin,
2007).

Those who care for trauma survivors are also vulnerable. First responders
and physical/mental health practitioners are at risk, particularly if they are
substance abusers (Institute of Medicine, 2003). See chapter 8 on vulnerable
populations for a more detailed discussion of the nuances of vulnerability that
many survivors face.

LETHALITY

The incidence of suicide, with lethality directed toward self, runs high enough
among survivors to warrant a separate assessment of risk. Studies have found
that close to one in five individuals (19%–19.2%) who experienced rape or military combat subsequently attempted suicide (Herman, 1992). Compare this to
one in 59 of the general population either attempting suicide or having a friend
or relative who did (Roberts & Yeager, 2005).

When assessing for suicide risk, we have evidence-based predictors to
consider. Research shows that adults over 65 are most likely to successfully
complete a suicide attempt. Chronic medical illness also poses a risk, with
Caucasian, elderly, medically ill males most at risk (Hillman, 2002).

Other suicide risk factors include suicidal thoughts; a suicide plan and the
means to carry it out; access to weapons; poor judgment or impulsivity, particularly if under the influence of substances that may impair judgment or
impulse control further; command hallucinations related to suicide; or other
people reporting that a survivor is suicidal (Roberts & Yeager, 2005). A history
of previous suicide attempts also indicates risk and the need for careful assessment (Hillman, 2002). In addition, survivors become more at risk when they
have histories of substance abuse; family histories of suicide; histories of child
abuse; and current stressors such as recent job loss, depression, ineffective coping including lack of supportive relationships and non-compliance with medication (Roberts & Yeager, 2005), and PTSD symptoms. The Beck Scale for

Suicide Ideation (SSI) is a useful assessment tool for determining risk (Roberts & Yeager, 2005). The Columbia-Suicide Severity Rating Scale (C-SSRS) can also be used for assessing suicidality (Posner et al., 2008).

We should carefully explore survivors' ideation, or the extent of their wish to die, when determining suicide risk, along with their intent to kill themselves and any plans for suicide. We should also consider the issues noted in this section when assessing the risk of self-harm, such as by cutting, and of violence toward others (Hillman, 2002).

Predictors of violence differ from those for suicide. Adolescent and young adult, substance abusing, emotionally labile and impulsive minority males have a higher risk, according to the literature, than other demographic groups (Wainrib & Bloch, 1998). Trauma survivors can be particularly vulnerable in this area, since they are often prone to aggressiveness resulting from high rates of trauma-related anger (McPherson-Sextona & Hostetler, 2009) and to difficulties with effective emotion regulation (Goelitz, 2009).

When assessing for lethality, it is important for social workers to be thorough and cautious. This includes assessing risk and asking a supervisor or colleague for help determining risk. The Danger Assessment checklist, for example, assesses risk of lethality in domestic violence situations. When assessing for lethality, erring on the side of safety and reporting concerns to authorities is essential both for the protection of those involved and to satisfy legal requirements (Gostin, 2000).

PROCESS OF REFERRING FOR AID

Once we have completed an assessment, we can determine the need for referrals. Social workers are particularly adept at this process because their focus on communities and systems within communities increases awareness of available services. The referral process includes not just determining need and obtaining referrals, but also working with survivors to utilize the referrals (Rosen, Matthieu, & Norris, 2009). This often entails follow-up with survivors.

Types of referrals made on behalf of survivors can include psychiatric, supportive counseling, legal, medical, job-related, day care, substance abuse including 12-step programs, counseling and self-help centers, churches, community centers, schools, law enforcement, entitlement-related, victim services and other community resources (A.R. Roberts & Roberts, 2005). Referral for shelters, including those for battered women, may also be required (Roberts, 2005a). Those in crises can particularly benefit from hotlines. Many provide 24-hour access, available any time that survivors feel unable to cope or need extra support. Types of hotlines available include child abuse, domestic violence, suicide prevention and general crisis intervention (Roberts, 2005a).

> **Tips**
>
> - *Use the Internet to locate referral sources* – International directories of hotlines, for instance, can be found at http://www.suicide.org/international-suicide-hotlines.html and https://togetherweare-strong.tumblr.com/helpline. The Internet provides access to many other referral sources as well. Use search engines by putting in keywords that include the services you are looking for and your geographic area. When you locate referral sources, ask them about others they recommend. Make up an Internet directory of services by bookmarking them and setting up folders to organize them by category. If you are unsure about how to do this, ask someone with computer expertise for help

Attention to schools, work places and to communities in general is also essential. Providing and/or encouraging outreach, education and referral via these venues increases access to care for those at risk. Encouraging and/or facilitating familial and community connectivity is important as well. Connection enables safety which is key for survivors' healing. This kind of connectivity is also an avenue of support and care for those in need (Institute of Medicine, 2003).

Case Study

Angela was a new client at an outpatient trauma clinic. Her intake was conducted utilizing the agency's standard intake questionnaire and centered around psychosocial history and current psychosocial state including symptoms, trauma history, history of mental illness, substance abuse and lethality. It was among the first I had done at the clinic. Others included assessments of individuals with intense trauma histories and symptoms of both PTSD and dissociation. I thought I was becoming proficient and was to a certain extent, but was also likely affected by the intensity of the interviews and of the numerous groups and clients I was working with.

Angela was sexually abused as a child and had several abusive romantic relationships as an adult, the most recent of which had ended recently. Her ex continued to harass and scare her. She was still in love with him, often waffling and considering going back to him. She reported a recent experience with him that had been both dramatic and harrowing, albeit filled with a passion that for her was alluring.

As she spoke she became more and more animated which I eventually recognized as anxiety and possibly dissociation. Unfortunately, by the time I did trauma memories had been triggered and she was panicking and looking for a quick fix. However, she was so worked up that it was difficult for her to focus on the grounding exercises we did and left the session in a state of arousal. She never returned for treatment despite what she described as, and appeared to be, a high level of motivation for treatment. Attempts were made to follow up, but she did not respond.

This case illustrates a common pitfall practitioners encounter when working with survivors. As discussed earlier in the chapter, setting the stage for the assessment and monitoring/managing the process as it progresses is crucial. As with many agency intakes, I had a specific amount of time allotted to complete it and there were clients and groups scheduled back-to-back directly after and throughout the day. This agency even had the practice of double booking because of a high rate of no shows so my day was packed. I was focused on getting through the interview within the timeframe.

Unfortunately, this did now allow enough time to adequately prepare Angela for the interview or to take regular pauses to monitor and manage the interview process. Queries that reminded her of trauma events increased her vulnerability so that subsequent questions jarred her. An example of this is that after reporting her childhood sexual abuse, Angela was raw and tearful. Therefore, admitting she had had multiple abusive relationships brought her instantly to tears. And the tears became sobs when she talked about her recent breakup and accompanying drama.

It was impossible for Angela to feel secure in this state or to respond to attempts cope. She was too wound up, no doubt experiencing flashbacks and dissociation. Her fear was in control at this point, not her motivation for treatment and health. Had the interview proceeded more sensitively, with (1) careful preparation and attention to areas of vulnerability, (2) information collection kept to the minimum required when it came to trauma so as not trigger her and 3) frequent pauses to assess her reactions in terms of hyperarousal and dissociation, the outcome may have been quite different, allowing Angela to obtain the care she so needed.

RESOURCES

Roberts, A.R. (Ed.). (2005). *Crisis intervention handbook: Assessment, treatment, and research* (3rd ed.). New York: Oxford University Press.

Wilson, J.P., & Keane, T.M. (Eds.). (2004). *Assessing psychological trauma and PTSD* (2nd ed.). New York: The Guilford Press.

ONLINE RESOURCES

Coping Assessment Tools:

The DBT-Ways of Coping Checklist (DBT-WCCL): http://depts.washington.edu/uwbrtc/wp-content/uploads/DBT-WCCL.pdf

The Resilience Scale: https://hr.un.org/sites/hr.un.org/files/The%20Resilience%20Scale%20%28Wagnild%20%26%20Young%29_0.pdf

The Strengths and Difficulties Questionnaire (SDQ): https://www.sdqinfo.com/py/sdqinfo/b3.py?language=Englishqz(USA)

DSM-V Assessment: https://www.psychiatry.org/psychiatrists/practice/dsm/educational-resources/assessment-measures

History of Stressful and Potentially Traumatic Events Assessment Tools:

The Stressful Life Events Screening Questionnaire (SLESQ): http://www.bharp.org/wp-content/uploads/2016/10/4-SLESQRevised.pdf

The Traumatic Events Questionnaire (TEQ): http://namvet.fatcow.com/traumatic-events-questionnaire-teq.html

The Traumatic Life Events Questionnaire (TLEC): http://namvet.fatcow.com/traumatic-life-events-questionnaire-tleq.html

The Traumatic Stress Schedule (TSS): http://namvet.fatcow.com/traumatic-stress-schedule-tss.html

Lethality Assessment Tools:

The Columbia-Suicide Severity Rating Scale (C-SSRS) with Safe-T: http://cssrs.columbia.edu/documents/safe-t-c-ssrs/

Danger Assessment: https://www.dangerassessment.org/uploads/DA_NewScoring_2019.pdf

Other Assessment Tools:

https://www.apa.org/ptsd-guideline/assessment/
https://istss.org/clinical-resources/assessing-trauma
https://www.ptsd.va.gov/professional/assessment/list_measures.asp

Find Support Groups:

https://www.mhanational.org/find-support-groups

Substance Abuse Assessment Tools:

https://www.integration.samhsa.gov/clinical-practice/screening-tools#drugs
https://www.drugabuse.gov/nidamed-medical-health-professionals/screening-tools-resources/chart-screening-tools

Trauma Assessment Tools:

https://www.ptsd.va.gov/professional/assessment/documents/PCL5_Standard_form.PDF
https://www.addictionsandrecovery.org/tools/post-traumatic-stress-disorder-test-pc-ptsd-5.pdf
https://www.ptsd.va.gov/professional/assessment/child/caps-ca.asp

Practice Exercises and Questions

- Imagine meeting with a potential trauma survivor and plan how to proceed with assessment
- Choose the assessment instruments to use as you interview a new client
- Explain why you chose those particular instruments
- Role-play an assessment process with a potential trauma survivor and evaluate the results, making recommendations for their care

Assessment Summary

Trauma History and PTSD

- Assess for trauma history and for PTSD
- Assess for safety and security
- Throughout assessment, take care to follow recommended guidelines

Strengths and Coping Skills

- Strengths and coping skills are key to safety and security
- Assessing for resilience, coping/social skills and strengths is important

Level of Distress

- A high level of distress increases vulnerability/risk and decreases safety
- Assessing distress includes determining whether basic needs are met
- Assessing survivors' needs, stressors and difficulties is also important

Specific Vulnerabilities

- Includes assessing for substance abuse, physical and mental illness, past trauma and current stress or trauma
- Being young, elderly or among the marginalized/underserved also creates vulnerability

Lethality

- Identify those at risk for self-harm or harm to others
- Important to err on the side of safety and report concerns to authorities if warranted

Chapter 14

Crisis Management

Crisis states ensue when survivors encounter dangerous or stressful situations they feel unable to cope with effectively (Roberts, 2005a). These include key times during the trajectory of the trauma recovery process. For example, when facing and acknowledging the trauma for the first time, sexual abuse survivors may become preoccupied with the abuse and flooded with memories, flashbacks and nightmares, creating an internal crisis that leaves them feeling out of control and off balance (Dinsmore, 1991). These crisis periods can occur right after the traumatic event, or years later if the memories are suppressed without healing occurring. Social workers and other professionals intervene at these times (Roberts, 2005a).

Crisis management requires an individualized approach that fits the situation. This means utilizing the social work premise of figuratively starting where clients are (Gelman & Mirabito, 2005), witnessing their internal struggles and attempts to adapt, in order to work with them to find the disrupted aspects of their lives and remedy them. Many people in crisis cannot identify this on their own, having experienced numerous stressors simultaneously. Patient exploration can help them to sort out their needs for support (McPherson-Sextona & Hostetler, 2009).

A case in point is Annette, a survivor of child abuse and intimate partner violence who experienced frequent crises and began most counseling sessions discussing the latest one. Since the crises were real, it took time to understand that the presenting problem was actually her inability to cope and to avoid re-traumatization by current stressful events so that she could handle difficulties in her life without them becoming crises. Diagnosed with a brain tumor, she feared for the safety of her family who lived amidst political unrest following a natural disaster. Her 16-year-old son left home and got involved with illegal activities. One of her abusers began calling her. These could all traumatize her, and without adequate coping skills, each became a crisis.

What constitutes a crisis varies, but most individuals in crisis feel helpless and out of control because current coping no longer remedies their experience. It is the job of the intervener to take control, without overpowering survivors, in order to help them re-establish safety and obtain the resources they need (McPherson-Sextona & Hostetler, 2009). With Annette, this meant not addressing each crisis in depth as it occurred, since this distracted from the real work of helping her create a safe and stable environment, both internally and externally, so that she could heal. The work became acknowledging the severity of the stressor and then reminding her of the need for balance and equilibrium, making this the focus of the intervention.

Definitions

- *Coping* – Process of dealing with difficulties, problem solving and adapting to the environment in order to manage stress and conflict effectively

---

In addition to starting where clients are by following their lead to decide what to address, practitioners need to take on various roles when intervening with survivors in crisis, focusing at the micro, mezzo or macro level and acting as case manager, educator, program developer, advocate or researcher, depending on the situation (Gelman & Mirabito, 2005). Examples of how social workers adapt their roles to client needs include their diverse functions during the September 11th disaster: creating a mental health clinic for survivors; providing financial support, job training and health insurance; educating community members about the effects of the traumatic event; as well as counseling survivors.

This chapter examines the ways in which social workers can aid trauma survivors facing crises. Topics covered include exploring the crisis intervention process and methodologies effective with survivors. Assessment and referral for aid are covered in the previous chapter.

TUNE IN TO CRISES

It helps for practitioners to tune in to their own experiences of crisis in order to understand survivors. Toward this end, search for times of crisis in your life when you felt out of control or upset. Remembering times when you seemed to have lost your internal compass and did not know where to turn for help will help you relate emotionally to survivors.

Crises come in many forms and can be set off by traumatic events, relationship issues, mental/physical illness, job conflict/loss, or feeling overburdened with a busy and demanding schedule. With crisis, we always feel unable to handle what is occurring. Even small stressors like missing a bus or breaking something accidentally can stack on the last straw that makes life feel unmanageable and leads to crisis.

As you locate examples of crisis in your life, remember to use coping and self-care to ensure that associated feelings do not overwhelm you and cause current or future stress. Avoid drawing on memories that might upset or traumatize you and refer to chapter 12 on self-care and chapter 1 on secondary trauma if coping with your memories becomes difficult.

Tips

- *Tune in to self* – Do a quick check within yourself for any physical, emotional and cognitive discomfort. Try to identify the source of any you find. Breathe into it or use other means to relax and nurture yourself. If the discomfort remains, remember you are carrying it with you so that it will not cause difficulty later.

Focus on the time of crisis you remember best and make a note of your emotional state as well as details of the crisis itself. What set it off? Was it a series of events or one stressor? Were you vulnerable at the time? Were you prepared for what happened? What did you do to cope and how did the crisis resolve itself? What was helpful, and what was not? The answers to these questions will help prepare you to work with survivors facing crisis.

CRISIS MANAGEMENT BACKGROUND

Caregivers have recognized crisis as potentially harmful since at least 400 BC when Hippocrates identified it as an issue (Roberts, 2005a). The first professional intervention center, however, was not established until 1906 (Roberts, 2005a). This center sought to prevent suicide, a form of crisis many survivors face. Increasing the prevalence of crisis intervention, suicide prevention became more widespread in the 1960s, primarily via telephone hotlines (Roberts, 2005a). The Community Reinvestment Act of 1963 also helped propel the growth of crisis facilities by requiring that comprehensive community mental health centers provide this type of emergency service in order to receive federal funding (Roberts, 2005a).

Statistics indicate the need for crisis intervention. In the United States alone, there are about 8.7 million intimate partner violence cases and 30,500 suicides a year. And more than 3,200 cancer diagnoses, 140 AIDS-related deaths, and 118 motor vehicle deaths occur each day. Compounding this, one in five children and teenagers have symptoms of psychiatric illness every year, and homicide ranked second as cause of death for 15- to 24-year-olds in 2000 (Roberts, 2005a).

Obviously, these events can cause crises for individuals and family members affected by them, potentially leading to acute stress or post-traumatic stress disorder (PTSD). An estimated minimum of 4.3 million and maximum of 35 to 45 million calls to crisis hotlines per year demonstrate that crisis intervention can help with processing of crisis, alleviating negative responses, and preventing these conditions (Roberts, 2005a). Despite these advances, healthcare services still often fail to assess patients presenting to them for the impact of crisis and trauma. Some studies indicate that as few as 50% of those exposed to potentially traumatic crises are assessed (Ursano & Engel, 2008). Social workers can help to fill this gap and assist those in need.

Definitions

- *Post-traumatic stress disorder (PTSD)* – A disorder resulting from exposure to traumatic events that causes symptoms lasting at least a month that include emotional responses of fear, horror or helplessness; flashbacks and/or nightmares of events; avoidance of reminders of the event; and increased arousal
- *Flashback* – Intrusive and involuntary re-experiencing of traumatic events through images, emotions or physical sensations
- *Hypervigilance* – A state of increased attention to the environment, in order to detect threat and prevent harm, that can increase anxiety, prevent sleep and cause fatigue

---

CRISIS INTERVENTION PROCESS

Crisis intervention is brief, time-limited, and active (Hillman, 2002). Crisis phone calls, for example, work most effectively when supportive structured interventionists determine the reasons why survivors call and help them to find coping they can do on their own to alleviate the feeling of crisis (McCann & Pearlman, 1990a). Social workers need to quickly establish rapport, and assess and refer survivors for aid, meeting the needs they have jointly identified. At times, this means providing less assistance than the situation seems to call for, because those in crisis only feel comfortable accepting help in limited areas.

Except in cases of imminent danger, providing for the basic needs requested can help more than we might realize. For example, a team of medical practitioners who wanted to treat his cancer saw Mr. Kasal in the hospital. He refused treatment and only wanted assistance with pain medication and health insurance to pay for it. These self-defined, crisis-related needs provided an opening for the social worker on the team to help restore balance in his life by getting him health insurance and other financial assistance for pain medication that the team prescribed. As a result of this crisis intervention, his life became more manageable and he later accepted more extensive help (Goelitz, 2003a).

Practitioners utilize a variety of crisis intervention methodologies when working with and assessing survivors for detrimental trauma impact after crises occur. You will find more detail in the section on crisis intervention methodologies below. However, most crisis interventions incorporate specific strategies or steps.

Roberts (2005a) describes these steps as the stages of crisis intervention and outlines them as: (1) assessing for safety and determining what needs require attention; (2) interacting considerately in order to establish safe connections; (3) determining key issues involved, including what set off the crises; (4) exploring related emotional difficulties; (5) evaluating current coping; (6) jointly coming up with a plan to augment coping and (7) arranging for follow-up as required.

Definitions

- *Safety* – State essential to trauma recovery and unique to each individual, in which: (1) risky behaviors, unhealthy relationships and negative emotions are reduced; and (2) a sense of well-being, trust, calm and positive coping are increased

---

Here is another, similar, but more trauma-focused view of the crisis interventions process (van der Kolk, McFarlane, & van der Hart, 1996): (1) stabilizing individuals in crisis; (2) helping them cope with flashbacks of the experience; (3) addressing disruptions to their cognitive schemas; (4) helping to establish safe relationships; (5) encouraging rejuvenation via good experiences and memories; and (6) focusing on restoring balance and rebuilding what has been broken internally and externally, including repairing physical damage to themselves and their property.

Definitions

- *Cognitive schemas* – Individuals' beliefs and thoughts about self and life, including faith in the world being a safe place and ideas about right and wrong

---

Both approaches emphasize establishing safety and balance, the importance of safe relationships and coping, and beginning the journey toward recovery. We must also assess individuals for detrimental trauma impacts and risk factors. See the chapter on assessment for more information on this.

CRISIS INTERVENTION METHODOLOGIES

Further research into the effectiveness of crisis intervention modalities is required prior to identifying whether most meet the standards of evidence-based practice (Roberts & Everly, 2006). One of the issues has been lack of standardization and manualization (step-by-step procedures documented in manuals accessible to practitioners) of treatment approaches. Psychological First Aid (PFA) is an example of a crisis intervention that has been determined to be an evidence-based practice (National Child Traumatic Stress Network, 2005).

PFA includes information-gathering techniques that facilitate rapid assessment of survivors' immediate concerns and utilizes evidence-informed supportive strategies in a flexible manner. The intervention is developmentally and culturally appropriate for those of various ages and backgrounds. It also includes handouts with important information that survivors can use over the course of their recovery process (National Child Traumatic Stress Network, 2005; Talbott, 2009). The US Departments of Veterans Affairs and Defense recommend PFA (2017).

In addition to PFA, best practices have emerged that social workers have utilized with diverse groups of trauma survivors. These include triage methodologies, such as the Mobile Crisis and the Assessment, Crisis Intervention, and Trauma Treatment (ACT) models; and brief mental health interventions, such as Psychological Debriefing (PD), intended to alleviate the likelihood of emotional issues occurring as a result of trauma (Roberts, 2005a; Talbott, 2009).

Critical Incident Stress Debriefing (CISD) is a form of PD that has become prevalent. It is a group-based intervention in which participants are encouraged to recall the crisis experience so that they can ventilate and normalize their reactions (Talbott, 2009). The results of studies conducted have been mixed regarding the efficacy of CISD, with some even showing a poorer outcome after this intervention (van der Kolk, McFarlane, & van der Hart, 1996). The US Departments of Veterans Affairs and Defense recommend against using CISD (2017).

The Solution Focused Approach is a brief crisis intervention strategy that has reports of success, but needs more study. It instructs practitioners to join survivors, asking them to define their issues and goals while using a "miracle or dream question" that helps them to imagine a solution that might seem unobtainable otherwise. Solutions and plans are then identified and the intervention is ended with future follow-up scheduled (Greene, Lee, Trask, & Rheinscheld, 2005).

The ACT model utilizes assessment and triage protocols as well as three crisis-oriented intervention practices. The triage assessment determines the need for emergency psychiatric care (Roberts, 2005b). Mobile Crisis, an intervention that provides support in the community for those in crisis by sending practitioners where help is needed, utilizes a similar form of triage assessment with the goal of preventing psychiatric hospitalization when appropriate (Ligon, 2005).

Other methodologies are also utilized in crisis situations. See the Resources section at the end of the chapter for further information. It is important for social workers to note that these crisis techniques are often not sufficiently preventative. Further treatment may be required to address cognitive disruptions caused by traumatic crises (McCann & Pearlman, 1990a).

Case Study

This case study illustrates how social work can focus on both the micro and macro levels when intervening with survivors of trauma. Juan was a young man in his 20s who survived the September 11th disaster. He attended a macro-level intervention for survivors who had lost their jobs as a result of the disaster. An informational meeting was held at which job training and health insurance were made available to eligible individuals as well as other resources such as psychoeducation about the effects of trauma. During the psychoeducation portion of the intervention, participants were told they could talk to social workers afterwards if they had further questions (Howard & Goelitz, 2004).

Juan approached a social worker after the meeting, asking for assistance in finding a place to live. By doing so, he was requesting a micro-level crisis intervention. The social worker paid close attention to his cues during the interview and, using crisis intervention techniques, was able to get him much-needed assistance as a result (Howard & Goelitz, 2004):

Juan:	Can you help find a place a live?
Social worker:	Did you lose your place because of the disaster?
Juan:	No. I have a place, but just don't want to go back. Sleeping on a friend's couch. Can't do that for long. *He makes very little eye contact as he talks.*
Social worker:	What made you leave your place? *Wondering if a crisis other than the September 11 disaster had occurred.*
Juan:	It's my boyfriend's place.
Social worker:	Did something happen between you that made you want to leave?
Juan:	We had a big fight. I can't go back. *He looks nervous and fingers a cast on his arm.*
Social worker:	What happened to your arm? *Probing for safety and risk factors.*
Juan:	I fell. *He looks away and down toward the ground.*
Social worker:	Did he do that to you, Juan? *Compassionately and with concern, establishing supportive rapport.*
Juan:	We were fighting and I pushed him first.
Social worker:	Did you hurt him?
Juan:	No, but I pushed him.

Social worker:	It's never okay for someone to hurt you, Juan. Do you feel like you're in danger now? Would he come after you? *Probing for risk and lethality factors.*
Juan:	He did once, but he doesn't know where I am now. It's all my fault. I should be hurt.
Social worker:	You seem mad at yourself. Do you ever think of hurting yourself? *Probing for suicidality.*
Juan:	Sometimes.
Social worker:	It sounds like you are having a hard time and could use some support and not just with finding a place. I'd like to hook you up with someone.
Juan:	Can you do that?

The social worker obtained an emergency appointment for Juan with a psychiatrist and therapist in a trauma-based mental health clinic nearby, letting him know that he would get psychological and emotional support as well as assistance finding a place to live. When asked whether he could contract for safety until the appointment the next day, he assured the social worker that he would be fine since he now knew he would get help. This survivor did not even know he wanted support beyond a place to live, but was relieved to have been given a higher level of support than he had requested.

RESOURCES

Roberts, A.R. (Ed.). (2005). *Crisis intervention handbook: Assessment, treatment, and research* (3rd ed.). New York: Oxford University Press.

ONLINE RESOURCES

https://www.mhanational.org/find-support-groups
National Child Traumatic Stress Network, & National Center for PTSD. (2005). *Psychological First Aid: Field operations guide.* https://learn.nctsn.org/course/index.php?categoryid=11

Practice Exercises and Questions

- The next time you have a client in distress, consider whether their situation seems to be a crisis. If you are unable to do so at the time, take a moment afterwards. You can also think of a past situation if none arises in the here and now

- Determine how to proceed with the client choosing techniques outlined in the chapter
- Explain why you chose the techniques to use
- Utilize the techniques or if unable to do so in the here and now with a client, role-play it with other practitioners

Crisis Management Summary

Tune in to Crisis

- *Creates sense of being out of control and helpless*
- *Safety and resources help to restore balance*

Defined

- *Crisis is loss of equilibrium due to stressor or trauma*
- *Requires individualized, person-in-environment assistance*
- *Interventions are focused on survivors' expressed needs*
- *Many roles used as social workers intervene at micro/macro/mezzo levels*

Process

- *Establish connection and determine focus of intervention*
- *Create safe environment for intervention to occur*
- *Work with survivors to ascertain stressors and goals*
- *Assess safety, coping, support systems and basic needs*
- *Process emotions related to what occurred*
- *Plan for augmentation of coping and steps toward goals*
- *Take steps toward goals (e.g., refer, advocate, organize)*
- *Follow up to ensure that survivors are no longer in crisis*

Chapter 15

Individual, Couples and Family Therapy

The prevalence of trauma means that most work with survivors at one time or another. Trauma is not always identified as an issue initially, but can surface in the course of therapy, sometimes taking therapists by surprise. When this occurs, many therapists encourage survivors to talk about what happened in detail, with the aim of promoting healing. Although this process may seem cathartic for survivors, it has its dangers. This chapter explores working effectively with survivors in therapy. Dealing with safety and trust issues by building secure therapeutic relationships, and working with partners and family members of survivors are also addressed.

TUNE IN TO INDIVIDUAL, COUPLES AND FAMILY THERAPY

In preparation for reading this chapter and working with survivors and their family members in therapy, tune in to the therapeutic process. Imagine how vulnerable survivors feel opening up in therapy after the pain of the traumatic event. Think about how it overwhelms them to encounter and share trauma-related feelings and recall the helplessness of the trauma experience.

Remember a time in your life when you felt vulnerable yourself or had a family member who did. Think about what made you or your family member feel either safe or more exposed at the time. Try to understand why these things helped or hurt. Imagine the kind of secure and supportive individuals you wished you had helping you and think about what characteristics would have made them so.

THE THERAPEUTIC RELATIONSHIP

Survivors need safe therapeutic relationships with professionals from whom they seek help. These include lawyers, medical staff, advocates and providers of concrete services. They also need safe relationships with individual, couples and family therapists. There are various hallmarks of therapeutic safety, including therapists who: (1) promote safety and trust; (2) establish trust; (3) become allies and (4) are sensitive to influences that erode safety and trust.

Effective trauma therapists are sensitive, supportive, warm and have positive regard for survivors (Seligman & Reichenberg, 2007). Constructivist self-development theory considers respect, information, connection and hope (RICH) fundamental to developing therapeutic relationships with survivors (Pearlman & Courtois, 2005). Effective therapeutic relationships with survivors are built upon respect, warmth, authenticity, empathy, concern, hope and the ability to withstand intense emotion (McCann & Pearlman, 1990a). This is the key component to a trauma-informed approach developed by Pearlman and others (Saakvitne, Gamble, Pearlman, & Lev, 2000) and called Risking Connection. It purports that the main ingredient for healing from trauma lies in the therapeutic relationship (Brown, Baker, & Wilcox, 2012).

Safety is crucial to the therapeutic relationship. Survivors need guidance on utilizing skills and resources that promote their safety. See chapter 10 on the importance of safety for more information. They also need help feeling safe enough during therapy sessions to experience and process intense trauma-related emotion (Bromberg, 2006).

Survivors need help developing safety and trust before discussing trauma memories, but this can take time. Therefore, the initial work needs to focus on building trust. This is particularly true for survivors of interpersonal trauma who have even more difficulty establishing trust in relationships (Rothschild, 2000).

Once trust is established, survivors have a powerful ally in therapy (Rothschild, 2000). Therefore, it is important to protect this collaborative relationship through awareness that survivors can easily be triggered or even retraumatized, especially when trauma memories/emotions are discussed (Seligman & Reichenberg, 2007). Moving too quickly or misjudging survivors' stability can cause problems and potentially damage the therapeutic relationship.

The therapeutic process requires constant reappraisal and, when needed, deceleration. Inadvertent therapeutic transgressions can trigger feelings of betrayal in survivors (Rothschild, 2000). Illustrating this, Jeanette, whose mother physically abused her as a child, became furious during her initial assessment at the use of wording that, to her, sounded like the clinician blamed her for the abuse. She never returned for treatment, despite all attempts to convince her otherwise.

Close attention to subtle messages from survivors helps to avoid triggering and lets therapists know when to slow down. Working collaboratively increases safety (Fabri, 2001). We empower survivors by supportively bearing witness to their traumatic experiences and reminding them they are in charge of the therapeutic process. This also emphasizes the importance of safety and demonstrates solidarity (Herman, 1992).

Being sensitive to power imbalances in the therapeutic relationship is also important. This can be difficult for survivors, particularly those who experienced human-designed trauma such as torture (Fabri, 2001). Responding genuinely during conflicts and anger, showing real emotion, talking about what occurred and taking responsibility for your part in it (Dalenberg, 2004), while negotiating and maintaining professional boundaries, all help maintain safety and trust (Pearlman & Courtois, 2005) and lessen the possibility of survivors experiencing power imbalances in the therapeutic relationship.

FACTORS TO CONSIDER

Effective trauma therapists are sensitive, flexible and attentive to the details of the therapeutic process and environment. These include: (1) physical space and boundaries in therapy; (2) the therapeutic process and being open to it, even when painful or difficult for the therapist and (3) working with unsuccessful interventions and non-compliance.

Physical space in therapy and other issues related to boundaries in the therapeutic relationship contribute to safety and trust. These include comfortable eye contact and surroundings, safe physical proximity and sensitivity with touch (Rothschild, 2000). Survivors can have difficulty with direct eye contact (see Chapter 11 on building safe relationships for information on how to work with this trust issue). Physical surroundings also influence how survivors feel. A pleasant, relaxed environment for therapy – for example, with plants, artwork and comfortable pillows – helps create a safe space for the therapeutic relationship to form (Goelitz & Stewart-Kahn, 2006/2007).

You may also need to address physical proximity. One client felt very anxious in therapy until he moved his seat further away from his therapist (Rothschild, 2000). Physical touch needs to be considered as well. Touch reassures some survivors, but may frighten others. One breast cancer patient undergoing chemotherapy was afraid of touch because of the germs she thought she might pick up. All these boundary issues matter.

Boundaries also matter when structuring client sessions. In terms of safety, it makes sense to do difficult work in the beginning of the session, exploration in the middle and to utilize the end of the session to help survivors stabilize and prepare to re-enter their lives (Herman, 1992). Generally, we want to keep stress levels manageable during sessions, ending with survivors' arousal level low (Rothschild, 2000). To this end, remind survivors that they control the process and can stop at any point (Graziano, 1997). Survivors may also need time to reorient after sessions, sitting in the waiting area, running water on their hands or going for a walk before they drive. Follow-up calls by social workers to survivors who leave their sessions feeling upset increase safety as well.

We also need to find ways to help survivors maintain safety between sessions. They need to know we are accessible. This includes availability for crisis or phone sessions and other means of communication (Graziano, 1997). One survivor, for example, benefited from periodic text messages asking how he was and reminding him of ways to cope. Providing tips on safety that survivors can use between sessions is also important. See Chapter 1 on secondary trauma and chapter 11 on building safe relationships for additional information on safe boundaries.

During therapy sessions, social workers help to heal survivors by bearing witness to their pain (Graziano, 1997). This can mean experiencing intense trauma emotions as we witness survivors' dissociation and the "nightmare" of their memories. Being fully present as a witness includes allowing painful feelings, while modeling how to maintain safety, even in the presence of strong emotion. This process helps to teach survivors to tolerate their own pain and integrate the trauma into their psyche (Bromberg, 2006). It also promotes trust and safety.

Transference and resistance often occur as trust develops and survivors encounter difficult territory in therapy (McCann & Pearlman, 1990a). Countering this, effective social workers do not judge survivors (or themselves) for non-compliance and ineffective interventions (Rothschild, 2000). Confrontation regarding non-compliance has the potential to retraumatize and must be done sensitively. Survivors also need to know that they are in control of therapy and can pick and choose among interventions (Graziano, 1997). Chapter 1 on secondary trauma provides information on transference in therapy.

TREATMENT APPROACHES

Survivors need flexibility in therapy, including using an eclectic mix of approaches, individualized for each situation and survivor (Rothschild, 2000). Mark, an adult survivor of childhood sexual abuse, for instance, often came late to sessions and failed to adhere to agreed-upon safe treatment plans, putting himself at risk. This generally occurred when he felt triggered and led to dissociation. His therapist acknowledged the transgressions, but also found ways to encourage him to fulfill their agreements. She made creative use of time as well so that Mark got the most out of his shortened sessions. This included suggesting he draw as he talked with her when he felt scared, dissociated, withdrawn and unable to make eye contact; doing 10 to 15 minutes of EMDR (Eye Movement Desensitization and Reprocessing), focused on safety; and using humor to help him relax and lighten up.

Definitions

- *Dissociation* – Disconnection from thoughts, memories or emotions that provides internal distance from reminders of traumatic events, but also prevents integration of trauma material and disrupts normal psychological functioning

Table 15.1 Dissociation Cues

Dissociation Cues		
Tuning out	Inattentive	Daydreaming
Falling asleep	Disoriented	"Spaced out," drifting away
Staring blankly	Emotionally flat or numb	Blinking or darting eyes
Missing what has been said	Avoiding eye contact	Slow to respond
Sitting still or stiffly	Out of touch with therapist	Making faces
Behavior suddenly changes	Disengaging	Soothing self, using coping

Source: Schiraldi, 2009

Recognizing and working with dissociation during therapy is essential. This requires re-establishing safety and helping survivors move away from the painful trauma memories and emotions that cause dissociated states (Rothschild, 2000). We identify dissociation through observation and survivors' reports of symptoms and can then work with them on reducing it. Activities requiring hand/eye coordination like playing catch with a pillow are effective antidotes. Here are some signs of dissociation you may observe during therapy (Table 15.1).

Survivors may also report symptoms of dissociation; or if you suspect it, query them regarding what they are experiencing. Ascertain the following symptoms by assessing survivors' reports (Table 15.2).

The goal, both during dissociation and throughout therapy, is to move away from the past, where trauma emotions and memories reside, and toward being fully present in the moment (van der Kolk, McFarlane, & van der Hart, 1996). Reducing dissociation and restoring equilibrium require conscious awareness of dissociation as it occurs. Safety also needs to be re-established. We therefore want to focus on interventions that increase stability before we can safely do any work with trauma material that may trigger dissociation (Seligman & Reichenberg, 2007). We also need to help survivors add to their repertoire of coping skills.

Constructivist self-development theory considers key survivor needs that can be addressed in therapy. Once addressed, these needs can add to equilibrium: Safety, trust, esteem, intimacy, control, self-worth, ability to tolerate emotions and

Table 15.2 Dissociation Reports

Dissociation Reports		
Life seems to be moving in slow motion	No pain when one would expect it	Observing, not participating
World is different, more or less intense, or like a dream	Self different, like someone else, not there, robotic	Feeling split between pre- and post-trauma self

Source: Schiraldi, 2009

connection to safe people (Pearlman & Courtois, 2005). Cognitive behavioral therapy (CBT) offers an approach that helps survivors work toward fulfilling these needs and that works well for both adults and children. For instance, studies show that Parent-Child Psychotherapy, a trauma-focused therapy that incorporates CBT, works well (Cohen, Kelleher, & Mannarino, 2008). See chapter 4 on family abuse and neglect for information on this modality.

Attachment theory/work, including observing survivors' abilities to attach to others and helping them to strengthen these skills, also helps (Pearlman & Courtois, 2005) because it builds trust and allows intimacy. Reparenting work can help as well, particularly for those traumatized during childhood. This developmental process works to achieve the feeling of being parented, without putting the therapist in the role of the parent, by finding meaning in what occurred, grieving, working with cut-off parts of the self (including child parts) and cognitively restructuring distorted beliefs such as the negative self-thoughts (Courtois, 2010) we see when survivors attack and blame themselves. Helping them to personalize, humanize and integrate split-off negative self-parts which they may have rejected post-trauma can promote healing (Kalsched, 1996).

Since trauma emotion has the potential to set off dissociation, helping survivors work with and regulate emotion is beneficial. Survivors often lose the ability to use emotion as an indicator of their personal experience because they are dissociated from their feelings. Having them identify feelings in their somatic states increases awareness and helps them to relearn this skill (van der Kolk, McFarlane, & van der Hart, 1996). This has the added benefit of increasing survivors' focus on their bodies, which many disconnect from post-trauma.

Awareness of bodily sensations also anchors survivors to the present moment and increases awareness of and intimacy with self. It can build dual awareness of past and present as well, enabling survivors to distinguish between their traumatic past somatic states and present moments in therapy. As always with any intervention, do not use this approach if it triggers trauma recall (Rothschild, 2000).

Although it may seem cathartic to do so, do not urge survivors to talk about what occurred until a safe equilibrium has been established and can be maintained. Many survivors become more symptomatic when they relive the trauma through discussion. In fact, crisis workers now tend to emphasize coping skills and only encourage sharing trauma experiences when it seems helpful (Carey, 2011).

COUPLES AND FAMILIES

Survivors can overcome the effects of trauma more effectively if they have secure connections with safe partners, family members and friends. This type of secure bond assists by soothing, comforting, providing hope, helping survivors make sense of what occurred, allowing them to grieve with loved ones and letting them know that they are "okay people" despite how trauma changed them. As an example of the impact of this intimate bond, a combat soldier became furious with his wife when she left him alone in the house after he returned from deployment. He told her he would never trust her again, so it was over between them. She did not understand until he explained that he was left alone, thought to be dead, after a priest gave him last rites in combat.

Another returning soldier chased a driver for miles at high speed, with his terrified wife in the car, after being cut off and forced onto the shoulder of the road. He later told his wife that the edges of roads are dangerous territory in Iraq. The discussion brought them closer and helped them to come up with ways to deal with this in the future (Johnson, 2008).

Emotion-focused therapy (EFT), a type of couples therapy that focuses on creating secure attachment, works well with distressed couples when one or both partners have experienced trauma (Johnson & Williams-Keeler, 1998). EFT is a short-term (12 to 20 sessions) approach that focuses on emotion and attachment issues. The treatment enhances couples' emotional responsiveness so that they form secure bonds (Johnson, 2008; Johnson & Williams-Keeler, 1998). This is a particularly important feat for survivors who have tremendous difficulty with intimacy and trust.

Family work can also help treat current trauma and prevent further trauma (Graziano, 1997). The fact that rape victims with optimal parenting had fewer trauma symptoms after the event highlights the importance of family bonds (Hauck, Schestatsky, Terra, Kruel, Ceitlin, 2007). Family work helps in more direct ways as well. In Iraq, an 11-year-old boy, Mohammed Ziara, had nightmares and did not do well in school after authorities arrested his father for arguing with neighbors. He feared they would torture or kill his father because he had seen news reports depicting this happening when police took people away. When teachers hit him for under-par work in class, he was scared to go to school. A social worker talked to him about the night of his father's arrest and worked with his parents and teachers, investigating the impact of these relationships on his trauma recovery. Among other things, she suggested they be gentle and compassionate with him. Mohammed began to feel better quickly as a result of her interventions (Leland, 2010). One study by social workers found that these kinds of interventions with survivor's families and social environments are essential when working with children and adolescents (Strand, Hansen, & Courtney, 2013).

Educating and supporting family members who may not understand survivors' experiences and symptoms are important components of working with trauma, particularly when recent. You will find several books for partners of sexually abused survivors listed in the Resources section at the end of the chapter. Secondary trauma can become an issue for these family members as well and should be assessed for. Safety within familial relationships should also be assessed as a means of helping survivors stay safe and secure.

Tips

- *Accessing safety of relationships* – Safe relationships are low-stress and positive, but also challenging, because people who are close and care often help us see ways to eliminate obstacles and grow. In safe relationships, it is alright to say no and set appropriate boundaries. It is also important to share concerns and fears because this helps create the strong connections that promote safety in relationships. Finally, the ability to laugh together even when facing difficult circumstances is essential to safe relationships

---

PERIODIC ASSESSMENT OF SYMPTOMS AND RISK FACTORS

Trauma survivors present to social workers with a variety of mental health disorders requiring attention, including depression, anxiety, stress disorders, dissociative disorders, somatoform responses, psychosis, substance abuse, post-traumatic stress disorder (PTSD) and borderline personality disorder (Briere & Scott, 2006). Associated risk factors can also put survivors in danger. A study funded by the National Institute of Mental Health and the National Institute on Drug Abuse, for instance, found significantly more risk of suicide with survivors of trauma with PTSD. This was true even after allowing for prior major depression, and substance abuse or dependence (Wilcox, Storr, & Breslau, 2009). Therefore, it is crucial to assess survivors periodically for symptoms and risk factors.

As symptoms and risk factors increase, you may need to recommend higher levels of treatment. This includes psychiatric medication, coping skills groups, substance abuse treatment, partial hospitalization programs and psychiatric hospitalization. See Chapter 14 on crisis management for more information on assessment.

Definitions

- *Post-traumatic stress disorder (PTSD)* – A disorder resulting from exposure to traumatic events that causes symptoms lasting at least a month that include emotional responses of fear, horror or helplessness; flashbacks and/or nightmares of events; avoidance of reminders of the event; and increased arousal

---

EVIDENCE-BASED PRACTICE

Individual and family trauma treatments utilized and investigated for efficacy by experts include supportive care and case management, psychodynamic therapy, psychopharmacology, CBT and psychological debriefing. CBT has attracted the most attention, proving effective for children, adolescents and adults (Cohen et al., 2008; La Greca & Silverman, 2009). Specific CBT interventions endorsed include exposure therapy, cognitive restructuring, cognitive processing, psychoeducation, parenting skills, relaxation, affect regulation, coping skills, narrative and three interventions discussed in the next chapter: Dialectical Behavioral Therapy (DBT), EMDR and hypnosis/guided imagery (American Psychiatric Association, 2004; Institute of Medicine, 2008; National Child Traumatic Stress Network, 2005).

Support, psychoeducation and case management are effective treatment approaches and avenues to further evidence-based psychotherapeutic treatment (American Psychiatric Association, 2004). Psychodynamic therapy, a psychotherapeutic approach, has been found to help with trauma-related work and relationship issues (American Psychiatric Association, 2004). Some, but not all, found Psychopharmacology effective, particularly when utilized in conjunction with other treatment approaches (American Psychiatric Association, 2004; Institute of Medicine, 2008). Psychological debriefing and other methods that encourage sharing of traumatic material were not found effective and even increased symptoms at times (American Psychiatric Association, 2004).

In terms of CBT interventions, exposure therapy has been found effective. It helps survivors confront trauma reminders that offer no current threat using (1) stress inoculation; (2) imagery rehearsal with survivors invoking trauma images and discussing them in therapy and (3) planned prolonged exposure to trauma images (Cahill & Foa, 2007; Carey, 2009). One report said this intervention needs to be done within a few hours of traumatic events. According to this report, we can help survivors retrieve trauma memories in order to confront and disengage associated fear during this timeframe, but if done later, the fear remains (Carey, 2009).

Other effective CBT techniques, such as cognitive restructuring and cognitive processing therapy (CPT), address beliefs that result from trauma. CPT has four main components (National Center for PTSD, 2011): (1) psychoeducation about trauma symptoms; (2) awareness of thoughts and feelings that for trauma survivors often include repetitive negative thoughts, such as what they could have done differently to avoid the trauma; (3) learning to question whether they should believe trauma-related negative thoughts and (4) understanding the changes often experienced by survivors in beliefs related to safety, trust, control, self-esteem and relationships.

Effective multifaceted CBT interventions that incorporate psychoeducation, coping skills, narrative and specific skills such as parenting, relaxation and affect regulation, include Psychological First Aid (PFA) and two modalities designed for children and parents: Parent-Child Interaction Therapy (PCIT) and Trauma-focused Cognitive Behavioral Therapy (TFCBT). We discuss these three evidence-based interventions in chapter 14 on crisis management, chapter 4 on family abuse and neglect. Coping skills, a component of these approaches that we discuss in chapter 12, have also generally been found to be effective. Although not universally endorsed as efficacious for trauma survivors, psychopharmacology is an important ingredient of treatment which

Case Study

Sandy and Joe were in couples therapy when Sandy revealed symptoms that affected their relations and indicated past sexual abuse:

Sandy:	I don't like to be touched. He knows that.
Social worker:	Really, why?
Sandy:	I've never liked it.
Social worker:	But we've hugged at the end of sessions and it didn't seem to bother you.
Sandy:	That's not about sex.
Social worker:	What's difficult about sex?
Joe:	I don't only touch you for sex. I like to be affectionate, but she always pulls away.
Sandy:	That's because you want sex.
Social worker:	Tell me about a time he touched you and you pulled away.
Sandy:	Yesterday I was washing dishes and he came up behind me and grabbed me. I didn't even know he was there. It scared me.
Joe:	That wasn't about sex at all.
Social worker:	It sounds to me like Joe coming up behind you triggered old memories and brought up strong emotions.
Sandy:	It's weird. I know on some level it must be him behind me, but I get so scared and confused.
Social worker:	I think it may remind you of something that happened to you when you were young.

The ensuing discussion revealed that Sandy had probably been sexually abused as a child and never realized it. Her sensitivity to touch was related to fear of the abuse and associated feelings so that she was unable to be truly intimate until she explored underlying trauma issues. She did this in individual therapy and her couples therapist assisted with the process by educating them about trauma and its effect on both of them, emphasizing the need for safety in their relationship.

we do not address extensively in this book because it is out of the scope of our expertise (American Psychiatric Association, 2004; Institute of Medicine, 2008). Survivors benefit from psychiatric medications and should be evaluated and treated by a psychiatrist when warranted. Examples include difficulty with sleep and/or nightmares; anxiety that gets in the way of functioning or of the therapeutic process and depression that overwhelms or leads to thoughts of self-harm.

RESOURCES

Briere, J., & Scott, C. (2006). *Principles of trauma therapy: A guide to symptoms, evaluation, and treatment*. Thousand Oaks, CA: Sage Publications.

Davis, L. (1991). *Allies in healing: When the person you love was sexually abused as a child*. New York: Harper Perennial.

Graber, K. (1991). *Ghosts in the bedroom*. Deerfield Beach, FL: Health Communications, Inc.

James, B. (1994). *Handbook for treatment of attachment-trauma problems in children*. New York: The Free Press.

Johnson, S.M., & Williams-Keeler, L. (1998). Creating healing relationships for couples dealing with trauma: The use of emotionally focused marital therapy. *Journal of Marital and Family Therapy*, *24(1)*, 25–40.

Pearlman, L.A., & Courtois, C.A. (2005). Clinical applications of the attachment formula: Relational treatment of complex trauma. *Journal of Traumatic Stress*, *18(5)*, 449–459.

ONLINE RESOURCES

National Center for PTSD: http://www.ptsd.va.gov/professional/pages/overview-treatment-research.asp; and http://www.ptsd.va.gov/professional/newsletters/research-quarterly/V19N3.pdf

National Child Traumatic Stress Network: Empirically supported treatments and promising practices: http://www.nctsnet.org/resources/topics/treatments-that-work/promising-practices

---

Practice Exercises and Questions

- Talk about why getting survivors to discuss and re-experience their trauma is not always therapeutic
- When and how can it be healing to talk about and re-experience the trauma?
- How are boundaries important when working with survivors? Give some examples
- Role-play introducing yourself to a new survivor client, keeping in mind the importance of the therapeutic relationship in healing
- Discuss a few treatment approaches, explaining why and how they work with survivors

---

Individual, Couples and Family Therapy Summary

Tune in to Individual, Couples and Family Therapy

- Survivors often feel vulnerable as they engage in therapy
- A secure and supportive therapeutic relationship is essential

The Therapeutic Relationship

- The therapist is an ally in treatment, promoting safety and trust
- Respect, information, connection and hope (RICH) are needed

Factors to Consider

- Eye contact, environment, proximity and the use of touch
- Session structure and support between sessions
- Social workers' ability to tolerate trauma emotions
- Ineffective interventions and non-compliance

Treatment Approaches

- Flexible approaches geared to specific individuals and situations
- Identifying and working with dissociation
- Increasing esteem, connection, affect tolerance and control
- Attachment work that increases the ability to bond with others
- Working with emotion through somatic states

Periodic Assessment of Symptoms and Risk Factors

- Assess for symptoms of psychiatric disorders and self-harm
- Refer for psychiatric assessment and medication
- Recommend higher levels of care such as hospitalization

Chapter 16

Group Therapy

The efficacy of support groups for breast cancer patients was among the things that drew me to social work. At the time, it was thought that these groups were so healing that they could even extend the lives of participants. Later studies invalidated these particular findings, but groups continue to be well known for the support they offer. Groups may not extend the lives of breast cancer patients, but they do help trauma survivors heal in other ways (Hudson, 2002).

Mutual aid, a major benefit of groups (Northen & Kurland, 2001), is a powerful force for survivors who feel alone with their suffering related to memories of traumatic events and associated emotions. Groups can also be forums for learning skills for coping with trauma (van der Kolk, McFarlane, & van der Hart, 1996). Therefore, groups have the potential to be an important component of survivors' recovery processes. This chapter discusses aspects of trauma groups that are important to social workers.

Definitions

- *Mutual aid* – Beneficial result of relationships formed within support groups as survivors realize their history and reactions are common and universal, rather than unique and dysfunctional, learning from each other's experiences and sharing coping techniques

---

TUNE IN TO TRAUMA GROUPS

Tune in to group experiences you have had during times of hardship. Remember the difficult or helpful aspects of the community offered by groups. Examples include a family gathering where your recent break-up was analyzed or a luncheon date with friends who wanted to know all about your car accident. People may have said that time heals or that things were not as bad as they seemed. You may have felt that these clichés invalidated your experience, preferring to hear others share about their own hardships and what helped them cope.

Remember also the feeling of being alone with your ordeal. You may have felt either: (1) less alone as you shared your sadness and pain with a group of people who cared or (2) more alone because no one seemed to comprehend what you were going through. Concentrate on what made the experiences different. Why did you feel less alone with some groups than with others? Some groups of people probably felt safer because you were close to them, but how well they listened, heard you and understood your experience may also have been significant.

As you locate examples of hardship, use coping and self-care (see chapter 12 on coping skills and self-care) to ensure that the stress of associated feelings is manageable. Avoid drawing on memories that are upsetting or traumatic.

BACKGROUND INFORMATION

Groups and the mutual aid they provide help participants in a number of ways. First, groups normalize the after-effects of trauma, reducing survivors' isolation as they share experiences (McCann & Pearlman, 1990a). In addition, they create a safe sense of community where, according to Blakley and Mehr (2008): (1) nurturing connections are made with others who understand; (2) members learn from each other about navigating recovery and (3) coping is enhanced. Finally, groups empower members as they help themselves and others, partaking in healing interactions that augment the sense of supportive community (Lee & Swenson, 1994).

Group members feel validated and their experiences are normalized when they share about their trauma and find similarities with other survivors. As they share, awareness of trauma-related thoughts or emotions and their current impact are often increased (van der Kolk, McFarlane, & van der Hart, 1996). Not only this, but groups can help survivors find the language and courage to talk about trauma emotions (van der Kolk, 1996) that may previously have been avoided.

Groups' safe supportive community is key, providing "a holding environment" (Blakley & Mehr, 2008, p. 243) in which survivors can make sense of what occurred and heal cognitive schemas. Positive coping is learned, modeled and reinforced (Blakley & Mehr, 2008), assuaging troublesome responses to trauma (van der Kolk, McFarlane, & van der Hart, 1996).

Definitions

- *Cognitive schemas* – Individuals' beliefs and thoughts about self and life, including faith in the world being a safe place and ideas about right and wrong

Groups help during times of stress, and trauma is stressful (Gitterman, 1994). Studies have found benefits for survivors, that often include decreased post-traumatic stress disorder (PTSD) symptoms, for, among others: (1) people with intellectual disabilities (Peckham, Howlett, & Corbett, 2007); (2) incarcerated youth (Ovaert, Cashel, & Sewell, 2003); (3) survivors of sexual abuse (Schiller & Zimmer, 1994); (4) children with PTSD (Nikulina et al., 2008); (5) survivors of the September 11th disaster (Howard & Goelitz, 2004); (6) breast cancer patients (Owen et al., 2005); (7) AIDS patients (Gabriel, 2007) and (8) Holocaust survivors (McCann & Pearlman, 1990a). Members are empowered by group benefits, which include mutual aid.

Groups also combat barriers to survivors obtaining help with trauma, providing assistance for marginalized individuals who may have no other supports. In rural areas where trauma treatment is difficult to locate (Blakley & Mehr, 2008), groups may be the only option. Groups generally increase access to support for survivors, reducing the effects of barriers to treatment such as a mental health stigma, lack of information about treatment or lack of trust in providers and financial issues (Weine et al., 2008).

SPECIAL CONSIDERATIONS

Things to consider when facilitating trauma groups include: (1) planning for survivors' special needs; (2) ensuring their safety as the group process potentially triggers trauma memories and (3) working to build connections with members so that the feeling of aloneness so prevalent among survivors is not amplified. Planning for their needs and ensuring their safety may include assessing prospective group members in order to determine their appropriateness for your group. This is particularly important for groups with experiential sharing, since some survivors lack the skills necessary to tolerate the emotional aspect of these groups. Other survivors may need the extra support of individual therapy (McCann & Pearlman, 1990a). If you are unsure about an individual's appropriateness for your group, talk with your supervisor before making a decision.

Planning, always important when facilitating groups, includes determining group purpose, membership, venue and scheduling. Since structure and clarity increase safety, these issues are key for survivors and must be well thought out. The purpose is primary because it determines other factors (Gitterman, 1994). If the purpose is informational and educative, for instance, group sizes can often be larger and one to three sessions may be sufficient; whereas groups with experiential sharing generally need small, intimate memberships and enough sessions to establish safety prior to sharing, and to process feelings and memories invoked after stories are told. Once the purpose is determined, we need to adhere to it so survivors know they will be kept safe. Turning an informational session into group therapy could be detrimental for survivors not prepared to hear and talk about traumatic events.

Planning considerations include: (1) session frequency/length – children, those in crisis, people who are cognitively impaired or physically sick often do better with frequent and short sessions; (2) group size – larger group sizes require more structure and rules, and smaller ones demand more individual sharing (Gitterman, 1994) and (3) venue – inviting and comfortable spaces contribute to safety (Goelitz & Stewart-Kahn, 2006/2007); and sitting in a circle, but around a table, may lessen feelings of exposure (Gitterman, 1994).

While facilitating groups, social workers need to be on the lookout for ways to protect members from graphic stories and from sharing in ways for which they are unprepared. We need to be more active when leading trauma groups than with other types of groups, continually guiding and containing members in order to ensure safety. This process builds trust with members, demonstrating that they are taken care of and protected. An example of the need to contain is when members remember forgotten/dissociated events during group sessions. Although this can be helpful to the healing process, it can also be harmful if facilitators do not keep members safe and allow them to feel in control of the process. Monitoring this includes managing the pace of groups, slowing things down when intensity increases, introducing coping as needed and ensuring members are connecting with and relating to one another, creating much-needed mutual aid (Blakley & Mehr, 2008; Herman, 1992).

TRAUMA GROUP DYNAMICS

Like families, groups develop dynamics to which social workers need to attend. Just as conflict within families decreases safety and warm supportive family relations heal, group dynamics affect the recovery process. Positive group dynamics can engender the supportive relations that mutual aid encourages and restore faith lost as a result of trauma.

Trauma issues related to "independence, power, dependency/trust" can cause conflict among group members (McCann & Pearlman, 1990, p. 273). Here is an example of a trauma group session where conflict was utilized to increase mutual aid and model safe interpersonal functioning:

Social worker: Even what you wear can be a way to cope after trauma. I see you have comfy clothes on, Ursula. Does that help?

Bob: Last week in group, one person had a baseball cap on and was sleeping.

June: *Angry.* I was the only one with a baseball cap and I was not sleeping.

Social worker:	Let's give Ursula a chance to answer. Also, remember that we need to keep the group safe for everyone and respecting each other by not criticizing helps safety. *Maintaining safe boundaries and inviting sharing despite the conflict.*
June:	I'm just saying I wasn't sleeping.
Bob:	I wasn't talking about you.
Social worker:	And Ursula, what about you?
Ursula:	*Looks down, no reply.*
Social worker:	It can be uncomfortable when there's conflict between people like now.
Ursula:	I'm sad today and just want to leave.
Social worker:	We hope you can stay. How have you been coping till now?
John:	Sometimes I leave places when I get upset.
Social worker:	Leaving can be good coping, especially when with unsafe people. *Several members, including John, nod.* How does it help, John?
John:	It gives me a chance to think.

Members shared ways of coping with trauma as a result of this interchange and in the midst of the discussion, Bob turned to June and apologized. She accepted the apology and later, when Bob talked about his grandson having cancer, she told him how sorry she was. Ultimately this exchange created new intimacy and trust, not just between June and Bob, but with all the members. It also gave the group a chance to practice coping with conflict in a real-life situation and to help each other in the process.

TYPES OF GROUPS

Types of groups for survivors include: (1) psychoeducational and cognitive behavioral therapy (CBT); (2) psychodynamic and supportive; (3) peer support and (4) telephone and online groups. Although some groups focus specifically on one methodology, many use a variety of approaches.

Psychoeducational groups can help survivors, providing information on trauma, common reactions and ways to cope. After the September 11th disaster, this type of group was offered for World Trade Center employees seeking health insurance, financial compensation and occupational resources, and was effective not only for this, but also as a means to screen for individuals at risk (Howard & Goelitz, 2004). Coping skills groups, a form of CBT group, are also effective, providing skills to alleviate trauma effects and promote safety (Najavits, 2002).

Once safety is established and survivors are stabilized, psychodynamic support groups, the type often offered through victim services and rape crisis centers, can be healing for those who want to share their stories (Gabriel, 2007). This methodology utilizes exposure/narrative therapy, with group members recounting what occurred and listening to others' stories. Survivors must be carefully screened and monitored to ensure continued safety since these groups are potentially triggering and re-traumatizing.

Peer groups can also be beneficial for survivors when safety is maintained. Examples include: (1) combat veteran rap groups whose members take responsibility for organizational issues, inviting professionals to participate and (2) rape survivor consciousness-raising groups that are geared toward social change rather than therapy (Herman, 1992). Twelve-step groups, such as those for survivors of sexual abuse, can also help.

Telephone groups address limited access to care; for example in rural areas (Morland, Greene, Rosen, Mauldin, & Frueh, 2009). Phone groups can also create a safe environment for survivors who participate from the comfort of their homes. The anonymity of these groups can help as well, allowing members to disclose more easily and alleviating awareness of differences among members (Goelitz, 2003b). Internet-based groups are valuable for similar reasons and have been found to reduce distress, facilitate development of strong therapeutic alliances (Knaevelsrud & Maercker, 2007) and reduce PTSD symptoms (Knaevelsrud, Böttche, Pietrzak, Freyberger, Kuwert, 2017). Online and telephone 12-step groups are also available for survivors.

SPECIFIC METHODOLOGIES

Seeking Safety and Psychological First Aid (PFA) are examples of group interventions that are evidence-based practices (Najavits, 2010; National Child Traumatic Stress Network, 2005; Talbott, 2009). Both combine several types of group modalities including psychoeducational, coping skills, CBT and supportive.

Seeking Safety is a manualized CBT treatment approach that was designed for addict and alcoholic survivors, but also works well for survivors with no substance abuse histories. It is present-focused and utilizes 25 practical group topics including relationships, coping with trauma triggers, establishing effective boundaries and detaching from and regulating emotions. Self-care and coping skills are emphasized since safety is the goal of this treatment. Concrete needs and interpersonal factors are also addressed (Najavits, 2002).

Another methodology, Critical Incident Stress Debriefing (CISD), and other forms of trauma debriefing have also been widely used with mixed results (van der Kolk, McFarlane, & van der Hart, 1996). See chapter 14 on crisis management for more information on CISD and PFA.

Case Study

In the third session of a cancer support group, Angie asked other members for help with an upcoming test for possible cancer recurrence. She shared this dream:

> She wakes up in an unfamiliar place where things are not as she would expect them to be. She is anxious and disoriented. As she looks out of the room, she can see rooms that look familiar but somehow not right. She also sees a door that seems ominous. She doesn't know where it leads. She gets more and more anxious as the dream goes on, until she locks multiple locks on the door of the room she is in, only to turn around and see her sister is in the room. She feels better with her sister's familiar presence.

The social worker facilitating the group encouraged Angie to focus on her sister's familiar presence at the end of the dream, helping her feel safety amidst the dream's anxiety. As Angie focused on it, the feeling of her sister grew stronger. She shared the comfort and safety she felt so clearly that other members felt it too and relaxed, creating mutual aid.

Then group members talked about their anxiety when Angie reported that she woke up in a strange place in the dream. They said it felt out of control and scary. With help from the social worker facilitating, they were able to feel both the anxiety and the comfort at the end of the dream, mimicking how their lives comprised both negative feelings related to cancer and good ones. Angie told them she felt reassured about the test and that she would use her sister's image to allay any anxiety she felt as she waited for her results. Other group members related this to their own lives and reported feeling reassured as well.

Angie's dream also introduced the theme of feeling out of control. Members discussed this in the next session, sharing their need to gain a feeling of control since it often felt as though cancer had taken over their lives. They expressed both hope about the future and fear of dying, supporting each other and healing in the process.

RESOURCES

Gitterman, A., & Shulman, L. (Eds.). (1994). *Mutual aid groups, vulnerable populations, and the life cycle* (2nd ed.). New York: Columbia University Press.

Najavits, L. (2002). *Seeking safety: A treatment manual for PTSD and substance abuse.* New York: Guilford Press. Retrieved from http://www.seekingsafety.org/

ONLINE RESOURCES

American Self-Help Group Clearinghouse: http://www.selfhelpgroups.org/
National Child Traumatic Stress Network, & National Center for PTSD. (2005). *Psychological First Aid: Field operations guide*: http://www.ptsd.va.gov/professional/manuals/psych-first-aid.asp

---

Practice Exercises and Questions

- When are different types of support groups appropriate for survivors?
- Explain why a clear group purpose is important
- Name and elaborate on some advantages to phone and online groups
- Role-play screening a survivor for a psychodynamic support group

---

Group Therapy Summary

Tune in to Trauma Groups

- *Feel safe and supported as others share hardship and coping*
- *Feel alone/disconnected if trauma is misunderstood by others*

Benefits of Groups

- *Supportive community, experiences shared and members empowered*
- *Increased coping and decreased trauma symptoms*
- *Accessible to many who have barriers to treatment*

Factors to Consider

- *Plan for special needs of trauma survivors*
- *Provide safety, including protecting members from harm*
- *Groups enable accessing of dissociated memories and feelings*
- *Members may need extra support such as psychotherapy*

Group Dynamics

- *Can evoke memories of traumatic family dynamics*
- *Power, dependency and control are crucial issues*
- *Conflict may develop, providing a learning tool*

Types of Groups

- *Psychoeducation, coping skills and CBT*
- *Psychodynamic and supportive, including exposure therapy*
- *Peer support, rap and 12-step groups*
- *Telephone and online support groups*

Chapter 17

Other Trauma Interventions

We can employ many supplemental treatment methods when working with trauma. Survivors may even discover beneficial techniques on their own. In fact, Alice Miller, a renowned psychoanalyst and trauma expert, investigated the lives of famous artists like Picasso and surmised they used their art to heal trauma histories (Miller, 1991). Creative approaches that promote recovery include psychodrama, dance, writing, music and art. Spirituality can also play a role, as can intentional physicality such as breathing, yoga and relaxation. Finally, there are psychotherapeutic interventions that are efficacious for many survivors. Eye movement desensitization and reprocessing (EMDR), guided imagery and hypnosis, dream work and Dialectical Behavioral Therapy (DBT) fall into this category. This chapter discusses these interventions and how to choose the most effective ones for each individual.

TUNE IN TO OTHER TRAUMA INTERVENTIONS

In preparation for reading this chapter and helping survivors find approaches that work for them, tune in to their unique needs, coupled with the myriad ways of expressing and dealing with suffering. Imagine survivors' responses when given choices about how to recover and their relief at knowing that if one technique does not work, another one will. Feel the hope that this entails.

Remember what heals you. Perhaps you pray, write in a journal, sing or dance to loud music. Picture these activities helping survivors. See yourself encouraging them to pursue them on their own, or perhaps with you. In some cases, refer them to more qualified professionals when a particular modality is needed.

EYE MOVEMENT DESENSITIZATION AND REPROCESSING

The International Society for Traumatic Stress Studies and the US Department of Veterans Affairs have found EMDR efficacious for treatment of trauma.

Meta-analysis also indicates its effectiveness as an intervention (Sharpless & Barber, 2011). Despite this, studies have had mixed results and there is insufficient evidence to declare it an evidence-based practice (Cahill & Foa, 2007; Institute of Medicine, 2008).

This manualized approach has eight structured phases utilized to desensitize and reprocess distressing trauma images and memories. The intervention alternately stimulates the left and right sides of the body as: (1) survivors' eyes move from side to side following clinicians' left-right-hand movements; (2) sound plays first in one ear and then the other or (3) tapping or a vibrating electronic device directly stimulates the left and right sides of the body, such as hands or knees.

The process helps survivors in these ways (Shapiro, 2001): (1) trauma experiences are relearned, and the brain stores the newly processed information in a healthy fashion that contrasts with fragmented storage of unprocessed trauma; (2) current distressing trauma triggers are desensitized and (3) coping is increased as EMDR strengthens and reinforces survivors' imagined safe places, resources and positive future outcomes.

EMDR eliminated symptoms for Charlotte, a survivor of an auto collision who had flashbacks and difficulty sleeping for weeks afterwards. She recalled what happened and her resulting inability to feel safe, while guided by her therapist as she moved her eyes from side to side. When asked how she felt leaving the wrecked car, she recalled a feeling of awe that she survived and was told to focus on this while doing EMDR. No longer experiencing flashbacks or sleep issues, she returned for one more EMDR session and afterwards felt no strong emotion when thinking of the event, even though she retained a healthy wariness of drivers who might not obey traffic signals (Naparstek, 2005).

A drawback of EMDR is the necessity for survivors to re-experience distressing trauma images and memories as they are desensitized and reprocessed. Some have been so overwhelmed by the feelings invoked by this modality that they are unwilling to continue using it. A new way of facilitating EMDR treatment called the Flash technique, has been found to alleviate this issue. It does not require the same exposure to trauma memories and thus seems to be better tolerated by most (Manfield, Lovett, Engel, & Manfield, 2017).

GUIDED IMAGERY AND HYPNOSIS

Hypnosis and guided imagery lead to a relaxed and open state of awareness that encourages general relaxation and helps survivors detach from trauma memories. Meta-analyses confirm the effectiveness of hypnosis, primarily as an adjunct treatment. One study, for instance, found that it decreased symptoms of post-traumatic stress disorder (PTSD), including sleep issues (Sharpless & Barber, 2011).

Guided imagery also works well. Research shows that it can heal physiological effects such as imbalance of the stress hormone cortisol, which is released during trauma and sometimes deficient in its aftermath (Naparstek, 2005). Imagery can be induced with music. With a method developed for cancer patients, for example, music produces a relaxed state, evoking images in survivors, while practitioners safely, supportively, and contemplatively guide their process (West, 2007).

A pediatrician with multiple myeloma, who almost died during bone marrow transplant treatment, eliminated his trauma symptoms (nightmares, poor sleep and feelings of detachment) by using guided imagery. He reported feeling moved, experiencing emotions he had avoided and grieving his multiple losses as he regularly imagined "invisible, kindly, protective helpers around him" (Naparstek, 2005, p. 7).

Definitions

- *Post-traumatic stress disorder (PTSD)* – A disorder resulting from exposure to traumatic events that causes symptoms lasting at least a month that include emotional responses of fear, horror or helplessness; flashbacks and/or nightmares of events; avoidance of reminders of the event; and increased arousal

---

DREAM WORK

Dream work can also contribute to survivors' healing process (Barasch, 2000; Barrett, 2002; Bosnak, 1996; Brunkow, 1996; Garfield, 1991; Lothane, 1983; Mindell, 1998). At times, nightmares let social workers know that survivors need help with increasing their safety. At others, discussion of dreams provides access to trauma emotions. Dreams can provide messages as well, often of hope as exemplified by this dream from a cancer patient, Alicia, whose dream increased her sense of inner strength:

> She wakes up in bed with a tiger sleeping with its head on her stomach. At first, she is afraid when she realizes how powerful it is. Then she knows that it is safe and marvels in its presence – how soft its fur is, how beautiful its coloring, how heavy it feels on her stomach. It feels like a healing presence. As she comes fully awake and comfortable with the tiger being there, it gets up and walks away.

The dream represented her ability to find strength in cancer, a powerful foe. Discussing the dream reinforced both her feeling of empowerment and the safe connection with her social worker (Goelitz, 2009).

Helping survivors find secure ways to process nightmares also contributes to the therapeutic alliance (Goelitz, 2009). Trauma nightmares with intense emotion can be an indication that recovery work needs to be done. This recurring dream discussed in chapter 10 on the importance of safety, for instance, signaled the triggering of past trauma:

> I'm in a big cavernous building with high walls and I am running. Running from someone – monsters or something else very scary. Every time I go down a hall I think, "This is the one," and then when I get closer, I see it is the same as the others, with still no way out.

This dream first occurred when the dreamer was abused as a child. It returned after invasive surgery, another trauma. Exploring this dream helped her understand that her experience had triggered a traumatic response. Knowing that helped her to change her perception of the dream from unknown terror into an explainable expression of trauma emotion (Goelitz, 2009).

DIALECTICAL BEHAVIORAL THERAPY

DBT is a cognitive behavioral therapy, based upon the Buddhist principles of mindfulness. Developed to treat borderline personality disorder (BPD), it is also effective with trauma, targeting issues that pertain to survivors (Reyes, Elhai, Ford, 2008). In fact, one version of DBT specifically applies to PTSD symptoms. Although extensive research with trauma survivors has not yet been done, the results look promising (Sharpless & Barber, 2011).

This manualized approach, utilized individually and in groups, teaches skills that many trauma survivors need: Interpersonal effectiveness, emotion regulation, distress tolerance and mindfulness (Linehan, 1993). By using these skills, they learn to tolerate emotion without stifling or intensifying it, managing problematic behaviors, including self-harm and substance abuse, and generally increasing their sense of balance and well-being. DBT also helps with dissociation, self-blame, shame, low self-esteem and the PTSD symptoms of flashbacks, nightmares and avoidance (Reyes et al., 2008).

Definitions

- *Avoidance* – Individuals staying away from people, places or activities, even when not dangerous, because they are reminders of trauma

---

A survivor of childhood abuse in her early 20s, Sarah, had been in and out of psychiatric hospitals since childhood. After a psychiatric hospitalization, she was referred to a DBT program. She grew to love it and the skills she learned there, traveling quite a distance for the group. As a result, she not only stayed out of the hospital, but began to function in ways she never could before: Building friendships, socializing and even making plans to move out of the group home where she lived.

BREATHING

When stressed, many survivors breathe shallowly, hyperventilate or even hold their breath unintentionally for a moment. Therefore, learning to breathe properly can have a calming effect, reducing the effects of trauma (Briere & Scott, 2006). Veterans with PTSD, for instance, had fewer symptoms of flashbacks, outbursts of anger and disturbed sleep (due to hyperarousal) when they used yogic breathing (Brown & Gerbarg, 2005). Watch survivors as you work with them. Notice when their breathing stops for a moment, or quickens. Help them become aware of their stress-induced changes in breathing and to use breath to gain peace of mind and reduce stress.

Definitions

- *Hyperarousal* – Heightened emotionality that can lead to agitation, anger, difficulty sleeping and/or hypervigilance

---

Tips

- *Breathe deeply from the abdomen* – Help survivors enhance their breathing. Have them put their hands on their abdomen. It should expand as they breathe in and contract as they breathe out. Do it with them, counting slowly. Talk with them about how this feels. Yogic breathing is also beneficial

---

YOGA

Yoga, another way to reduce trauma symptoms, significantly decreased PTSD symptoms after eight 75-minute sessions, according to the results of a study testing its efficacy (van der Kolk, 2006). Not only that, but participants made comments like "I learned to be able to focus and sense where my body was" (van der Kolk, 2006, pp. 286–287), an important accomplishment since many survivors lose touch with their bodies. Yoga offers flexibility as well. Interventions can be directed toward specific symptoms. For example, yoga interventions can be utilized to decrease hyperarousal and dissociation or to increase affect regulation (Hopper, Emerson, Levine, Cope, & van der Kolk, 2011).

RELAXATION

Practitioners' use of relaxation as a method for coping with trauma-related fear and anxiety is not new. It is particularly beneficial when used in conjunction with other treatments (Sharpless & Barber, 2011). The most important factors in relaxation are: (1) being in a quiet place; (2) using something to relax the mind such as repeating a word over and over silently or out loud; (3) not being active and (4) feeling physically comfortable. However, relaxation can be used anywhere, empowering survivors as it provides a tool that they will always have, and it is effective for children as well as adults (Klein, 2008).

Progressive muscle relaxation, for example, decreases the arousal caused by trauma and facilitates processing of trauma material. Survivors tighten and release their muscles, starting with the head and working down to the feet (Briere & Scott, 2006). Effective for children and adults, it works better for adolescents if they imagine their muscles relaxing because they often find tensing and releasing too difficult. Children, on the other hand, also benefit from progressively moving each body part, first quickly and then as slowly as possible. Some children learn what it means to slow down from doing this exercise (Klein, 2008).

Ask survivors to describe their reactions to the methods described in this chapter. For some, relaxing feels vulnerable and can increase their anxiety rather than reducing it. Remind survivors to use only the methods that work for them.

PSYCHODRAMA

According to Kellermann (2000), psychodrama, an effective treatment for survivors, has the following therapeutic features: (1) replaying what occurred; (2) making sense of the traumatic event; (3) releasing negative trauma emotion; (4) finding and acting out new, more positive endings to their experiences; (5) feeling supported and (6) using rituals for healing. This methodology combines psychotherapy with aspects of the theater such as role-play and improvisation.

Because psychodrama uses imagination and play, it is a good technique to use with children. For example, it was used with a group of children who lost their parents during the September 11th disaster. Once their facilitator had worked with them to build a secure environment, they played "monster." The child playing the monster acted out the horrific deaths they imagined, eating its victims' limbs. The facilitator then helped them create a safe place under a table, after which they came out together and defeated the monster (Haen, 2008).

DANCE

Dance/movement therapy is effective treatment for people with trauma experiences such as cancer and abuse. According to one study (Leseho & Maxwell, 2010), women reported the following outcomes from dance: (1) empowerment, including taking ownership of and having gratitude for their bodies; (2) transformation and healing; for example, by expressing emotion through dance and (3) finding a connection to themselves and a spiritual presence in life. One survivor described it this way: "The dancing ... is who I am minus all the trauma ... and when I dance ... it's like something comes alive in me that goes right to the cell of my being ... a space inside of me that's connected to the deepest level" (Leseho & Maxwell, 2010, p. 28).

WRITING

Alice Walker, a Pulitzer Prize winner and survivor of child abuse, said she wrote as a result of her suffering as a child. She described writing as life-saving and began by making up stories to comfort herself as a child (Desalvo, 2000). Writing can come in many forms, including journaling and poetry, and survivors do not need to be accomplished writers to attain healing from the process.

Survivors should exercise care when writing about trauma because the process can retraumatize them as they re-enter their experiences through a narrative. The writing is best done with a clear plan in mind and under the guidance of a professional. Sometimes telling stories in a fictional way, with imaginary characters, helps create a safe distance. This can also provide a valuable tool when survivors ask themselves what the protagonist would feel and discover their own lost trauma-related feelings (Desalvo, 2000).

MUSIC

Music is healing for survivors in a variety of ways. Singing, for example, helps them connect with their bodies because sustaining musical notes requires deep breathing. The deep breathing is relaxing and grounding. The creative aspects of singing are also important, providing a way to express emotion and thoughts related to trauma experiences (Austin, 2006).

Illustrating this, Bruce Springsteen and the E Street Band used music and song to convey the pain of the September 11th disaster. Their album *The Rising* expressed powerful emotions, such as anger and fear. It also provided the healing message that, through connecting with others, horror and loss are transcended (Weingarten, 2004).

ART

Art is also healing. Children with traumatic grief, for example, often feel a loss of control which, combined with trauma symptoms, can hinder grieving. Having the opportunity to choose how to express feelings through art can alleviate this and help them make sense of what occurred. This is particularly valuable for those too young to understand and articulate their emotions (Edgar-Bailey & Kress, 2010).

Art can be used in family work as well. In family therapy, for instance, 4-year-old Julia drew her mother shooting her and her sister and then killing herself when asked to draw anything she wanted. She then repeatedly asked her father why her mother did this and why she survived. These questions were the starting point for a discussion that her father had avoided until that time, enabling Julia to express herself and providing healing for them both (Klorer, 2006).

SPIRITUALITY

Surveys show that spirituality increases coping for those affected by trauma, also aiding the recovery process. Trauma destroys survivors' sense of safety and erodes their faith. As evidenced by studies, such as one in which Israeli adolescents used prayer to cope with traumatic stress related to the possibility of missile attacks during the Persian Gulf War (1990–1991), spirituality bolsters faith and increases coping, often helping survivors find meaning related to what occurred and even promoting post-traumatic growth (PTG), as opposed to PTSD, as a result (Weaver, Flannelly, Garbarino, Figley, Flannelly, 2003). See Chapter 6 on life-threatening illness for more information on PTG.

Definitions

- *Post-traumatic growth (PTG)* – Condition resulting from exposure to traumatic events that causes symptoms that include the ability to see trauma from positive perspectives, to find benefit in it, to attach meaning to it that makes sense and inspires and to make constructive and helpful behavioral changes as a result

---

Spiritual and religious ceremonies can particularly help survivors. Memorials, for instance, allow survivors to remember, grieve and feel gratitude for those lost in wars or disasters. Rituals and other healing traditions drawn from survivors' cultures can also help (Turner, McFarlane & van der Kolk, 1996). According to shamanic tradition, for example, retrieving souls that were separated from survivors' bodies as a result of what occurred heals trauma. This is done for both survivors and the community because it is believed that illness and trauma affect the community as a whole, not just individuals, an idea that can further increase survivors' sense of connectivity and safety (Levine, 1997).

CHOOSING INTERVENTIONS FOR TRAUMA RECOVERY

The most important factor in choosing interventions, besides safety, is client interest. For instance, art therapy can be a good choice for survivors who use art as a means of coping with stress. Other considerations for each modality are discussed below. To ensure safety, survivors should work with practitioners with knowledge of trauma.

EMDR is a relatively short-term treatment method that works well for a variety of survivors, including combat veterans (keeping in mind physical constraints from injuries), adolescents and children. However, survivors with multiple trauma events and adult survivors of childhood trauma do not respond as well as others; and those with comorbid issues, such as substance abuse, and risk factors, such as suicidality, should be assessed carefully prior to treatment (Foa, Keane, Friedman, & Cohen, 2010). EMDR has a meditative quality that some people like, but it helps even those who aren't attracted to that. Rene tried it because she had anxiety stemming from childhood trauma that improved with anti-depressants, but she did not want to take them any longer due to weight gain. She was very motivated for treatment as a result and did well.

Hypnosis has been found beneficial for survivors experiencing the PTSD symptoms of dissociation and nightmares. It is also useful as they work with distressing memories, creating a sense of separateness from the memories and helping them manage associated emotion. We do not recommend it for survivors who do not respond to hypnotic suggestion or resist the process. It is also not the best choice for survivors who have low blood pressure or sleepiness since it relaxes. In addition, victims of crimes should use hypnosis cautiously and with legal advice, because memories obtained during hypnosis have been contested in court (Foa et al., 2010).

Dream work is not appropriate for all survivors and needs to be done safely when utilized. Since nightmares are often replays of traumatic events, accessing them can trigger memories and cause further distress. Despite this, the frequency of nightmares after trauma encourages utilizing them as conduits to trauma emotions. Using reassuring images as anchors often allows safe access to dream emotions (Goelitz, 2001a, 2001b).

Definitions

- *Dissociation* – Disconnection from thoughts, memories or emotions that provides internal distance from reminders of traumatic events but also prevents integration of trauma material and disrupts normal psychological functioning

---

DBT teaches skills effective for a broad range of survivors, particularly those at risk of suicide (Sharpless & Barber, 2011). It can reduce other self-harm behaviors, including substance abuse and PTSD symptoms of avoidance, flash-backs, nightmares and dissociation. It is also helps establish the safety needed to function well and work with trauma issues (Reyes et al., 2008).

Intentional physicality should be utilized in ways that fit each survivor. For those with breathing issues, such as from lung cancer, breathing techniques may accentuate this, increasing anxiety rather than lessening it. Help survivors be conscious of how techniques affect them, letting them know that choosing effective methods is an individual matter. Illustrating this, progressive muscle relaxation can increase arousal or cause dissociation for some survivors. Others are unable to relax using this method. It may not work well, for instance, for those who have chronic flashbacks (Briere & Scott, 2006).

Although efficacy has not yet been determined through research, creative approaches are considered effective when done with trained professionals, in con-junction with other trauma treatment and with the consent of survivors. Providing an avenue for exposure therapy, cognitive restructuring of what occurred, stress reduction and empowerment, these approaches are non-verbal and access memory differently from verbal techniques (Foa et al., 2010), making them a good vehicle for those unable or unwilling to talk directly about what happened.

Spirituality is an approach that is appropriate for many survivors. Some say they have no spiritual beliefs, but it is unusual for individuals not to have a life philosophy, reason for living or belief system that is their brand of spirituality. This can include a sense of connection to community and family, appreciation for creativity or nature, love of animals or universal love. When I worked in hospice, Alfred insisted he believed in nothing, but reported having visits from dead loved ones when he was dying. These visits, which may have been dreams or delirium-induced hallucinations, comforted him as he died and provided him with a sense of purpose and a spiritual connection with the afterlife he was moving toward.

Case Study

Genevieve and Natasha were members of a poetry group for trauma survivors at The Women's Health Project. The format of the group was that the leader read a poem chosen from the literature or by a group member. Group members discussed it and then spent time writing and sharing their own poems in response.

The members were women ranging in age from 30 to 60 years old. They were fiercely protective of the group and of each other, having become close as they wrote together and told their trauma stories through their poems. They had experienced much loss and shared strong emotion during the group, including anger and sadness. They even cried for each other. Out of this emotion grew hope and their poems reflected it:

. . . The Face of Darkness

Light will reveal itself . . .
In all its glory Strength, and Praise
The Light will Come
The Light will Cleanse
The Light will heal
And, Will you receive it
With a closed mind?
A metal door blocking the light
And all you see are Rays around it?
Or will you be awakened?
Into the light – And eclipse the Darkness
When Next, It too, Arrives

Genevieve André

Continuance

When Cassie died I was surprised – yet not
For little mice do come and go
While my life must continue on.
I mourned her death. I held her and I cried
But not for long. The other mice live on
And ask for my attention.
And so to them I turn.
When my soul died I didn't understand
I hadn't had it for so very long
Then little dreams and hopes and wishes gone
I mourn its death. I hold myself and cry
I know I'll do this till the day I die
But – I live on, and though it hurts to know
It hurts to feel, to love, to trust, to be.
The present is asking for my attention.
And so to it I must turn

Natasha Millikan

These group members not only gave permission for their poems to be used in academic publications, but also asked for their names to be included. Proud of their work, they want it to be shared so it can help others as it helped them.

RESOURCES

Barrett, D. (Ed.). (1996). *Trauma and dreams.* Cambridge, MA: Harvard University Press.

Hopper, E., Emerson, D., Levine, P.A., Cope, S., & van der Kolk, B.A. (2011). *Overcoming trauma through yoga: Reclaiming your body.* Boston: North Atlantic Books.

Linehan, M.M. (1993). *Skills training manual for treating borderline personality disorder.* New York: Guilford Press.

Malchiodi, C.A. (Ed.). (2008). *Creative interventions with traumatized children.* New York: Guilford Press.

Naparstek, B. (2005). *Invisible heroes: Survivors of trauma and how they heal.* New York: Bantam.

Shapiro, F. (2001). *Eye movement desensitization and reprocessing: Basic principles, protocols, and procedures* (2nd ed.). New York: Guilford Press.

Practice Exercises and Questions

- Name several of the interventions discussed in the chapter
- When and why would these interventions be appropriate?
- When and why would these interventions be contraindicated?
- Role-play talking with a survivor about how to choose an intervention

---

Other Trauma Interventions Summary

Tune in to Other Trauma Interventions

- *Think about what helps your healing process*
- *Imagine the relief of knowing there are choices for healing*

Psychotherapeutic Interventions

- *Eye movement desensitization and reprocessing (EMDR)*
- *Guided imagery, dream work and psychodrama*
- *Dialectical Behavioral Therapy (DBT)*

Intentional Physicality

- *Breathing, yoga, relaxation and dance.*
- *Writing, music and art*

Spirituality

- *Meditation, prayer, ritual and spiritual readings*

Choosing Interventions for Trauma Recovery

- *First consider survivor interest and safety*
- *Then consider:*
- *physical limitations or predispositions*
- *blocks, fears or curiosity related to modalities*
- *types of coping that have helped in the past*
- *survivor age and cultural background*

Healing Trauma on a Macro Level

Part V

Healing Trauma on a Macro Level

Chapter 18

Program Development

The National Association of Social Workers' Code of Ethics principles of service and social justice (National Association of Social Workers, 2017) call for us to "elevate" others' needs above our own and fight to change systems that oppress. History is littered with examples of our efforts in this area. The first abused child taken from her home and placed in a safe environment formed the basis for child welfare program development. This example also illustrates how even social workers who are direct service providers have a role in program development. Front-line clinicians are crucial to improving service delivery and increasing survivor satisfaction. This includes addressing survivors' special needs for security. Because trauma destroys well-being, all trauma focused care must help survivors create a sense of safety.

Definitions

- *Safety* – State essential to trauma recovery and unique to each individual, in which: (1) risky behaviors, unhealthy relationships and negative emotions are reduced and (2) a sense of well-being, trust, calm and positive coping are increased

---

This chapter highlights key aspects of trauma program development. It summarizes basic program development theory, using examples to illustrate the process. The chapter also seeks to explain the unique challenges of developing programs for survivors and the key role of survivor safety in service delivery.

SAFETY FIRST

Trauma destroys the sense of safety that is crucial to healthy human experience. Without it, survivors' are fraught with worry. Everyday living is often experienced as terrifying and can be difficult to manage. Many systems that survivors interact with, including medical, social services, mental health and justice, do not attend to this. Noting that a large number of mental health consumers are survivors, Harris and Fallot (2001) discuss the mental health system's failure to address their needs, suggesting a paradigm shift in order to refocus the system on trauma and the importance of safety. An example of failing to consider safety first occurred when a trauma-based mental health program with a city-wide service area built its main offices in a high-crime neighborhood because rent was low. Travel to this location scared clients, causing a decreased sense of safety. Another example is providers who do not always ask about or understand trauma despite its high rate of incidence.

Court systems, can be among the organizations survivors interact with that do not address trauma. In court, it is not unusual that victims of traumatic crimes wait in the same courtroom or waiting area as their perpetrators. Integrated Domestic Violence (IDV) Courts, which are designed to hear all legal matters related to domestic violence, now require separate waiting areas for victims. Even these progressive courtrooms, however, often unwittingly fail to protect survivors as they tackle one of the most difficult aspects of healing – confronting the perpetrator in the justice system (Levy, Ross, & Guthrie, 2008). For example, when working as a victim advocate in an IDV courtroom, one practitioner walked survivors to the train, while telling the abusive partner to go back to the courtroom and wait, because, though survivors were well protected inside the courtroom, they were typically not protected on their way to lunch or home.

Children's Advocacy Centers work with child survivors of abuse to prepare them for court, reduce the number of times the child is interviewed about the abuse, and advocate for testimony to be conducted in chambers with the offender elsewhere, when allowed by law (Finkelhor, Cross, & Cantor, 2006). This attention to survivors' needs is a crucial step in the right direction. Other systems need to incorporate similar measures, ensuring survivors' protection and safety as they interact with systems designed to support them.

TRAUMA INFORMED CARE

Trauma informed care (TIC) addresses survivors' needs for protection and security by: (1) focusing on issues of safety and trust and (2) ensuring services promote growth and healing without triggering past trauma. These principles of TIC: Safety, choice, collaboration, trustworthiness and empowerment, operate when programs provide care via healthy professional relationships not reminiscent of past trauma, empowering survivors by promoting post-traumatic growth (PTG) (Levenson, 2017).

The results of care that is not trauma informed are evident and wreck havoc on organizations. Not only can clients be inadvertently triggered by professional

> **Definitions**
>
> * *Post-traumatic growth (PTG)* – Condition resulting from exposure to traumatic events that causes symptoms that include the ability to see trauma from positive perspectives, to find benefit in it, to attach meaning to it that makes sense and inspires and to make constructive and helpful behavioral changes as a result

relationships that mimic those with abusers, but the triggering can spread to staff as well until it infiltrates the organization as a whole. Examples of this include clients who do not feel seen or heard by social workers who, burdened by large caseloads and burned out by survivors' trauma stories, rush through interviews without truly connecting (Bloom, 2010).

The organizational stress this creates can lead to more dysfunction, potentially traumatizing clients even more. The "Sanctuary Model" was developed to take trauma informed care to another level, addressing this issue and providing organizational healing (Bloom, 2010). An organizational self-assessment and planning protocol has been developed to aid this process and can be utilized with existing organizations and when planning for new programs (Harris & Fallot, 2001). This and other forms of trauma-focused care have become so prevalent that institutions such as Substance Abuse and Mental Health Services Administration (SAMHSA) and American Psychological Association (APA) have developed guidelines and competencies to address them, demonstrating the need for other organizations in the field to follow their example and emphasizing the importance of keeping a focus on program development (American Psychological Association, 2015; Substance Abuse and Mental Health Services Administration, 2014).

PROGRAM DEVELOPMENT THEORY AND STAGES

The process of program development involves four phases: (1) problem analysis and needs assessment, through which we determine the type and extent of need for new or modified programs; (2) development of a program rationale, where we create a program hypothesis, mission, goal and objectives; (3) program implementation, which involves putting the ideas into action and (4) program evaluation and monitoring, which it is particularly important to address soon after the program is implemented in order to ensure that the new program is effective (Kettner, Moroney, & Martin, 2016).

The trauma-based program example outlined below illustrates key concepts in program development at each stage of the process. As is noted, the input of frontline staff and survivors is key to keeping pertinent issues at the forefront during the development process. For more information regarding program development theory and phases, see the Resources section at the end of the chapter.

In this program example, a lack of appropriate mental health resources for military in an area with many returning from active service was identified as a gap in services. Data was collected and analyzed, literature and best-practice research reviewed, and input from stakeholders solicited. The needs assessment identified a reticence to use existing mental health resources. It was hypothesized that this was due to a combination of fear and a lack of support/understanding of mental healthcare within the military culture of the community, pointing to a need for culturally sensitive resources.

This directive program goal – to promote understanding of mental health services in the military community so that more traumatized veterans seek needed services – and this measurable program objective – to increase utilization of evidence-based mental health services by veterans who served in active duty 50% by January of next year – were developed. Developers, staff and stakeholders designed specific activities based on program goals/objectives and set up timelines for each based on staff ability/readiness, balanced with the need for services. These included (1) mental health service providers developing relationships within the community and (2) creating forums for stakeholder education on mental healthcare. Among the stakeholders were military support systems, chaplain programs and other existing and trusted community support structures.

Evaluation was also planned for with questionnaires handed to members of support groups and digital tracking systems designed to generate evaluation reports. For example, one real-time evaluation was the expansion of a group developed for military men and women parenting young children. When it grew from four to sixteen members in the first group cycle, another staff member was located to start a second group.

TRAUMA PROGRAM DEVELOPMENT ISSUES

There are specific program development issues to address when working with trauma survivors such as the need to involve stakeholder groups. Stakeholders are individuals or groups of people who have a vested interest in the success of the program, including clinicians, survivors, funders, referring agencies and community members, among others. Clinicians are tasked with voicing the needs of survivors as well as ensuring that the needs assessment process does not trigger survivors who participate.

Outside stakeholders such as potential funders and trauma experts lend research support, reality checks as to what is fundable, and information on best practices in the field to ensure that new programs do not make the mistakes of their predecessors. This assures limited resources are used well and effectively.

A FIELD DIVIDED

When there are a variety of specialized programs addressing different types of trauma it can make it difficult for survivors with multiple trauma experiences to have their needs met by one program. Examples include programs for survivors of specific disaster such as September 11th, domestic violence survivors with criminal court cases, and children exposed to domestic violence. The divided and specific nature of trauma programs, while an asset in many circumstances, can also lead to a disconnected, disorganized and internally competitive field. Social workers find themselves at the doors of the local, state and federal governments, sometimes as allies, but often as competitors for necessary legislative change and funding.

In order to put the well-being and healing of survivors above each program's self-interest and to advocate for social justice, an increased understanding of the array of programs designed to serve survivors is needed as well as a focus on working collaboratively. One example of this is the field of family violence, which includes child abuse, intimate partner violence and elder abuse. Though there has been progress, historically programs addressing the needs in each area competed for limited resources and were often adversaries, despite the fact that any form of violence in the home can negatively impact all family members (Ehrensaft, 2008). To address this issue, representatives from these specialties came together in one jurisdiction and formed a council that meets regularly to support communication, partnership and shared advocacy, advancing the causes of all.

As an upside to the division of programs for survivors, social workers have learned from each program about the varying needs of survivors of different kinds of trauma and cultures. In the domestic violence movement, for example, workers discovered the danger of diagnosing survivors with depression or even post-traumatic stress disorder (PTSD). In some courtrooms, batterers use these diagnoses to argue that survivors are unfit parents. Though judges have become more aware of these tactics, survivors may still lose their children or have their children exposed to unsafe visitation as a result. Without programs targeted to the needs of survivors of domestic violence, social workers would be unaware of the danger of giving a client a diagnosis in these situations.

In sum, learning from experiences of other programs and combining with other programs where appropriate, can help serve trauma survivors' broader needs. Collaborative projects funded through joint proposals or by co-locating related services to provide a holistic continuum of care for survivors are two examples of models for combining programs and services. When it is not appropriate to combine services, advocating for survivors of trauma with one voice reduces competition for dollars and legislative changes.

Definitions

*   *Post-traumatic stress disorder (PTSD)* – A disorder resulting from exposure to traumatic events that causes symptoms lasting at least a month that include emotional responses of fear, horror or helplessness; flashbacks and/or nightmares of events; avoidance of reminders of the event; and increased arousal

---

Tips

*   Consider where clients are most often referred. Determine whether funding or advocacy efforts could be improved through partnership. Broach the issue with a colleague at the potential partner program, keeping in mind that although partnership creates a stronger coalition that is more likely to lead to needed change, it also requires compromise

---

PARTNERSHIPS, WHOLE-CLIENT APPROACH, ONE-STOP SHOPPING

When designing programs, developers understand that survivors of trauma have complex and layered needs. Many survivors have experienced more than one form of trauma (Bayard, Williams, Saunders, & Fitzgerald, 2008; Herman, 1992). And survivors often note that certain programs meet their mental health needs or address specific traumatic experiences, but do not help with obtaining medication or housing. In addition, going from one program to the next, retelling their trauma stories, can be overwhelming. One way to support the safety of survivors is "one-stop shopping," as with the Family Justice Center (FJC) model which embraces a whole-client approach. FJCs, Children's Advocacy Centers and other models that address multiple needs under one roof, represent multidisciplinary partnerships between potential players in a survivor's life, including district attorneys, law enforcement, lawyers, case managers, job training support, medical assistance and mental health experts (for more information, see the FJC and National Children's Alliance websites in the Resources section at the end of the chapter). One-stop models that include multiple agencies housed under one roof also allow for increased cultural sensitivity and linguistic competence as they bring together agencies with varied cultural roots.

For those programs that cannot be housed under one roof, partnerships with other providers are essential for survivors. For example, a program for survivors of trauma worked with a substance abuse and a job training program at the same hospital to meet their survivors' needs. They also sought the support of trained volunteer case managers to work with survivors' entitlement benefits and concrete service needs in order to ensure that the program worked with the whole person, not just one of the presenting issues.

Multidisciplinary partnerships and one-stop shopping models require work in order to maintain effective inter-agency relationships, but in the end survivors' needs are met more comprehensively and this creates needed safety (Lew et al., 2007). In the case of The Children's Program (see case study at end of chapter), survivors' children were referred by case managers who worked down the hall from The Children's Program staff. During the referral process, case managers, whom the survivors already trusted, walked the survivors down the hall and introduced them to a member of the children's staff so that trust, safety and client information could transfer to the newest member of the survivor's support team. This process worked despite team members working for different organizations (A. Stewart-Kahn, personal communication, March 1, 2007).

Tips

- When partnering with non-trauma-focused organizations to meet clients' comprehensive needs more effectively, ensure that partner agencies have been adequately trained on trauma issues, symptoms and ways to support survivors

---

PROGRAM FLEXIBILITY

Developers must stay sensitive to survivors' sense of safety, understanding that questions asked to identify unmet needs can be triggering for survivors. For example, one program developer asked a group of survivors which aspects of their trauma still felt the most "unhealed." This is what transpired:

Program developer: As we develop programs to support you, we would like to know which parts of your trauma experience still feel the most unhealed.
Group: *Long silence.*
Survivor 1: Well, that's difficult to talk about.
Group: *Continued silence.*
Survivor 2: For me, it's that any time I see a child at a playground, I feel a sense of terror that someone is going to hurt him. *Silence.* It's gotten so that I walk blocks out of my way to avoid schools and playgrounds. *Beginning to cry.*
Program developer: I'm sorry, I didn't mean to upset you.

While the facilitator intended to obtain information that would aid development of a program that could meet survivors' complex needs, her questions caused survivors to dissociate or become overwhelmed with emotions as they focused on the scariest part of their experiences (A. Stewart-Kahn, personal communication, March 1, 2007). As with every aspect of program development for survivors, flexibility and patience are important (Goodman & Brown, 2008). Survivors might have a higher rate of missed appointments due to their situations, and programs that give up on them quickly will not meet their needs. Likewise, survivors might need to stop a data collection interview or clinical session before it is complete if they feel unsafe. This reality requires flexibility in the program development process.

EVIDENCE-BASED PROGRAMS

Increasingly, social workers feel pressure from funders and other stakeholders to use evidence-based practice. While evidence-based practices represent an important step forward in the field because they can bring valuable information that allows programs to ensure quality programming, program developers face two challenges. First, these models are often expensive and labor-intensive, making it difficult for social service organizations to afford the associated staffing and training unless they find additional funding. Second, program developers need to balance the pressure to adopt evidence-based models with the needs of survivors.

While some models provide a good fit for the needs of the developer's specific population, others do not. Each model requires careful research to ensure appropriateness. One abuse prevention organization solved these two challenges by carefully researching various evidence-based models that related to their clients' needs. They decided on one called Triple P – Positive Parenting Program® (Triple, n.d.) and worked with local government partners, participating in a pilot program in which the government paid for the training in exchange for the organization participating in research that would ensure the model was appropriate in the setting before introducing it to other similar organizations.

Tips

- If the cost of purchasing an evidence-based model is too high, consider seeking funding in partnership with the developers of the evidence-based model. This provides the benefit of increased funding and a new setting for research on the model for the developers and access to the evidence-based model and research grants typically not available for the service provider

SPECIAL CONSIDERATIONS

While some trauma-based programs focus on chronic societal issues such as gang violence, others focus on time sensitive issues such as the aftermath of disaster. Traumatic issues are by their nature crises that require immediate attention so social workers must respond rapidly to meet the needs of survivors. Despite this time pressure, the program development process requires a painstaking and thorough step-by-step process to ensure services chosen for implementation optimally fit the needs being addressed. In addition, survivors must be kept safe at all times. In one unfortunate example, a post-earthquake trauma program did not screen volunteers who cared for children while their parents dealt with the damage of the earthquake. As a result, a predator, who no doubt noted and took advantage of the chaotic planning, sexually abused many of the children.

As discussed throughout this book, working with survivors of trauma can be both inspiring and draining (see chapter 1 on secondary trauma for more information). Because of this, it is essential that program developers consider issues of staff support and self-care. During the needs assessment phase, facilitators can also consider the needs of the program staff. For example, will staff need additional supervision or training, given the nature of the work? Do current supervisors need additional training in order to provide effective clinical supervision and support to direct service staff? These factors bear consideration when starting a new trauma-based program.

TRAUMA PROGRAM DEVELOPMENT PITFALLS

Stretching for funding is a common program development pitfall. Access to funding improves with a comprehensive program development process because funders are more likely to allocate resources to well-thought-out programs. Concise, thorough explanations help funders understand what went into development. The funding proposal is also important (see the Resources section at the end of the chapter for more information on proposal writing).

Funding creates additional issues where survivors are concerned. Scarcity of funds and competition can cause developers to squeeze program ideals into funding streams not appropriate for planned services. When this happens, pressure from funders may lead to dilution of program goals. Open and honest conversations with potential funders ensures understanding of program objectives and full disclosure funding.

In the case of The Children's Program (see case study at end of chapter), funders wanted short-term counseling so that more clients could be served. Staff determined that the four-to eight-session treatment initially discussed with funders was not clinically appropriate for survivors with serious trauma issues and could, in fact, compromise safety. Managers told funders they could not fulfill contract requirements because of changes necessary to the service model, but agreed to expand educational outreach in order to meet funder's goals (A. Stewart-Kahn, personal communication, March 1, 2007).

Mission Creep can also cause problems. Program developers run the risk of losing sight of their original mission as they get caught up in meeting survivors' needs, at times offering services outside the realm of what they can support. This "mission creep" undermines the organization, as organizations that spread themselves too thin often experience staff morale or funding issues. Over-extending trauma workers can make it difficult to create and maintain the self-care environment critical to protecting them from secondary trauma. When one organization hired paraprofessional case managers to work with survivors of crime who needed both concrete and mental health assistance, the case managers found themselves attempting to provide mental health support without sufficient training or supervision. Turnover at the organization became a problem and staff experienced vicarious trauma. As a result, clients' needs were not met (A. Stewart-Kahn, personal communication, March 1, 2007).

Another issue is that staff members may be anxious about the evaluation phase of the development process. To alleviate anxiety, it is essential that program developers and managers articulate how evaluation helps improve services. Also key is keeping the door open for questions and concerns from stakeholders (Gazelle, Buxbaum, & Daniels, 2001; Kettner et al., 2016).

Tips

- Navigating staff concerns can become tricky. Anxiety can be alleviated by reiterating that program evaluation is about evaluating the program model performance, not staff performance
- Ignoring the work required during evaluation by front-line workers is not productive. Instead, acknowledging extra work, such as digitizing case records (often a first step in developing evaluation systems), but pointing out that work can be eliminated once the learning curve ends, can help with morale

---

The appropriateness of communication with funders, press and other interested parties should also be considered. These parties, who may help obtain future funding and increase understanding of trauma in the community, often want to hear survivors' stories. However, if survivors are pushed to talk to media or funders prematurely, their safety can be compromised and healing may stall or regress. Members of the media, for example, may not understand trauma issues and inadvertently ask questions that re-trigger traumatic experiences.

Instead, survivors further along in the recovery process could be interviewed or stories that protect the identity of survivors could be compiled, painting a picture for funders and other stakeholders of the trauma experience. The key question to keep in mind when making decisions about survivors and the media is: Will talking to funders or media be part of the survivor's healing process? If not, the answer to a request from the media must always be no, despite pressure to the contrary.

Tips

• One agency developed a "Speakers Bureau" for interested survivors who were deemed safe enough to do so. Survivors received training on media and public speaking, so they could tell their stories in a way that could be understood by listeners. Survivors were also supported during the process

---

Case Study

The Sanctuary for Families Children's Program (The Children's Program) at the FJC of New York City in Brooklyn was created in response to a need for services for children of FJC clients. Its program development process is an example of effective problem analysis. Had developers defined the *program need* as clinical intervention for child survivors of family trauma in Brooklyn, they would have limited options for program design to specific mental health interventions. Instead, the program utilized a relatively quick needs assessment process that led to defining the problem as a dearth of services for Brooklyn children exposed to and impacted by family violence, as well as a lack of understanding in the Brooklyn community of the impact of exposure to violence on children (A. Stewart-Kahn, personal communication, March 1, 2007).

During the *needs assessment*, program developers talked with advocates at the FJC to learn about child survivors' needs. Developers added their feedback to data from current literature related to the impact of family violence on children and best practices along with other data collected by the agency (A. Stewart-Kahn, personal communication, March 1, 2007). The literature affirmed the dangers of exposure to violence (Edwards et al., 2005). After collecting data, program developers sought the input of adult and child survivors. Advocates and survivors became an informal stakeholder group for this program development process.

After developers established the *problem/need*, they attempted to understand what societal and familial situations led to these issues. As a result of this process, developers understood the chain of events that brought survivors to their door, creating a *program hypothesis* that enabled intervention along that chain, not just at the end point. Specifically, the program identified key FJC referral sources and created a prevention-oriented training seminar for school counselors, teachers, early childhood educators, after-school program staff and other community members. The training clarified the impact of violence on children and taught ways to assist families facing trauma issues. Developers also created a clinical intervention that combined concrete service provision (including crisis financial assistance, support with housing searches, referrals for needed programs, etc.); advocacy with schools, courts and other systems; and non-directive and directive play therapy (A. Stewart-Kahn, personal communication, March 1, 2007).

Additionally, according to the needs assessment, family members who survive violence together often feel isolated from each other and find it difficult to communicate their shared experiences of abuse. With this understanding, developers utilized a best-practice model to create support groups for parents and children who had survived trauma and linked these groups together in an isolation-reducing format. (Peled & Davis, 1995; A. Stewart-Kahn, personal communication, March 1, 2007).

Based on The Children's Program problem analysis and hypothesis, goals and objectives were determined and funder's suggestions incorporated. The objectives for the first twelve months of programming included:

- Conduct outreach with 1,000 key community members in order to educate them about the incidence and impact of family trauma and train them on how to support family members
- Conduct family-based support groups for adult and children survivors (40 clients in total), in which survivors learn about domestic violence and its impacts, develop safety through peer support, become less isolated and gain insight
- Create individual treatment plans for children whose needs are not met within the group context (45 children in total), for example individual therapy, advocacy, family work, educational/developmental assessment, case management and concrete services (A. Stewart-Kahn, personal communication, March 1, 2007)

Developers returned to stakeholders to review program goals and objectives. Stakeholders noted that objectives would require cultural sensitivity, given the racial and ethnic diversity of the geographic location, and that there might be families for whom coming to the Center would be neither safe nor feasible. As a result, developers added the objective of creating a seamless web of community-based referrals for survivors not able to physically access The Children's Program services, or in need of cultural or linguistic support not available in the program. Developers also created a cross-training program with many of the referral providers to educate them specifically about domestic violence and educated program staff about specific cultural issues (A. Stewart-Kahn, personal communication, March 1, 2007).

Initial service monitoring for evaluation purposes revealed underfunding. Workers interviewed during the needs assessment thought 1% to 5% of survivors on their caseloads would seek services for their children. Instead, over 40% did because other survivors told them the program was safe. The two counselors originally funded to staff the program could not meet this need. Program managers and the host FJC site used this data to seek additional funding, interns and other support in order to expand the program (A. Stewart-Kahn, personal communication, March 1, 2007).

Developers also addressed client satisfaction early on. Group evaluations indicated the group cycle was too short. Clinicians agreed that trauma response could be too severe for one session a week. Select members began to attend two sessions per week, especially during crisis (A. Stewart-Kahn, personal communication, March 1, 2007). While many organizations do not have the means for complex program evaluation, every organization can implement basic evaluation and monitoring of programs. This example shows it is an essential part of the development process.

Tips

- When creating a program objective, ensure it is specific, time-limited and measurable before making promises to funders or other stake-holders. Ask: When can this objective be reached and how will I know when this has been achieved? If you can answer these two questions, your objective is appropriate

---

RESOURCES

Kettner, P.M., Moroney, R.M., & Martin, L.L. (2016). *Designing and managing programs: An effectiveness-based approach.* Thousand Oaks, CA: Sage.

Yuen, F.K., Terao, K.L., & Schmidt, A.M. (2013). *Effective grant writing and program evaluation for human service professionals.* Hoboken, NJ: John Wiley & Sons.

ONLINE RESOURCES

Family Justice Center: http://www.familyjusticecenter.org/

National Children's Alliance: http://www.nationalchildrensalliance.org/

Substance Abuse and Mental Health Services Administration. *SAMHSA's Concept of Trauma and Guidance for a Trauma-Informed Approach.* https://store.samhsa.gov/product/ SAMHSA-s-Concept-of-Trauma-and-Guidance-for-a-Trauma-Informed-Approach/ SMA14-4884

Practice Exercises and Questions

- Discuss examples of the importance of considering survivor safety during program development
- List and summarize the stages of program development
- Why is it important to include stakeholders and survivors in the process of program development?
- Describe pitfalls that can be encountered during the program development process
- Why is program evaluation important and what can happen if it does not occur?

Program Development Summary

Follow Four Program Development Steps

- *Needs assessment and problem analysis*
- *Development of rationale, goals and objectives*
- *Implementation*
- *Evaluation*

Program Development Issues Specific to Trauma Programs

- *Include all stakeholders in the process, particularly survivors*
- *Address whole-client needs, creating safety through partnerships with other agencies and one-stop shopping models*
- *Promptly and flexibly respond to survivors' needs whenever possible*
- *Consider evidence-based models and whether they are a good fit for the needs of your population*
- *Start with support for staff. The earlier support issues are considered, the more likely staff will avoid secondary trauma*

Avoid Program Development Pitfalls

*   *Stretching for funding*
*   *Mission creep*
*   *Staff fear of evaluation*
*   *Involving survivors in press/communication when appropriate*

Chapter 19

Advocating for Survivors

Being a social worker often requires going "beyond the clinical walls" (Gomez & Yassen, 2007, p. 260), providing case management, referrals, accompaniment to appointments and advocacy. This chapter discusses, in the context of working with trauma survivors, the history of social work and advocacy, advocacy steps and pitfalls and both micro (or case) advocacy and macro (or cause) advocacy.

Disempowerment is generally at the core of trauma's impact (Herman, 1992; Levy Simon, 2004) and advocacy is designed to address this. Further, social justice, the goal of most advocacy efforts, is a core value of social work practice according to the National Association of Social Workers' Code of Ethics (National Association of Social Workers, 2017) and advocacy is one of social workers' cardinal roles (Hepworth, R.H. Rooney, Rooney, Strom-Gottfried, & Larsen, 2010).

TUNE IN TO POWERLESSNESS

Social workers are challenged by their work with survivors. It can be tiring, frustrating and difficult. This is compounded by a sense of powerlessness due to inability to (1) make the system respond to clients' needs as it should, (2) ensure their safety or (3) wave a magic wand and create healing. This same sense of powerlessness is generally felt even more profoundly by survivors.

Definitions

- *Powerlessness or disempowerment* – A feeling that may result from experiencing or working with trauma and involving the belief or reality that one is unable to take control or make changes in one's life
- *Empowerment* – A feeling that can result through the healing process from trauma in which the survivor gains or regains a sense of control

---

To tune in to powerlessness, first, imagine the end of a long, difficult work day. Two clients did not attend their appointments and you are worried about them. Other clients seem to have taken steps backwards and your supervisor had to cancel supervision due to a budget meeting where she hopes to help avoid drastic funding cuts. It is likely you feel a combination of anger, worry, fatigue, stress and hopelessness and you may also feel disempowered or powerless.

You will ideally use self-care techniques, support systems and other resources to refresh yourself at the end of this day. Since these are resources many survivors do not have, they often feel disempowered. Advocacy is designed to help clients – and, in turn, social workers – respond proactively and effectively to feelings of disempowerment and powerlessness.

MICRO-LEVEL ADVOCACY WITH SURVIVORS

Social workers are uniquely poised to engage in micro-level advocacy (Freddolino, Moxley, & Hyduk, 2004; Levy Simon, 2004; Mickelson, 1995). If an individual is experiencing injustice or lack of access to services and you are able to remedy this, then you are prepared for micro-level advocacy. Micro-level advocacy may include things like going with a client to court, a referral source or even a supermarket. This unique use of the self (i.e., working with clients outside the typical clinical context) can be challenging as it changes professional boundaries. Despite this, micro-level advocacy, has been an integral part of social works' history (Mickelson, 1995).

Definitions

- *Micro-level advocacy* – Working with individuals or small groups to help them create change in their lives through interventions with the systems (i.e., social service and government service delivery and response systems) around them. The goals of this practice are to both change systems and increase survivors' sense of empowerment

---

THEORY AND PRINCIPLES

Some have written specifically about micro-level advocacy with survivors (Gomez & Yassen, 2007; Hays, Green, Orr, & Flowers, 2007; Kelley, Schwerin, Farrar, & Lane, 2005; Tam, 2007) and others have outlined theories, structures and principles that can be applied to traumatized individuals (Bateman, 2000; Friedman, 2004; Lens, 2005; Schneider & Lester, 2001). All agree that the work is done in partnership, with social workers guiding rather than leading these initiatives (Hays, Green, Orr, & Flowers, 2007).

Summarizing advocacy frameworks from the literature in the context of trauma interventions, four key messages emerge (Bateman, 2000; Friedman,

2004; Gomez & Yassen, 2007; Hays et al., 2007; Kelley et al., 2005; Lens, 2005; Schneider & Lester, 2001; Tam, 2007). First, advocacy, like any social work tool, should begin with assessment and setting an objective. Assessment questions include: What problem is the client facing and would micro-level advocacy remedy it? Is the survivor is in a safe enough emotional state to pursue this objective and work toward empowerment? Assessing for anxiety, depression and a sense of empowerment versus hopelessness is also critical to this process.

Tips

- When assessing whether clients are prepared for the challenges involved with advocacy work, apply clinical skills. For example, consider clients' levels of emotional and physical safety by asking if they feel safe discussing their stories with new people and if they feel safe in general. Ask clients if there is anything they try to stop thinking about (but cannot), if they have nightmares often or if they often feel "worried," assessing for PTSD-related symptoms

---

Second, discerning who is in control of situations and has the power to make changes is particularly relevant for survivors whose sense of power may have been obliterated. These conversations are not only important to advocacy, but can also be therapeutic. For example, Janet, a survivor of stranger rape, felt intimidated about talking with the assistant district attorney (ADA) prosecuting her case. As they prepared for her to meet the ADA, her social worker learned Janet had difficulty disagreeing with males she did not know. Working on this issues as she interacted with the ADA helped Janet regain a sense of empowerment with men. She said, "Eventually, I told him what I wanted and he actually listened. I realized this was a surprise to me because I'd tried so hard to reason with [the attacker] and he just wouldn't listen. I'm thinking I can try and talk with that professor now about my grade."

Tips

- Survivors often face "power holders" who have the ability to change their lives. For example, a welfare worker could decide to designate them a crime victim and grant a work waiver as they heal. Social workers can (1) help survivors by therapeutically discussing the imbalances in order to prepare for frustration, anger or fear arising when self-advocating and (2) by sharing information/experiences about specific power holders they may encounter, including approaches that have worked with them in the past

---

Third, understanding leverage is an essential component in micro-level advocacy (Bateman, 2000). For example, in the aftermath of trauma, survivors who lose their sense of power may be revictimized by the systems designed to protect them. Understanding their rights as survivors gives them leverage that is essential to advocacy. This discussion between the aforementioned rape victim, Janet, and her social worker demonstrates the importance of leverage:

Janet:	Why would he [ADA] talk to me? I need to talk to him for more than the five minutes he gives me on the phone, but I don't know how to make him take the time. He has so many cases and he keeps telling me that he isn't *my* lawyer, he is the lawyer for the people of the state of Arizona. I'm not quite sure what that means, but I'm the victim here, right?
Social worker:	It sounds like you feel frustrated that the person who holds all the power to move your case forward against your attacker isn't really listening to you.
Janet:	YES! I feel frustrated. Of course I'm frustrated, but I don't know what to do since it doesn't seem like he has to pay any attention to me if he doesn't want to.
Social worker:	We need to figure out how to get him to spend some time with you so you can explain your issues. I think that ADAs working in this locality are required to document at least one hour of time with the crime victim before making a decision about how to proceed.
Janet:	Really? Well there is no way he has spent one hour with me.
Social worker:	Do you think you could explain to him that you learned this information and would like to set up a 45-minute meeting to discuss your point of view which he can document in his case record as time he spent with the crime victim?
Janet:	Can we practice before I call? I think that helped last time.
Social worker:	Of course we can. This information may give you a bit of leverage in the situation and practicing in advance might help you feel more confident.

MICRO-LEVEL ADVOCACY TECHNIQUES AND POTENTIAL PITFALLS WITH SURVIVORS

Since healthy relationships are crucial to survivors' healing, it is essential for social workers doing micro-level advocacy with survivors to attend to relationships and collaboration (Cohen, de la Vega, & Watson, 2001; Finkelstein et al., 2005; Hays et al., 2007). Paternalism and/or taking over for clients during the advocacy process is a common pitfall (Kiselica & Robinson, 2001; Mickelson, 1995) as is "rescuing" survivors in challenging advocacy situations.

For example, during difficult conversations with a "power holders," social workers may jump in and speak on behalf of survivors, rather than stay silently supportive and debrief later.

One way to avoid this pitfall is to ensure clarity in advance regarding your role in a advocacy meeting. Ask yourself and your client if you are there to support, lead the meeting or in some other capacity. Consider setting up signals for your client to utilize if they are feeling overwhelmed or anxious during the meeting and need your intervention. If you have established this, ensure that you stick to it despite wanting to help your client when the meeting appears difficult for him or her.

Tips

- Since (1) the role of advocate is often difficult to navigate and (2) issues of rescue fantasies, power dynamics, secondary trauma and professional boundaries can come up for social workers. Seek regular supervision when conducting advocacy work with survivors of trauma.

Some survivors appear ready to take back their power through advocacy. Others need considerable support in this process. Narrative approaches are one way support can be provided. Through storytelling, survivors are encouraged to "rewrite" their own experiences to include moments when they felt powerful or utilized survivor skills rather than feeling disempowered (Roberts & Hamilton, 2010). This narrative work can be conducted with children through book projects or sand trays (Gil, 2006); and with adults through journaling, group work, reading stories of survival or other creative techniques (Freeman & Combs, 1996). See the Resources section at the end of the chapter to learn more about narrative therapy techniques and approaches.

Since the ability to tell one's story is a crucial aspect of self-advocacy, survivors' storytelling is often the first step in advocacy work. For example, one program worked with a survivor to write, rewrite and practice her story of domestic violence and her children's abuse prior to testifying before the local city council on a city budgeting issue that would have an impact on the funding of the program in which she received therapy. Over the course of this process, the victim's story changed from victim to survivor and she noted after her testimony, "that it felt like the finale in this big play I've been in. I told them what really happened so now if they don't fund us, they know the real deal."

Some programs teach skills by utilizing speech coaches, writing teachers and other often pro bono support. Social workers working with clients can teach and model advocacy storytelling skills by putting the call on speaker phone when they are making a referral so the survivor can hear the interaction. The social worker and survivor can then debrief regarding the call afterwards to see if the survivor has any questions or concerns. The following is an inter-action with one survivor, Eleanor, who listened in on a call between her social worker and her attorney:

Eleanor: She doesn't listen to me the way she just listened to you ... why do you think that is? I guess I need to learn to speak my mind, but it's really scary because she has a fancy office and so little time for me.

Social worker: Sounds like there were a lot of things going on for you when you listened in on that call, including how to make someone listen to your story and how you want to tell your story. The idea of telling your story to someone who has so much power can be really scary.

Eleanor: Yes. I wish I could tell it just like you did on the phone.

Social worker: Well, it's sort of a different situation because I'm telling your story on your behalf on that call so the emotions are really different. I wonder if there is a way for us to help you tell your story to your lawyer that feels safe and so she will listen.

Eleanor: Maybe.

Social worker: I was thinking we could start by you telling me your story and pretending I'm the lawyer. We can write it down today so you can practice it in a safe place. When you come back next week, we can practice again and then, when you are ready, we can think about calling the lawyer together, but this time having you tell the story.

Eleanor: I have to admit it scares me, but I would love to make her lis-ten the way you just did ... I think that would feel really good.

Several weeks later, Eleanor was able to tell her story to her lawyer in person without the social worker present, and advocated for herself in the process: "She looked at her watch before we even got started and I said, 'I know you are very busy, but I need five more minutes of your time today' and she stopped looking at her watch and listened!"

Finally, we recommend processing advocacy interventions with both survi-vors and supervisors. With supervisors, we can share specifics about the advo-cacy outcomes that could be helpful in the future – such as when an essential social agency intakes new clients; or when to submit an application so a worker with a better understanding of trauma reviews it. With survivors, processing the experience can be healing. For example, a former child soldier, who experienced severe anxiety when talking with doctors about his medical needs, learned that he was able to articulate his needs if he took someone with to appointments, and planned for it in advance with his social worker. His confidence began to build as he processed this and realized that doctors were on his side rather than on the side of the militia as was the case in his country of origin.

Case Study

A hospital-based rape crisis program hired social workers to respond 24/7 to rape survivors presenting at the hospital. Jesse, a 14-year-old male, was brought to the pediatric emergency room (ER) after being raped by a worker in his group home setting. The social worker responding felt he was calmer than she would have expected, until she learned he had been raped multiple times and went into the foster care system due to molestation by his stepfather. Understanding his experiences with multiple, complex traumas might contribute to varied reactions, including the apparent calm with which he presented, the worker proceeded carefully.

Rape crisis programs ensure clients' needs and rights are met while in the ER and that they receive care afterwards. The social worker advocated on a micro level with nurses and doctors sharing his trauma experiences (with Jesse's permission) and ensuring his medical needs were met and that processes were fully explained to him. Unfortunately, an assistant responsible for getting Jesse clothing so that his soiled ones could be used as evidence told the social worker he did not believe Jesse's story and mocked traits of Jesse's that he said were "faggy." She intervened with the assistant, reminding him of his role. This went well until it came time to find Jesse underwear and the assistant said, "Do you even wear underwear?"

Jesse responded by shrinking into the corner of the room and mumbling curses at the assistant. The social worker suspected this was a protective reaction, but was unsure, from an advocacy perspective, about whether to intervene and take over for Jesse or leave him to manage the situation himself, given his obvious resilience and strength. She decided to intervene in a way that kept Jesse involved. Asking the assistant to step out of the room, she debriefed with Jesse about his feelings, his goals while interacting with the assistant, and how he wanted to handle it. Jesse said, "I want to respond to that asshole about my boxers." They quickly role-played the language he would use and asked the assistant to return.

Jesse said, "Sir, I would appreciate it if you would help me by doing your job and getting me the clothes I need so I can go home. I don't particularly care what you think of me, but I do need my clothes and it's been a very long night." The assistant brought his clothes and the social worker debriefed with Jesse afterwards. The next day, she discussed the case with her supervisor and discovered the assistant had been written up for similar interactions with male victims in the ER. They agreed this should be added to his record while protecting Jesse's confidentiality.

MACRO-LEVEL ADVOCACY WITH SURVIVORS OF TRAUMA

Macro-level advocacy, like its micro-level counterpart, has many names including class advocacy, cause advocacy, political activism, systems advocacy, community advocacy, group advocacy and citizens advocacy, and is defined by Schneider and Lester (2001) as "promoting changes in policies and practices affecting all persons in a certain group or class" (p. 196). In the case of trauma survivors, it is social workers' role to seek to improve policies and practices that affect them. Indeed, Herman (1992) reminds us that without political activism, our understanding and response to trauma would not be what it is today. For example, advocates working to ensure that the US military fully acknowledges the impact of war trauma on soldiers are conducting macro-level advocacy with and for survivors of trauma; and at the same time are advancing public understanding of the impact of war trauma.

Definitions

- *Macro-level advocacy* – Working with a population or sub-population of survivors to encourage or demand changes in practices and policies affecting them

---

Social workers have historically been involved in this form of intervention (Gomez & Yassen, 2007; Kiselica & Robinson, 2001; Mickelson, 1995) and (M.S. Sherraden, Slosar and Sherraden (2002)) argue that ethically social workers can and should take the lead as major players in high-level policy development and reform – a form of macro-level advocacy. Beyond historical and ethical reasons the goal of advocating for survivors is to work toward social justice and healing.

Advocates from other professions, such as lawyers pursuing class-action lawsuits on behalf of survivors, can have different mandates than those of social workers. Lawyer's responsibilities, for example, do not require attending to healing, increasing the need for social workers. In addition, one author suggests that advocacy work can be good self-care, potentially reducing secondary trauma for social workers working in the field by allowing them to positively harness survivors' painful stories for constructive change (Hesse, 2002).

THEORY, STAGES AND PRINCIPLES

Macro-level advocacy has distinct and intentional stages that include: (1) setting objectives; (2) selecting a target audience; (3) defining the problem and determining possible solutions; (4) developing an action plan and assembling a project team; (5) conducting the intervention and (6) evaluating the process (Fisher & Penny, 1996; Friedman, 2004; Schneider & Lester, 2001).

An example of this is if survivors and social workers jointly determine that using police cars to transport children in foster care is unnecessarily stigmatizing and/or re-traumatizing, the advocacy objective can be defined as creating a policy and/or agreement with local law enforcement and protective services to ensure children are transported in unmarked vehicles whenever safety is not an issue. The target audience might be police supervisors and protective services employees and, if necessary to reach advocacy goals, the larger public, who might be rallied to apply pressure for change. The problem can be defined as a lack of understanding on the part of government employees of the impact on traumatized children of riding in police cars.

Action planning might involve bringing in a foster youth advocacy organization or similar entity to research the problem and work with social workers and their individual foster youth clients to develop a strategy and intervention. Groups like California Youth Connection often have advocates train foster youth to speak publicly about their concerns as part of their empowerment process (California Youth Connection, 2010). Adding these types of advocates to the team provides resources and increases partnership.

The intervention phase might involve brainstorming with government employees to develop a new policy, which can be reviewed by the locality's attorney and signed by the heads of police and protective services. The final step is evaluating what did and did not work. In this phase, it is important to learn from the process and to ensure adequate support and safety for survivors.

TECHNIQUES OF MACRO-LEVEL ADVOCACY WITH TRAUMA SURVIVORS

Specific macro-level advocacy techniques utilized with survivors include community organizing, collaboration with other organizations and survivors, background research and information sharing, message development, message delivery – for example to thought leaders, mass media and lobbyists – and legislative advocacy (Fairbank & Gerrity, 2007; Schneider & Lester, 2001). One such case was that before 2005, abuse cases documented by Child Protective Services in New York City were entered in the system under the name of the mother of the abused child. This process was followed whether or not the mother was the alleged perpetrator of the abuse. When the mother was not the abuser, particularly when she was a victim of trauma herself, the fact that the abuse case was in her name felt disempowering and unfair to mothers. This led to petitioning the New York City Council to change the policy so that cases were entered in the name of the abuser (Voices of Women Organizing Project, 2006).

Another macro-level technique is to conduct background research before beginning advocacy efforts (Friedman, 2004). An example could be to read and share this book with others. Social workers considering how to advocate for survivors of life-threatening illness, for example, can use this as a resource for information, statistics and subsequent development of public communications about the issue.

Finally, social workers and survivors have an important role to play in legislative advocacy. Developing collaborations with organizations charged with legislative advocacy and other experts can bring together skills and increase the likelihood of success (Schneider & Lester, 2001). A political refugee organization, for instance, pooled resources with other local organizations to pay for a part-time lobbyist in their state capital. This lobbyist kept the consortium informed of crucial upcoming legislation such as potential changes in funding for refugee organizations and, when advocacy was deemed necessary, helped craft legislative advocacy strategies.

PITFALLS IN CONDUCTING MACRO-LEVEL ADVOCACY WITH TRAUMA SURVIVORS

There are specific areas to avoid when conducting macro-level advocacy work (Schneider & Lester, 2001). First, it is essential to define and hold to advocacy objectives. Losing them as outside pressures are applied (Cohen, de la Vega, & Watson, 2001; Friedman, 2004) can undermine the success of advocacy efforts.

Tips

- Once your advocacy objective is drafted, consider posting it at your desk and the desks of other participants. Review it often and consider reading it out loud or including it in the agenda of any related meetings. These steps will help you stay focused as advocacy proceeds

---

It can also be difficult to feel successful in macro-level advocacy work, especially when politics are involved, as it is often about compromise. So even when the objective is reached, it may not feel like a victory. Processing this with involved survivors and colleagues is important. Similarly, prepare survivors and colleagues for losses and make plans to advance your cause again (Schneider & Lester, 2001).

Further, macro-level advocacy can be expensive if done comprehensively and it can be difficult to raise needed funds (Malekoff, 2000). Social workers may need to think creatively about funding. For example, foundations or donors who are not interested in direct services may fund this type of work. It is also important to understand the rules about tax deductions on advocacy-related dollars in your locality when raising money in this arena in order to avoid

potential penalties, as there are generally limits on the amount of direct advocacy work non-profit organizations are allowed to conduct with tax-exempt
dollars.

An additional and common pitfall arises when allies in the advocacy process disagree. An example of this is controversy related to whether advocating
for benefits for veterans' families should be included in initiatives designed
to benefit veterans. One group felt that if they kept their objectives narrow
and demanded benefits for veterans only, they would be more likely to suc-
ceed. A group advocating for survivors of those killed in action noted that
these individuals needed the same benefits, causing disputes within the alliance. Returning to the original purpose of the alliance, "to ensure the veterans,
families and children suffering from PTSD developed as a result of serving in
the US military receive full care and benefits," helped to guide this group to
resolution.

Finally, if working in partnership with survivors, as is recommended in
both micro-and macro-level advocacy, it is essential to ensure the objective
and intervention serve not only the organizational mission, but also, more
importantly, the healing of survivors. If testifying before the city council is
overwhelming for the survivors involved in your project, cancel the testimony
and develop an alternative such as letter writing that will help survivors safely
express their experiences and needs.

Tips

- Consider creative advocacy strategies that safely involve survivors. If
  survivors are comfortable sharing about their experiences in public,
  they can speak to media and government officials and at rallies and
  other events. If they prefer to participate more privately, consider
  letter writing, petition organizing or even making posters for rallies
  they do not yet feel safe enough to attend

Case Study

An organization that values macro-level advocacy for its ability to create
change, healing and support for staff did not have significant resources
to spend in this arena. They decided, however, to dedicate resources to
developing an advocacy platform each year. These platforms, formed by a
committee made up of staff, board members and survivors, generally contained three to five political advocacy issues that related to their clients,
survivors of domestic violence. One year, the organization focused on:

(1) housing options and policies that created economic independence for survivors; (2) equal access to family court orders of protection for teen, elder and gay and lesbian survivors of domestic violence and (3) a new human trafficking law.

Throughout the year, the advocacy campaign used various opportunities including media, advocacy days at the state capital, discussion and education forums and class-action litigation with pro bono support to advance their advocacy agenda.

Interestingly, much of the advocacy work was done in addition to the staff's normal work responsibilities, but many found the time and energy to get involved despite busy schedules. After a trip to the state capital, one colleague said, "I'm not sure I've ever felt more tired or more empowered at the same time." The two clients of the organization that went on this trip received significant support before attending, throughout the day, and as debriefed afterwards. The clients came because, as gay men who were victims of domestic violence, they had been turned away from family court when seeking restraining orders, and it was important to their own healing to ensure this did not happen to others. Their presence was essential in making the organization's advocacy agenda clear to elected officials.

RESOURCES

Freeman, A., & Combs, G. (1996). *Narrative therapy*. New York: WW Norton & Company.

Lens, V. (2005). Advocacy and argumentation in the public arena: A guide for social workers. *Social Work, 50*, 231–238.

Schneider, R.L., & Lester, L. (2001). *Social work advocacy*. Belmont, CA: Brooks/Cole Thomson Learning.

Practice Exercises and Questions

- Role-play planning Jesse's discussion with the ER assistant (from the first case study) and debriefing after
- Describe an advocacy effort you could apply to past or present social work, identifying whether it would be a micro or macro level effort
- Outline the processes of the effort described above, being careful to include any steps outlined in the chapter
- List some of the pitfalls of macro level advocacy and how to avoid them
- Talk about why advocacy is important for all social workers

Advocating for Survivors Summary

Tune in to Disempowerment

- *A major goal of advocacy is to increase survivors' sense of power, eliminating the disempowerment many feel*
- *Advocacy work can also benefit social workers by increasing their sense of power and decreasing the risk of secondary trauma*

Micro-level Advocacy

- Stages of micro-level advocacy include:
- *collaborating with survivors*
- *preparing survivors to tell their stories as an aid to advocacy*
- *evaluating and processing the efforts with survivors*

Macro-level Advocacy

- *Stages of macro-level advocacy include forethought, planning and procurement of partners and resources.*

Macro-Level Advocacy Pitfalls

- *Macro-level advocacy pitfalls include:*
- *losing the objective part way through the process*
- *failing to define success*
- *high cost of advocacy efforts*
- *disagreements among allies*
- *failing to ensure objective are geared toward survivors' healing*

Chapter 20

Prevention and Community Organizing

"To win the war against trauma, there must not only be effective interventions but also prevention" (Bryant-Davis, 2005, p. 176). This requires being "radical enough to believe that every human being deserves safety, justice, and equality" (p. 175), which can make preventing trauma and its short- and long-term impact possible. In this chapter, ways social workers can participate in prevention work are outlined.

TUNE IN TO THE IMPORTANCE OF PREVENTION

Imagine a world with no traumatic events. A parent about to hit her child receives support and stays her hand; two countries on the verge of war find resolution, preventing generations of trauma and suffering; a government learns to adequately prepare in advance of natural disaster so that, while the storm still comes, the impact is lessened and the community remains whole and supported.

Now consider times you have prevented events that could have caused trauma by reaching out to stop someone about to step front of a car, calling the police when you heard neighbors violently arguing, attending a peace rally or educating your friends and family about the impact of trauma after reading this book. Because of its incremental nature, experiencing one trauma can put individuals at risk for future trauma (Finkelhor, 2008; van der Kolk, McFarlane, & Weisaeth, 1996). Thus, preventing any one trauma can have a significant impact.

INTEGRATING PREVENTION THEORY
WITH UNDERSTANDING OF TRAUMA

Efforts to prevent disease, violence and psychological impairment can be found in many fields including medicine, public health, education and social work. In fact, given the complex nature of trauma, preventing it typically requires multidisciplinary approaches. But how does what we know about prevention intersect with our knowledge of trauma? Feldner, Monson and Friedman (2007) argue that prevention efforts lacking a grounding in an understanding of trauma have limited impact.

In fields such as public health that address prevention of disease, efforts typically fall into three categories – primary, secondary and tertiary. Primary prevention targets individuals not known to have experienced an event in order to prepare or "inoculate" them (Ursano, Grieger, & McCarroll, 1996; Whitaker et al., 2006). An example of this is an educational bullying program for children. Secondary prevention is generally defined as early identification and treatment of risk factors or symptoms in order to limit disability (Ursano et al., 1996). Providing support for police officers involved in a shooting event falls into this category. Using a different kind of approach, tertiary prevention attempts to rehabilitate or prevent chronic disability in those who have already experienced trauma (Ursano et al., 1996). This includes evidence-based therapy programs for individuals with post-traumatic stress disorder (PTSD). Most trauma-related research has been linked to the tertiary prevention but primary and secondary prevention research is also emerging (Feldner et al., 2007; Kenny, Capri, Thakkar-Kolar, Ryan, & Runyon, 2008; Ursano et al., 1996; Whitaker et al., 2006).

Definitions

- *Primary prevention* – Targets individuals who have not experienced an event; can be viewed as preparation before an event or "inoculation"
- *Secondary prevention* – Early identification and treatment of risk factors or symptoms, in order to limit development of a disorder
- *Tertiary prevention* – Attempts to rehabilitate or prevent chronic disability in those who have experienced an event and its deleterious impact

---

While primary, secondary and tertiary prevention is widely accepted in the field of disease prevention, Gordon (1983) proposed an alternative classification of prevention based on costs and benefits of delivering interventions (Feldner et al., 2007). In this typology, (1) "universal" intervention refers to interventions applied to a population regardless of risk of developing a disorder; (2) "selective" intervention targets individuals at risk of developing a disorder or of experiencing an event and (3) "indicated" intervention is targeted at individuals who have a known vulnerability for a disorder, but are currently asymptomatic (Feldner et al., 2007). Social workers should be aware of both typologies and consider their fit in particular contexts.

> **Definitions**
>
> - *Universal intervention* – refers to interventions applied to a whole population regardless of their risk for developing a disorder
> - *Selective intervention* – targets individuals deemed at risk for developing a disorder or experiencing an event, but who show no signs of that disorder
> - *Indicated intervention* – targets individuals with increased vulnerability for a disorder, but who are currently asymptomatic

MAKING THE CASE FOR PREVENTION EFFORTS

Few would argue that if society could prevent events that cause trauma and their short- and long-term impact, it should do so. But in times of tight resources where issues compete for funders' time and attention, understanding the importance of preventing the effects of trauma is critical.

First, trauma is not something that just a few individuals experience. Most people in the West are expected to encounter at least one traumatic event during their lives (Briere & Scott, 2006) and studies of the US population indicate that between 55% and 69% of individuals are exposed to at least one traumatic event in their lifetimes (Feldner et al., 2007; Kessler, Sonnega, Bromet, Hughes, & Nelson, 1995; Norris, 1992). The Adverse Childhood Experiences (ACEs) Study, a collaboration between the Centers for Disease Control and Prevention (CDC) and Kaiser Permanente, looks at distinct adverse childhood events and their outcomes and finds even more about why prevention is important. In what has become a world wide effort, ACEs, and even more so multiple ACEs, have been tied to (1) risky health behaviors, (2) chronic health conditions, (3) low life potential and (4) early death, underscoring the need for prevention efforts (Anda, Butchart, Felitti, & Brown, 2010).

Second, research indicates that prevention is cost-effective (Ursano et al., 1996). For example, investing in child abuse prevention programs – such as parent education and safety programs designed to make children less vulnerable to abuse – yields a 19:1 cost savings (i.e., for every dollar spent, 19 dollars are saved by keeping children safe and preventing the long-term impact of abuse) (Caldwell, 1992). Therefore, much of the pain we witness, such as that shared in this book, can be avoided if sufficient resources were invested in preventing trauma.

Beyond arguments for the impact and cost-effectiveness of prevention efforts, efforts to prevent the effects of trauma are in keeping with social work principles calling for empowerment of the disenfranchised (National Association of Social Workers, 2017) because trauma is disproportionately felt by the disenfranchised (Bryant-Davis, 2005; Feldner et al., 2007). For example, individuals caught in the same subway bombing in Europe, experience it differently – those with resources and a strong support network will likely fare better than individuals who do not have access to support, health and mental healthcare and who may, due to historical disenfranchisement, fear seeking support from available resources.

Finally, one author passionately argues that efforts to prevent the impact of psychological trauma on a child watching his or her home destroyed by war would contribute to world peace. This is true, he says, because a major cause of violence between sub-populations (e.g., ethnic, religious or national groups) is "unresolved and buried psychological trauma in childhood" (Taylor, 1998, p. 175).

PREVENTING EVENTS THAT CAUSE TRAUMA

Primary or universal prevention – the eradication of traumatic events – is the ideal prevention mechanism. Unfortunately, there is less information in the literature about these techniques regarding trauma; instead research efforts have focused on secondary or indicated prevention as well as tertiary techniques (Ursano et al., 1996). There are, however, some programs designed to protect the entire population from exposure to trauma. Programming in the area of primary or universal prevention tends to focus on community organizing and education, examples of which are discussed below.

COMMUNITY EDUCATION

In the field of intimate partner violence (IPV), many programs that serve survivors now also work with teens, providing education on what constitutes healthy relationships. The goal is to empower youth in order to prevent abuse (National Resource Center on Domestic Violence, 2002; Whitaker et al., 2006). This makes sense since a review of primary prevention programs targeting IPV found that those that provide the most comprehensive curriculum to the widest audience of young people and caregivers are the most effective (Whitaker et al., 2006).

Wolfe et al. (2003) evaluated one such program, the Youth Relationships Project. The efficacious model, implemented by social workers and other community professionals, delivers a total of 36 hours of education over a four-month period and focuses on alternatives to aggression-based interpersonal relations and gender-based role expectation. The curriculum includes education and awareness, skills development and social action.

The field of childhood sexual abuse has also historically been a focus of primary prevention community education. There are many curricula available that educate children and their support networks about child safety. Some of these programs, such as "Talking about Touching" from the Committee for

Children or "Darkness to Light" have developed strong evidence bases that support their effectiveness (Kenny et al., 2008). Research indicates that children can learn, understand and perform new skills needed to prevent victimization in simulated scenarios, but further research is needed to determine if they prevent abuse population-wide as is hoped (Finkelhor, 2009).

Lessons from community-established education programs may prove helpful to prevention planning. These lessons include the importance of: Repeating skills trainings multiple times with the same audience to ensure integration; targeting multiple access points including schools, homes, community forums and religious institutions; designing curricula that are culturally sensitive; and creating partnerships between disciplines – e.g., social workers, educators, medical providers, academic institutions (Kenny et al., 2008).

COMMUNITY ORGANIZING

Community organizing is a central area of practice for social workers including many who focus on the prevention of trauma and its impact. The Flint Youth Violence Prevention Center in Flint, Michigan (hereafter called "the Center"), for example, created a strategy that mobilized community representatives to prevent youth violence. Specifically, the Center worked with diverse stakeholders – hospital emergency departments, school systems and community-based service providers – to support, coordinate and evaluate the creation of youth violence prevention methodologies that fit their populations. Broad education curriculum and web-based tools, for example, were offered to youth who came to the emergency department for violence-related issues. Lessons from the project indicate that (1) community-level interventions, while extremely labor-intensive, are critical to successful youth violence prevention programs and (2) collaborative partnerships central to community organizing and advocacy efforts can effectively rally communities to address complex problems like youth violence (Griffith et al., 2008).

PREVENTING THE SHORT- AND LONG-TERM IMPACT OF TRAUMATIC EVENTS

More attention has been paid to preventing *the impact* of trauma either by using primary prevention strategies (i.e., before exposure occurs, but with a focus on preventing the impact rather than the event) or secondary prevention strategies, including early/acute intervention strategies. These strategies are reviewed below.

Prevention of traumatic stress is a way of preventing the impact of trauma. Raphael, Wilson, Meldron and McFarlane (1996), for instance, highlight strategies targeted at professionals and volunteers involved with disaster-relief efforts. These include training; creating teams with varied levels of experience; group/organizational leadership; management of meaning, exposure, fatigue, sleep and exhaustion; buddy care; national social supports and caretakers; educating on disaster stress; educating healthcare providers; and screening. In addition, prevention of vicarious trauma is receiving attention in the literature. A few central strategies are outlined below.

Definitions

* *Vicarious traumatization* — Results from numerous exposures to clients' trauma material, causing disruption of cognitive schemas and distortion of memory so that practitioners take on clients' trauma memories and related emotions

---

TRAINING

Research indicates that advanced training has a positive impact on preventing the danger of exposure to traumatic events from natural or man-made disasters. For example, in a study of employee survivors of a fire at a paint factory, responses both during the disaster and in the long term varied dramatically; good disaster-response behavior and positive long-term outcomes were correlated with a high level of prior disaster training/experience. In this case, employees had received general disaster-preparedness training which may have readied them so that they maintained better control of cognitive responses to the incident (Raphael et al., 1996).

Similar impacts of general traumatic event training are not, however, always apparent. If, for example, the duration of the events is ongoing, such as when living in a violent household, general training has little demonstrated impact. It is not only that training is important, but also that training and preparedness match the magnitude and type of trauma experienced (Raphael et al., 1996).

GROUP/ORGANIZATIONAL LEADERSHIP

Effective leadership during and after a disaster or other form of traumatic incident has also been noted to have a positive impact on the prevention of traumatic impact (Raphael et al., 1996). Leaders shoulder a moral and ethical responsibility to support their employees, maintain high standards of physical safety in the case of disaster response, and model a good emotional response to trauma, including connecting with mental health providers and supporting the need of their workers/employees for mental health support. For example, a social worker trained in Psychological First Aid (PFA) (see below for more information) made a decision to travel to New Orleans in the days following Hurricane Katrina.

Though the social worker had no leadership role to play in the disaster response, she was paired by the American Red Cross with a police captain responsible for limiting chaos and looting in a sector of the city. The social worker supported the captain, encouraging him to talk with his officers and emphasize the importance of rest and downtime despite the amount of work to be done, while she provided mental health consultation and PFA techniques to the squad to which she was assigned. In this role, the social worker was able to support the natural leader so that he could best support those in his command.

EDUCATION AND PREVENTION OF VICARIOUS TRAUMA

While relief workers and other first responders should be educated on the impact of working in trauma zones, this is often not a priority due to lack of time and resources. Indeed, many professionals working with trauma are given little time to learn about or discuss the strain they experience or to receive support for themselves. Because those responding to trauma – whether it be natural disaster, interpersonal violence or other forms – can also become "victims" of vicarious trauma, they should be educated on its impact (Bell, Kulkarni, & Dalton, 2003; Raphael et al., 1996).

Beyond education, Bell et al. (2003) argue that broad changes – such as in organizational culture, workload, group support, supervision, self-care and work environment – effectively prevent vicarious trauma in staff and volunteers. While some examples of these changes may be cost-prohibitive for agencies, such as changing health insurance to support intensive mental health services for staff, others are easier to institute and, in the long run, can have a positive impact on the effectiveness of workers. For example, one trauma program wanted to address the high turnover rate and burnout in its team. Case workers requested a supervision group, and the social worker on the team was asked to lead it. The supervision group met only monthly, but workers were encouraged to bring topics and focus on self-care and mutual support. The social worker advocated for the group to continue when upper management required that more cases be seen per day. The manager of the program thought that cutting the group might save some time for workers to see clients, but eventually understood that the group improved productivity overall. For more information on vicarious trauma, see chapter 1.

EARLY/ACUTE INTERVENTION STRATEGIES

Efforts have been made historically to address trauma's impact. Attention to trauma responses post-September 11th in the United States, for instance, led to increased research on best-practice, early intervention strategies. This research indicates that previously accepted forms of early intervention, such as Critical Incident Stress Debriefing – a group approach that focuses on sharing trauma experiences, normalizing stress reactions and on positive coping (Mitchell, 1983) – have little documented effect and may be detrimental (Briere & Scott, 2006). Proximity, Immediacy and Expectancy, a model used by the military because of its positive impact on soldiers with low-risk factors and high resilience, was also found to be detrimental for some, specifically those overwhelmed by their traumatic experience (Jones & Wessely, 2003).

Another widely accepted early intervention, PFA, was developed by the National Child Traumatic Stress Network and the National Center for PTSD. It focuses on concrete solutions in the immediate aftermath of a trauma and encourages practitioners to allow survivors to talk about their experiences only as much as they want to, without pushing for the deeper processing prior models encouraged (Vernberg et al., 2008). It is an evidence-based, manualized approach and is widely available to providers and first responders in multiple languages. Social workers are encouraged to receive this training. For more information, see the Resources section at the end of the chapter.

FUTURE DIRECTIONS

Significant advances are being made in the prevention of traumatic events and of short- and long-term trauma impact. Authors in this field recommend that given high levels of trauma exposure, future research and programming should focus on risk and protective factors, screening after traumatic events and on how responses might vary for different forms of trauma in order to help those working in the prevention field target their interventions more effectively. They further suggest that future prevention strategies put more emphasis on education, information processing, memory and psychobiology (i.e., biological functions protecting those exposed to trauma from developing PTSD), as they believe these are key processes involved in outcome (Feldner et al., 2007; Raphael et al., 1996).

Case Study

Trauma prevention strategies must comprehensively address all areas of prevention – primary, secondary, tertiary or universal, selective, indicated – if it is to have any hope of succeeding. One example of this is the San Francisco Child Abuse Prevention Center (SFCAPC), which has, since the mid-1970s, targeted known risk factors for child abuse and promoted protective factors with varied and tiered responses. Currently, SFCAPC works to prevent child abuse and neglect in three ways: (1) direct services to support healthy families; (2) community education to empower providers, children and caregivers to understand, prevent and respond to child abuse and (3) strategic partnerships, public awareness campaigns and community organizing designed to improve community systems that prevent and respond to abuse incidents.

Components of these efforts which address the full spectrum of prevention efforts – primary, secondary and tertiary – include: (1) a 24-hour parental stress hotline designed to support parents by reducing isolation and increasing positive coping; (2) a Child Safety Awareness program which uses an evidence-informed curriculum in public schools to educate children on how to keep themselves safe from sexual abuse and on how to seek help if needed and (3) the ongoing development of strategic partnerships that advance prevention in the community. One example of the latter is the development of a Children's Advocacy Center in San Francisco.

Program evaluation is currently underway at SFCAPC. Early results indicate lower levels of parental stress and mental health issues as a result of involvement in the program. Children educated in the community maintain 85% of the curriculum provided and anecdotal evidence indicates that a child who received this curriculum was able to spot a potential perpetrator outside the schoolyard fence and ran to tell the teacher rather than let him photograph her and a friend. Effectively evaluating the true preventive impacts of these programs is a complex and ongoing process at SFCAPC.

RESOURCES

Bell, H., Kulkarni, S., & Dalton, L. (2003). Organizational prevention of vicarious trauma. *Families in Society: The Journal of Contemporary Human Services, 84*(4), 463–470.

ONLINE RESOURCES

Adverse Childhood Experiences (ACEs)
https://www.cdc.gov/violenceprevention/acestudy/about_ace.html
Psychological First Aid: For more information or to access the field manual, visit: https://www.nctsn.org/treatments-and-practices/psychological-first-aid-and-skills-for-psychological-recovery/about-pfa

Practice Exercises and Questions

- Give examples of when and how you would use secondary prevention efforts rather than primary or tertiary and why
- What are some prevention efforts you could see yourself engaged in or that you have been engaged in the past? Elaborate
- Outline the processes of the efforts described above, being careful to include any steps outlined in the chapter
- Role-play talking with management about the importance of efforts to prevent vicarious trauma in the workplace

Prevention and Community Organizing Summary

Basic Prevention Theory

- *There are various ways to break down prevention:*
- *primary prevention efforts focus on the whole population*
- *secondary efforts focus on those at high risk for trauma*
- *tertiary efforts focus on those who have been exposed to trauma in an effort to prevent the short- and long-term impact*

Preventing Events That Cause Trauma

- *Community organization and education provide individuals with skills and information that can prevent trauma*

Preventing Short- and Long-term Impacts of Traumatic Events

- *Preventing the short-term impact of trauma focuses on support and concrete services, utilizing models such as Psychological First Aid*
- *Preventing the long-term impact of trauma is the treatment of trauma*

Sample Trauma Course Syllabus

COURSE DESCRIPTION

This course is designed to provide a framework for practice with individuals, families, organizations and communities who are coping with trauma. The coursework presented will enhance the skills and knowledge base of all students and will be particularly useful to students interested in working with survivors of trauma. Trauma is surrounded by a complex set of issues that will be addressed, including treatment choices, sociocultural forces that shape care provision and coping, multicultural perspectives on trauma, psychosocial challenges and secondary stresses connected with this type of work. Social work skills vital to this work will be examined including psychosocial assessment, crisis intervention, supportive care, psychoeducation, psychosocial intervention, advocacy, program development and prevention/community organizing. Values and ethics in practice will be discussed as they relate to the role of social workers in a rapidly changing environment in which awareness of the short and long term effects of trauma is increasing. At least two guest speakers will present on their areas of expertise.

Course Objectives:

By the end of this course, students should be able to:

- Understand the impact of trauma on individuals, families, communities and organizations
- Articulate their own personal and culturally based beliefs about trauma and evaluate the impact of these on the helping process
- Understand the common psychosocial challenges, adaptive tasks and treatment/symptom management issues that clients often face when coping with trauma
- Establish familiarity with literature related to psychosocial issues of trauma

- Understand the meaning and significance of different culturally-based forms of client's belief systems and coping mechanisms during the recovery process
- Demonstrate an understanding of social work interventions with empirical evidence of effectiveness in assisting clients coping with trauma
- Grasp the fundamentals of ethical dilemmas inherent in trauma work
- Learn about the effects of vicarious trauma during the helping process. Understand how to watch out for, avoid, identify and treat vicarious trauma when it occurs

STUDENT EVALUATION

Since professional dialogue and reflection are an important component of this course, regular and timely attendance at each class is essential. In addition to physical presence, students are expected to read assignments for each class and to be prepared to engage in a thoughtful and critical discussion of these as well as related fieldwork experiences during class. An assessment of class participation will be incorporated into the student's final grade. Several written assignments are also required. These include:

- A 3 page personal or professional experience with trauma, due week #2
- Two 2 page responses to the readings in a journal format, due weeks #5
- An 8–10 page paper, due week #10
- An in class group project presentation demonstrating a trauma intervention due week #12

The first paper is intended to encourage students to reflect upon their own experiences with trauma. It also requires a brief analysis of how these experiences may impact their work with clients coping with traumatic events. The second and third papers offer students an opportunity to reflect on the readings in their own words with informal references included. At least eight readings should be mentioned in each. The final paper provides students with an opportunity to critically apply what they have learned from class materials (i.e., readings, videos, discussions) to a specific "case" from their own practice. If no such case exists in a student's practice, an appropriate case will be provided. This paper should include an annotated bibliography with at least ten references. The final class group presentation provides students with an opportunity to apply what they have learned about how to intervene with this population, demonstrating an intervention of their choice.

Exemplary papers and presentations reflect not only students' ability to utilize class materials to challenge themselves as practitioners, but also their willingness to contribute to the ongoing development of empirical knowledge and practice wisdom by sharing ideas and experiences.

REQUIRED READING

The required readings are comprised of:
  Readings from a text on reserve in the library or available for purchase at Amazon.com and other mail order venues –

Goelitz, A. (2020). *From trauma to healing: A social worker's guide to working with survivors* (2nd ed.). New York: Routledge.

* 20 chapters from text
* 9 websites

SESSION OUTLINE AND READING LIST

WEEK 1
TOPIC: Stresses and Rewards of Working with This Population

* Introduction to course
* You can be affected too – secondary trauma
* Practitioner bias and vulnerability
* Setting appropriate professional boundaries
* Self-care for the professional
* Case study at the end of chapter 1 in the text

REQUIRED READING

Goelitz, A. (2020). *From trauma to healing: A social worker's guide to working with survivors* (2nd ed., chapters 1 and 2). New York: Routledge.

OPTIONAL READINGS

Brown, L.S. (2009). Cultural competence: A new way of looking at integration in psychotherapy. *Journal of Psychotherapy Integration, 19*(4), 340–353.
Rothschild, B.A. (2006). *Help for the helper: The psychophysiology of compassion fatigue and vicarious trauma* (entire book, chapters 1 and 5 in particular). New York: WW Norton & Company.
Saakvitne, K., & Pearlman, L.A. (1996). *Transforming the pain: A workbook on vicarious traumatization* (entire book, chapters 4 and 5 in particular). New York: WW Norton & Company.

WEEK 2   (Trauma history paper due)
TOPIC: Overview of Working with Trauma Survivors

* Introduction
* Experiential sharing on trauma history papers

- Types of traumatic events
- Witnessing trauma
- Role-play, fish bowl style with opportunity to ask for time outs for class assistance, from your practice experience with this population or from one of the cases in the text chapters. When determining how to approach the client you choose to role-play, consider not only care for your client but also for yourself and the impact on loved ones and community members

REQUIRED READING

Goelitz, A. (2020). *From trauma to healing: A social worker's guide to working with survivors* (2nd ed., chapters 3, 5 and 7). New York: Routledge.

OPTIONAL READINGS

Bragin, M. (2014). Clinical social work with survivors of disaster and terrorism. In J. Brandell (Ed.), *Essentials of clinical social work* (pp. 366–401). London: SAGE Publications. Available for download at https://www.cswe.org/getattachment/ac73b154-b499-4d52-aa40-0a479141afd6/Clinical-Social-Work-in-Situations-of-Disaster-(1).aspx

Briere, J., & Scott, C. (2006). *Principles of trauma therapy: A guide to symptoms, evaluation, and treatment*. Thousand Oaks, CA: Sage Publications.

Tehrani, N. (Ed.). (2001). *Managing trauma in the workplace: Supporting workers and organisations*. New York: Routledge.

Tick, E. (2005). *War and the soul*. Wheaton, IL: Quest Books.

Weingarten, K. (2004). *Common shock: Witnessing violence every day – how we are harmed, how we can heal*. New York: New American Library.

WEEK 3
TOPIC: Life-threatening Illness

- Supportive care to patients and family
- Concrete services, referrals and discharge planning
- Patient advocacy
- Financial considerations
- The future of end-of-life care
- Role-play, fish bowl style with opportunity to ask for time outs for class assistance – critical incident with a patient recently diagnosed with cancer

REQUIRED READING

Goelitz, A. (2020). *From trauma to healing: A social worker's guide to working with survivors* (2nd ed., chapter 6). New York: Routledge.

OPTIONAL READINGS

Clark, E. (2004). The future of social work in end-of-life care: A call to action. In J. Berzoff, & P. Silverman (Eds.), *Living with dying: A handbook for end-of-life healthcare practitioners* (pp. 838–847). New York: Columbia University Press.

Goelitz, A. (2003). Suicidal ideation at end-of-life: The palliative care team's role. *Palliative and Supportive Care, 1*, 275–278.

Otis-Green, S., & Rutland, C. (2004). Marginalization at end of life. In J. Berzoff, & P. Silverman (Eds.), *Living with dying: A handbook for end-of-life healthcare practitioners* (pp. 462–481). New York: Columbia University Press.

Van Fleet, S. (2000). Relaxation and imagery for symptom management: Improving patient assessment and individualizing treatment. *Oncology Nursing Forum, 27*(3), 501–510.

Wilber, K. (2000). What kind of help really helps? In *Grace and grit* (2nd ed., pp. 242–252). Boston, MA: Shambhala.

WEEK 4 (1st Readings journal paper due)
TOPIC: Family Abuse and Neglect

- Overview
- Intimate partner violence
- Child abuse/neglect
- Abuse/neglect of the elderly and disabled
- Class discussion on how children, adults, the elderly and the disabled react differently to family violence

REQUIRED READINGS

Goelitz, A. (2020). *From trauma to healing: A social worker's guide to working with survivors* (2nd ed., chapter 4). New York: Routledge.

Child Welfare Information Gateway. Signs & Symptoms of Child Abuse/Neglect: https://www.childwelfare.gov/pubPDFs/whatiscan.pdf

HelpGuide. Signs & Symptoms of Domestic Violence: https://www.helpguide.org/articles/abuse/domestic-violence-and-abuse.htm/

HelpGuide. Signs & Symptoms of Elder Abuse/Neglect: https://www.helpguide.org/articles/abuse/elder-abuse-and-neglect.htm Power and Control Wheel developed by the Domestic Violence Intervention Project in Duluth, Minnesota: http://www.theduluthmodel.org

WEEK 5
TOPIC: Cultural Considerations/Vulnerable Populations

- Culture and socio-economic status
- Race, ethnicity, religion, class and education level
- Age, gender, disabilities, psychological issues, substance abuse
- Marginalization increases vulnerability and risk of harm from trauma

- Includes poverty, lack of education and work, prejudice, immigration
- Small group and class discussions on practice exercises in chapter 8 on vulnerability and the last 2 in chapter 9 on safety

REQUIRED READINGS

Goelitz, A. (2020). *From trauma to healing: A social worker's guide to working with survivors* (2nd ed., chapters 8 and 9). New York: Routledge.

The National Child Traumatic Stress Network recommendations: http://www.nctsn.org/nctsn_assets/pdfs/culture_and_trauma_brief_v2n3_LatinoHispanicChildren.pdf

OPTIONAL READINGS

Weiss, T., & Berge, R. (Eds.). (2010). *Posttraumatic growth and culturally competent practice: Lessons learned from around the globe.* Hoboken, NJ: Wiley.

WEEK 6
TOPIC: The Importance of Safety

- Stress created by trauma
- Freeze flight fight freeze faint response
- Importance of safety
- Building safe relationships
- Coping skills and self-care
- Small group exercise – finding your class partners' coping strengths

REQUIRED READINGS

Goelitz, A. (2020). *From trauma to healing: A social worker's guide to working with survivors* (2nd ed., chapters 10, 11 and 12). New York: Routledge.

Najavits, L. (2010). Seeking Safety: http://www.seekingsafety.org/

OPTIONAL READINGS

Davis, L. (1991). *Allies in healing: When the person you love was sexually abused as a child.* New York: Harper Perennial.

Herman, J.L. (1992). *Trauma and recovery.* New York: Basic Books.

Nix, A., & Fine, S. (Writers) (2007). *War dance.* In A. Hecht (Producer): ThinkFilm.

van der Kolk, B.A. (2014). *The body keeps the score: Brain, mind, and body in the healing of trauma.* New York: Viking.

WEEK 7   (2nd Readings journal paper due)
TOPIC: Assessment/Crisis Intervention

- Assessment including assessment tools
- Crisis intervention
- Identifying risk for harm to self or others
- Application of assessment questions to specific case(s) from your work

OPTIONAL READINGS

Walsh-Burke, K. (2004). Assessing mental health risk in End-of-life care. In J. Berzoff & P. Silverman (Eds.), *Living with dying: A handbook for end-of-life healthcare practitioners* (pp. 360–379). New York: Columbia University Press.

WEEK 8
TOPIC: Psychosocial Interventions – Part I

- Communication
- Individual, group and family work
- Cognitive behavioral techniques
- Psychoeducation
- Group exercise simulating a support group

REQUIRED READINGS

Goelitz, A. (2020). *From trauma to healing: A social worker's guide to working with survivors* (2nd ed., chapters 13 and 14). New York: Routledge.

Goelitz, A. (2020). *From trauma to healing: A social worker's guide to working with survivors* (2nd ed., chapters 15 and 16). New York: Routledge.

National Center for PTSD: http://www.ptsd.va.gov/professional/pages/overview-treatment-research.asp; and http://www.ptsd.va.gov/professional/newsletters/research-quarterly/V19N3.pdf

National Child Traumatic Stress Network: Empirically supported treatments and promising practices: http://www.nctsnet.org/resources/topics/treatments-that-work/promising-practices

OPTIONAL READINGS

Briere, J., & Scott, C. (2006). *Principles of trauma therapy: A guide to symptoms, evaluation, and treatment.* Thousand Oaks, CA: Sage Publications.

Gitterman, A., & Shulman, L. (Eds.). (1994). *Mutual aid groups, vulnerable populations, and the life cycle* (2nd ed.). New York: Columbia University Press.

WEEK 9   (8–10 page paper due)
TOPIC: Psychosocial Interventions – Part II

- Hypnosis and guided imagery
- EMDR including Flash method
- Relaxation and meditation

- Creative arts
- Class exercise self hypnosis

REQUIRED READING

Goelitz, A. (2020). *From trauma to healing: A social worker's guide to working with survivors* (2nd ed., chapter 17). New York: Routledge.

OPTIONAL READINGS

Barrett, D. (Ed.). (1996). *Trauma and dreams.* Cambridge, MA: Harvard University Press.

Hopper, E., Emerson, D., Levine, P.A., Cope, S., & van der Kolk, B.A. (2011). *Overcoming trauma through yoga: Reclaiming your body.* Boston: North Atlantic Books.

Linehan, M.M. (1993). *Skills training manual for treating borderline personality disorder.* New York: Guilford Press.

Malchiodi, C.A. (Ed.). (2008). *Creative interventions with traumatized children.* New York: Guilford Press.

Naparstek, B. (2005). *Invisible heroes: Survivors of trauma and how they heal.* New York: Bantam.

Shapiro, F. (2001). *Eye movement desensitization and reprocessing: Basic principles, protocols, and procedures* (2nd ed.). New York: Guilford Press.

WEEK 10
TOPIC: Advocating for Survivors

- Micro-level advocacy
- Macro-level advocacy
- Macro-level advocacy pitfalls
- Class discussion regarding micro or macro-level advocacy efforts you could apply to past or present social work

REQUIRED READING

Goelitz, A. (2020). *From trauma to healing: A social worker's guide to working with survivors* (2nd ed., chapter 19). New York: Routledge.

OPTIONAL READINGS

Lens, V. (2005). Advocacy and argumentation in the public arena: A guide for social workers. *Social Work, 50,* 231–238.

Schneider, R.L., & Lester, L. (2001). *Social work advocacy.* Belmont, CA: Brooks/Cole Thomson Learning.

WEEK 11
TOPIC: Prevention and Community Organizing

- Prevention theory
- Preventing events that cause trauma
- Preventing impact of trauma events
- Discussion regarding prevention efforts you could see yourself engaged in or that you have been engaged in the past

REQUIRED READINGS

Goelitz, A. (2020). *From trauma to healing: A social worker's guide to working with survivors* (2nd ed., chapter 20). New York: Routledge.

Adverse Childhood Experiences (ACEs) https://www.cdc.gov/violenceprevention/acestudy/about_ace.html

OPTIONAL READINGS

Bell, H., Kulkarni, S., & Dalton, L. (2003). Organizational prevention of vicarious trauma. *Families in Society: The Journal of Contemporary Human Services, 84*(4), 463–470.

Raphael, B., Wilson, J., Meldrum, L., & McFarlane, A.C. (1996). Acute prevention interventions. In B.A. van der Kolk, A.C. McFarlane, & L. Weisaeth (Eds.), *Traumatic stress: The effects of overwhelming experience on mind, body, and society* (pp. 463–480). New York: Guilford Press.

WEEK 12 (Group project demonstrating an intervention due)
TOPIC: Program Development

- Program development steps
- Issues specific to trauma programs
- Program development pitfalls
- Group project presentations

REQUIRED READING

Goelitz, A. (2020). *From trauma to healing: A social worker's guide to working with survivors* (2nd ed., chapter 18). New York: Routledge.

OPTIONAL READINGS

Kettner, P.M., Moroney, R.M., & Martin, L.L. (2016). *Designing and managing programs: An effectiveness-based approach*. Thousand Oaks, CA: Sage.

Yuen, F.K., Terao, K.L., & Schmidt, A.M. (2013). *Effective grant writing and program evaluation for human service professionals*. Hoboken, NJ: John Wiley & Sons.

References

Aarts, P.G.H., & Op den Velde, W. (1996). Prior traumatization and the process of aging: Theory and clinical implications. In B. A. van der Kolk, A. C. McFarlane, & L. Weisaeth (Eds.), *Traumatic stress: The effects of overwhelming experience on mind, body, and society* (pp. 359–377). New York: Guilford Press.

Alderfer, M.A., Navsaria, N., & Kazak, A.E. (2009). Family functioning and posttraumatic stress disorder in adolescent survivors of childhood cancer. *Journal of Family Psychology*, *23*(5), 717–725.

Alim, T.N., Feder, A., Graves, R.E., Wang, Y., Weaver, J., & Westphal, M. et al. (2008). Trauma, resilience, and recovery in a high-risk African-American population. *The American Journal of Psychiatry*, *165*(12), 1566–1575.

Alexander, W. (2012). Pharmacotherapy for Post-traumatic Stress Disorder In Combat Veterans: Focus on Antidepressants and Atypical Antipsychotic Agents. *P & T: A Peer-reviewed Journal for Formulary Management*, *37*(1), 32–38.

Altilio, T. (2004). Pain and symptom management: An essential role for social work. In J. Berzoff, & P. Silverman (Eds.), *Living with dying: A handbook for end-of-life healthcare practitioners* (pp. 380–408). New York: Columbia University Press.

American Psychiatric Association. (2000). *Diagnostic and statistical manual of mental disorders: DSMIV-TR* (4th ed., updated). Washington, DC: American Psychiatric Association.

American Psychiatric Association. (2004). *Practice guideline for the treatment of patients with acute stress disorder and posttraumatic stress disorder*. Arlington, VA: American Psychiatric Association.

American Psychiatric Association. (2013). *Diagnostic and statistical manual of mental disorders: DSMIV* (4th ed.). Washington, DC: American Psychiatric Association.

American Psychological Association. (2015). *Guidelines on Trauma Competencies for Education and Training*. Retrieved September 23, 2018 from http://www.apa.org/ed/resources/trauma-competencies-training.pdf

American Psychological Association. (2017). Ethical principles of psychologists and code of conduct. Retrieved February 3, 2020, from https://www.apa.org/ethics/code/

Anda, R.F., Butchart, A., Felitti, V.J., & Brown, D.W. (2010). Building a framework for global surveillance of the public health implications of adverse childhood experiences. *American Journal of Preventive Medicine*, *39*(1), 93–98.

Ashford, J.B., Lecroy, C.W., & Lortie, K.L. (2001). *Human behavior in the social environment: A multidimensional perspective*. Belmont, CA: Wadsworth.

Association for Play Therapy. (2007). Clinical lessons learned from trauma survivors and their traumatic play. *Play Therapy*. Retrieved March 30, 2010 from http://www.a4pt.org/download.cfm?ID=22578

Austin, D. (2006). Songs of self: Vocal psychotherapy for adults traumatized as children. In L. Carey (Ed.), *Expressive and creative arts methods for trauma survivors* (pp. 133–152). London and Philadelphia: Jessica Kingsley Publishers.

Ayalon, O. (1998). Community healing for children traumatized by war. *International Review of Psychiatry, 10*, 224–233.

Baladerian, N.J. (2009). Domestic violence and individuals with disabilities: Reflections on research and practice. *Journal of Aggression, Maltreatment & Trauma, 18*, 153–161.

Baladerian, N.J. (2013). Abuse of People with Mental Illness and Developmental Disabilities, *Keynote Presentation*, Charleston, WV: Behavior Health Conference with WVDHS/DMH. Retrieved July 1, 2019 from http://dhhr.wv.gov/bhhf/Documents/2013%20IBHC%20Presentations/Day%203%20Workshops/Healing%20the%20Trauma.pdf

Baladerian, N., Coleman, T., & Stream, J. (2013) *Findings from the 2012 Survey on Abuse of People with Disabilities*. Retrieved March 18, 2019 from http://www.disabilityandabuse.org/survey/findings.pdf

Barasch, M. (2000). *Healing dreams*. New York: Riverhead Books.

Barker, R.L. (1999). *Social work dictionary*. Washington, DC: NASW Press.

Barrett, D. (2002). The "Royal Road" becomes a shrewd shortcut: The use of dreams in focused treatment. *Journal of Cognitive Psychotherapy, 16(1)*, 55–64.

Bateman, N. (2000). *Advocacy skills: A handbook for human service professionals*. Philadelphia: Jessica Kingsley Publishers.

Bayard, V.L., Williams, L.M., Saunders, B.E., & Fitzgerald, M.M. (2008). The complexity of trauma types in the lives of women in families referred for family violence: Multiple mediators of mental health. *American Journal of Orthopsychiatry, 78(4)*, 394–404.

Behrendt, A., & Moritz, S. (2005). Posttraumatic stress disorder and memory problems after female genital mutilation. *American Journal of Psychiatry, 162*, 1000–1002.

Belicki, K., & Cuddy, M. (1996). Identifying sexual trauma histories from patterns of sleep and dreams. In D. Barrett (Ed.), *Trauma and dreams* (pp. 46–55). Cambridge, MA: Harvard University Press.

Bell, H. (2003). Strengths and secondary trauma in family violence work. *Social Work, 48(4)*, 513–522.

Bell, H., Kulkarni, S., & Dalton, L. (2003). Organizational prevention of vicarious trauma. *Families in Society: The Journal of Contemporary Human Services, 84(4)*, 463–470.

Bernal, G., & Saez-Santiago, E. (2006). Culturally centered psychological interventions. *Journal of Community Psychology, 34(2)*, 121–132.

Blancato, R. (2012). History of the elder justice act. *Public Policy & Aging Report, 22(1)*, 17–21.

Blakley, T., & Mehr, N. (2008). Common ground: The development of a support group for survivors of homicide loss in a rural community. *Social Work with Groups, 31(3/4)*, 239–254.

Bloom, S. (2010). Organizational stress as a barrier to trauma-informed service delivery. In M. Becker, & B.A. Levin (Eds.), *Public health perspective of Women's mental health* (pp. 295–311). New York: Springer.

Bloom, S. (2011). Sanctuary: An operating system for living organisations. In N. Tehrani (Ed.), *Managing trauma in the workplace: Supporting workers and organisations* (pp. 235–251). New York: Routledge.

Blount, R.L., Simons, L.E., Devine, K.A., Jaaniste, T., Cohen, L.L., Chambers, C.T. et al. (2008). Evidence-based assessment of coping and stress in pediatric psychology. *Journal of Pediatric Psychology*, *33*(9), 1021–1045. Retrieved December 28, 2019 from https://doi.org/10.1093/jpepsy/jsm071

Blum, D., Clark, E.J., & Marcusen, C.P. (2001). Oncology social work in the 21st century. In M.M. Lauria, E.J. Clark, J.F. Hermann, & N.M. Stearns (Eds.), *Social work in oncology: Supporting survivors, families and caregivers* (pp. 45–71). Atlanta, GA: American Cancer Society.

Bogat, G.A., DeJonghe, E., Levendosky, A.A., Davidson, W.S., & von Eye, A. (2006). Trauma symptoms among infants exposed to intimate partner violence. *Child Abuse and Neglect*, *30*, 109–125.

Boggs, S.R., Eyberg, S.M., Edwards, D., Rayfield, A., Jacobs, J., Bagner, D. et al. (2004). Outcomes of parent–child interaction therapy: A comparison of dropouts and treatment completers one or three years after treatment. *Child and Family Behavior Therapy*, *26*(4), 1–22.

Boothby, N., Crawford, J., & Halperin, J. (2006). Mozambique child soldier life outcome study: Lessons learned in rehabilitation and reintegration efforts. *Global Public Health*, *1*(1), 87–107.

Bosnak, R. (1996). *Tracks in the wilderness of dreaming*. New York: Dell Publishing.

Bowles, R., & Mehraby, N. (2007). Lost in limbo: Cultural dimensions in psychotherapy and supervision with a temporary protection visa holder from Afghanistan. In B. Drozdek & J.P. Wilson (Eds.), *Voices of trauma: Treating psychological trauma across cultures (International and Cultural Psychology series)* (pp. 295–320). New York: Springer.

Boyer, P.S. (2001). Domestic violence. *The Oxford companion to United States history*. Oxford: Oxford University Press.

Bracken, P. (2002). *Trauma: Culture, meaning and philosophy*. London and Philadelphia: Wiley.

Bragin, M. (2014). Clinical social work with survivors of disaster and terrorism. In J. Brandell (Ed.), *Essentials of clinical social work* (pp. 366–401). London: Sage Publications.

Brave Heart, M.Y.H. (2007). The impact of historical trauma: The example of the native community. In M. Bussey & J. Bula Wise (Eds.), *Trauma transformed: An empowerment response* (pp. 176–193). New York: Columbia University Press.

Briere, J., & Scott, C. (2006). *Principles of trauma therapy: A guide to symptoms, evaluation, and treatment*. Thousand Oaks, CA: Sage Publications.

Bromberg, P. (2006). *Awakening the dreamer: Clinical journeys*. Mahwah, NJ: The Analytic Press.

Bronson, P., & Merryman, A. (2009). *Nurture shock: New thinking about children*. New York: Hachette Book Group.

Brooks, B., & Siegel, P.M. (1996). *The scared child: Helping kids overcome traumatic events*. New York: John Wiley & Sons, Inc.

Brown, L.S. (2008). *Cultural competence in trauma therapy: Beyond the flashback*. Washington DC: American Psychological Association.

Brown, L.S. (2009a). Cultural competence: A new way of looking at integration in psychotherapy. *Journal of Psychotherapy Integration*, *19*(4), 340–353.

Brown, L.S. (2009b). Cultural competence. In C.A. Courtois, J.D. Ford, B.A. van der Kolk, & J.L. Herman (Eds.), *Treating complex traumatic stress disorders: An evidence-based guide* (pp. 166–182). New York: Guilford Press.

Brown, R.P., & Gerbarg, P.L. (2005). Sudarshan Kriya yogic breathing in the treatment of stress, anxiety, and depression: Part II – Clinical applications and guidelines. *Journal of Alternative and Complementary Medicine*, *11*(4), 711–717.

Brown, S.M., Baker, C.N., & Wilcox, P. (2012). Risking connection trauma training: A pathway toward trauma-informed care in child congregate care settings. *Psychological Trauma: Theory, Research, Practice, and Policy, 4*(5), 507–515.

Brunkow, K. (1996). Working with dreams of survivors of violence: Facilitating crisis intervention with a psychoanalytical approach. In J. Edward & J. Sanville (Eds.), *Fostering healing and growth: A psychoanalytical social work approach* (pp. 212–225). Northvale, NJ: Jason Aronson, Inc.

Bryant-Davis, T. (2005). *Thriving in the wake of trauma.* Lanham, MD: AltaMira Press.

Bryant-Davis, T., & Wong, E.C. (2013). Faith to move mountains: Religious coping, spirituality, and interpersonal trauma recovery. *American Psychologist, 68*(8), 675–684.

Cahill, S.P., & Foa, E.B. (2007). PTSD: Treatment efficacy and future directions. *Psychiatric Times, 24*(3), 32–34.

Caldwell, R. (1992). The cost of child abuse vs. child abuse prevention: Michigan's experience. Retrieved September 4, 2010 from http://www.msu.edu/user/bob/cost.html

California Youth Connection. (2010). Home page. Retrieved June 28, 2010 from http://www.calyouthconn.org/site/cyc/

Callahan, C. (2010). Combat-related mental health disorders: The case for resiliency in the long war. *Journal of the American Osteopathic Association, 110*(9), 520–527.

Calley, N.G. (2009). Comprehensive program development in mental health counseling: Design, implementation and evaluation. *Journal of Mental Health Counseling, 21*(1), 9–21.

Carey, B. (2009, December 10). Study suggests methods and timing to treat fears. *The New York Times*, p. A28.

Carey, B. (2011, July 29). Sept. 11 revealed psychology's limits, review finds. *The New York Times*, p. A18.

Carlson, E.B., Furby, L., Armstrong, J., & Shlaes, J. (1997). A conceptual framework for the long-term psychological effects of traumatic childhood abuse. *Child Maltreatment, 2*, 272–295.

Carmona, R.H. (2005). Surgeon General's workshop on making prevention of child maltreatment a national priority: Implementing innovations of a public health approach. Retrieved October 19, 2012 from http://137.187.25.243/topics/childmaltreatment/

Carver, C.S. (2001). Affect and the functional bases of behavior: On the dimensional structure of affective experience. *Personality and Social Psychology Review, 5*, 345–356.

Centers for Disease Control and Prevention. (2003). HHS study finds life expectancy in the U.S. rose to 77.2 years in 2001. Retrieved October 13, 2012 from http://www.cdc.gov/nchs/pressroom/03news/lifeex.htm

Centers for Disease Control and Prevention. (2006). *Understanding child maltreatment: Fact sheet.* Retrieved January 15, 2010 from http://www.cdc.gov/violenceprevention/pdf/CM-factsheeta.pdf

Centers for Disease Control and Prevention. (2008). Adverse health conditions and health risk behaviors associated with intimate partner violence. *Morbidity and Mortality Weekly Report.* Retrieved November 11, 2009 from www.cdc.gov/mmwr/preview/mmwrhtml/mm5705a1.htm

Center for Substance Abuse Treatment (US). (2014). Trauma-Informed Care in Behavioral Health Services. Rockville, MD. Retrieved December 15, 2019 from https://www.ncbi.nlm.nih.gov/books/NBK207188/

Chalfant, A.M., Bryant, R.A., & Fulcher, G. (2004). Posttraumatic stress disorder following diagnosis of multiple sclerosis. *Journal of Traumatic Stress, 17*(5), 423–428.

Chan, C.L.W., Chan, T.H.Y., & Ng, S.M. (2006). The Strength-Focused and Meaning-Oriented Approach to Resilience and Transformation (SMART): A body–mind–spirit approach to trauma management. *Social Work in Health Care*, 43(2/3), 9–36.

Charlton, M., Kiliethermes, M., Tallant, B., Taverne, A., & Tishelman, A. (2004). National Child Traumatic Stress Network Adapted Trauma Treatment Standards Work Group. Subgroup on developmental disability. Retrieved January 27, 2012 from http://www.nctsn.org/sites/default/files/assets/pdfs/traumatic_stress_developmental_disabilities_final.pdf

Charney, D. (2004). Psychobiological mechanisms of resilience and vulnerability: Implications for successful adaptation to extreme stress. *The American Journal of Psychiatry*, 161(2), 195–216.

Chemtob, C.M., Nakashima, J., Hamada, R.S., & Carlson, J.G. (2002). Brief treatment for elementary school children with disaster-related posttraumatic stress disorder: A field study. *Journal of Clinical Psychology*, 58, 99–112.

Chemtob, C.M., Nomura, Y., & Abramovitz, R.A. (2008). Impact of conjoined exposure to the World Trade Center attacks and to other traumatic events on the behavioral problems of preschool children. *Archives of Pediatrics & Adolescent Medicine*, 162(2), 126–133.

Chetty, S., Friedman, A.R., Taravosh-Lahn, K., Kirbu, E.D., Mirescu, C., Guo, F. et al. (2014). Stress and glucocorticoids promote oligodendrogenesis in the adult hippocampus. *Mol Psychiatry*, 10(12), 1275–1283.

Child Welfare Information Gateway. (2008). Long-term consequences of child abuse and neglect: Fact sheet. Retrieved January 15, 2010 from www.childwelfare.gov/pubs/factsheets/long_term_consequences.cfm

Chung, M.C., Berger, Z., Jones, R., & Rudd, H. (2008). Posttraumatic stress and co-morbidity following myocardial infarction among older patients: The role of coping. *Aging & Mental Health*, 12(1), 124–133.

Cohen, D., de la Vega, R., & Watson, G. (2001). *Advocacy for social justice: A global action and reflection guide*. Bloomfield, CT: Kumarian Press, Inc.

Cohen, J.A., Deblinger, E., Mannarino, A.P., & Steer, R.A. (2004). A multisite, randomized control trial for children with sexual abuse-related PTSD symptoms. *Journal of the American Academy of Child and Adolescent Psychiatry*, 43, 393–402.

Cohen, J.A., Kelleher, K.J., & Mannarino, A.P. (2008). Identifying, treating, and referring traumatized children: The role of pediatric providers. *Archives of Pediatric and Adolescent Medicine*, 162(5), 447–452.

Cohen, J.A., & Mannarino, A.P. (2008). Trauma-focused cognitive behavioural therapy for children and parents. *Child and Adolescent Mental Health*, 13(4), 158–162.

Collins, S.E., Clifasefi, S.L., Logan, D.E., Samples, L.S., Somers, J.M., & Marlatt, G.A. (2012). Current status, historical highlights, and basic principles of harm reduction. In G.A. Marlatt, M.E. Larimer, & K. Witkiewitz (Eds.), *Harm reduction: Pragmatic strategies for managing high-risk behaviors* (2nd ed., pp. 3–35). New York: Guilford Press.

Conradi, L., Hendricks, A., & Merino, C. (2007). Preliminary adaptations for working with traumatized Latino/Hispanic children and their families. *Culture and Trauma Brief*, 2(3). Retrieved November 30, 2011 from http://www.nctsn.org/nctsn_assets/pdfs/culture_and_trauma_brief_v2n3_LatinoHispanicChildren.pdf

Cordova, M.J., Giese-Davis, J., Golant, M., Kronenwetter, C., Chang, V., & Spiegel, D. (2007). Breast cancer as trauma: Posttraumatic stress and posttraumatic growth. *Journal of Clinical Psychology in Medical Settings*, 14(4), 308–319.

Costin, L.B. (1991). Unraveling the Mary Ellen legend: Origins of the "Cruelty" movement. *Social Services Review*, 65(2), 203–223.

Courtois, C.A. (2010). *Healing the incest wound: Adult survivors in therapy* (2nd ed.). New York: W. W. Norton & Company.

Cunningham, M. (2003). Impact of trauma work on social work clinicians: Empirical findings. *Social Work, 48*(4), 451–459.

Cwikel, J., & Behar, L. (1999). Organizing social work services with adult cancer patients: Integrating empirical research. *Social Work in Health Care, 28*(3), 55–76.

Dalenberg, C.J. (2004). Maintaining the safe and effective therapeutic relationship in the context of distrust and anger: Countertransference and complex trauma. *Psychotherapy: Theory, Research, Practice, Training, 41*(4), 438–447.

Dane, B. (2000). Child welfare workers: An innovative approach for interacting with secondary trauma. *Journal of Social Work Education, 36*(1), 27–38.

Davis, A. (2008). Interpersonal and physical dating violence among teens. The National Council on Crime and Delinquency Focus. Retrieved October 30, 2009 from http://www.nccd-crc.org/nccd/pubs/Dating%20Violence%20Among%20Teens.pdf

Davis, L. (1991). *Allies in healing: when the person you love was sexually abused as a child.* New York: Harper Perennial.

Del Rio, N. (2004). A framework for multicultural end-of-life care: Enhancing social work practice. In J. Berzoff & P. Silverman (Eds.), *Living with dying: A handbook for end-of-life healthcare practitioners* (pp. 489–461). New York: Columbia University Press.

Department of Veterans Affairs & Department of Defense (2017). *VA/DoD clinical practice guideline for the management of post-traumatic stress.* Washington, DC: Veterans Health Administration, Department of Veterans Affairs and Health Affairs, Department of Defense. Office of Quality and Performance publication 10Q-CPG/PTSD-04. Retrieved November 18, 2019 from https://www.healthquality.va.gov/guidelines/MH/ptsd/VADoDPTSDCPGFinal.pdf

Desai, R.A., Harpaz-Rotem, I., Najavits, L.M., & Rosenheck, R.A. (2008). Impact of the seeking safety program on clinical outcomes among homeless female veterans with psychiatric disorders. *Psychiatric Services, 59*(9), 996–1003.

Desalvo, L. (2000). *Writing as a way of healing: How telling our stories transforms our lives.* Boston: Beacon Press.

Devine, D., Parker, P.A., Fouladi, R.T., & Cohen, L. (2003). The association between social support, intrusive thoughts, avoidance, and adjustment following an experimental cancer treatment. *Psycho-Oncology, 12*(5), 453–462.

de Vries, M.W. (1996). Trauma in cultural perspective. In B.A. van der Kolk, A.C. McFarlane, & L. Weisaeth (Eds.), *Traumatic stress: The effects of overwhelming experience on mind, body, and society* (pp. 398–413). New York: Guilford Press.

Dinsmore, C. (1991). *From surviving to thriving: Incest, feminism, and recovery.* Albany: State University of New York Press.

Disability Rights International: Kenyan Association for the Intellectually Handicapped. (September 27, 2018). *Infanticide and Abuse: Killing and confinement of children with disabilities in Kenya.*

Dominguez, R.Z., Nelke, C.F., & Perry, B.D. (2006). Sexual abuse of children. American Academy of Experts in Traumatic Stress website. Retrieved April 24, 2010 from http://www.aaets.org/article124.htm

Dutton, M.A., Orloff, L.E., & Hass, A. (2000). Characteristics of help-seeking behaviors, resources and service needs of battered immigrant Latinas. *Georgetown Journal on Poverty Law & Policy, 2*(2), 245–305.

Dziegielewski, S.F., & Sumner, K. (2005). An examination of the U.S. Response to bioterrorism: Handling the threat and aftermath through crisis intervention. In A.R. Roberts (Ed.), *Crisis intervention handbook: Assessment, treatment, and research* (3rd ed., pp. 262–278). New York: Oxford University Press.

Edgar-Bailey, M., & Kress, V.E. (2010). Resolving child and adolescent traumatic grief: Creative techniques and interventions. *Journal of Creativity in Mental Health*, 5(2), 158–176.

Edwards, A., & Lutzker, J.R. (2008). Iterations of the SafeCare® model. An evidence-based child maltreatment prevention program. *Behavior Modification*, 32, 736–756.

Edwards, V.J., Anda, R.F., Dube, S.R., Dong, M., Chapman, D.F., & Felitti, V.J. (2005). The wide-ranging health consequences of adverse childhood experiences. In K. Kendall-Tackett & S. Giacomoni (Eds.), *Victimization of children and youth: Patterns of abuse, response strategies* (pp. 178–197). Kingston, NJ: Civic Research Institute.

Ehrensaft, M.K. (2008). Intimate partner violence: Persistence of myths and implications for intervention. *Children and Youth Services Review*, 30, 276–286.

Elklit, A., & Kurdahl, S. (2013). The psychological reactions after witnessing a killing in public in a Danish high school. *European Journal of Psychotraumatology*, 4, 10.3402/ejpt. v4i0.19826. https://doi.org/10.3402/ejpt.v4i0.19826.

Episode 133 – Elaine Hammond: Burnout and Self-Care in Social Work. (2013, December 9). *inSocialWork® Podcast Series*. [Audio Podcast] Retrieved from http://insocialwork.org/episode.asp?ep=133

Episode 137 – Eda Kauffman: Clinical Supervision: Integrating a Trauma-Informed Lens. (2014, February 17). *inSocialWork® Podcast Series*. [Audio Podcast] Retrieved from http://insocialwork.org/episode.asp?ep=137

Evans, A. (2018). #MeToo: A study on sexual assault as reported in the New York Times. *Occam's Razor, 8*, Article 3. Retrieved August 18, 2019 from https://cedar.wwu.edu/orwwu/vol8/iss1/3

Evans, S.E., Davies, C., & DiLillo, D. (2008). Exposure to domestic violence: A meta-analysis of child adolescent outcomes. *Aggression and Violent behavior*, 13, 131–140.

Fabri, M.R. (2001). Reconstructing safety: Adjustments to the therapeutic frame in the treatment of survivors of political torture. *Professional Psychology: Research and Practice*, 32(5), 452–457.

Fairbank, J.A., & Gerrity, E.T. (2007). Making trauma intervention principles public policy: Commentary on "Five Essential Elements of Immediate and MidTerm Mass Trauma Intervention: Empirical Evidence" by Hobfoll, Watson et al.. *Psychiatry Interpersonal & Biological Processes*, 70(4), 316–319.

Fang, L., & Chen, T. (2004). Outreach and education to deal with cultural resistance to mental health services. In N. Webb (Ed.), *Mass trauma and violence* (pp. 234–255). New York: The Guilford Press.

Farrell, D.P. (2009). Sexual abuse perpetrated by Roman Catholic priests and religious. *Mental Health, Religion & Culture*, 12(1), 39–53.

Farwell, N., & Cole, J.B. (2001–2002). Community as a context of healing: Psychosocial recovery of children affected by war and political violence. *International Journal of Mental Health*, 30(4), 19–41.

Feldman Barrett, L., Gross, J.J., Conner, T., & Benvenuto, M. (2001). Knowing what you're feeling and knowing what to do about it: Mapping the relation between emotion differentiation and emotion regulation. *Cognition and Emotion*, 15, 713–724.

Feldner, M.T., Monson, C.M., & Friedman, M.J. (2007). A critical analysis of approaches to targeted PTSD prevention: Current status and theoretically derived future directions. *Behavior Modification, 31(1)*, 80–116.

Figley, C.R. (2002). Compassion fatigue: Psychotherapists' chronic lack of self care. *JCLP/In Session, 58(11)*, 1433–1441.

Finkelhor, D. (1984). *Child sexual abuse: New theory and research*. New York: Free Press.

Finkelhor, D. (1986). *Sourcebook on child sexual abuse*. Beverly Hills, CA: Sage.

Finkelhor, D. (2008). *Childhood victimization: Violence, crime and abuse in the lives of young people*. New York: Oxford University Press.

Finkelhor, D. (2009). The prevention of childhood sexual abuse. *The Future of Children, 19(2)*, 169–194.

Finkelhor, D., Cross, T.P., & Cantor, E.N. (2006). How the justice system responds to juvenile victims: A comprehensive model. *Juvenile Justice Bulletin, NCJ210951*, 1–12. Washington, DC: Office of Juvenile Justice & Delinquency Prevention.

Finkelstein, N., Rechberger, E., Russell, L., Van De Mark, N.R., Noether, C.D., O'Keefe, M. et al. (2005). Building resilience in children of mothers who have co-occurring disorders and histories of violence. *Journal of Behavioral Health Services & Research, 32(2)*, 141–154.

Fisher, W.A., & Penny, D.J. (1996). Mental health service recipients: The role in shaping organizational policy. *Administration and Policy in Mental Health, 23(6)*, 547–553.

Foa, E. (2001). The Child PTSD Symptom Scale. Retrieved March 17, 2012 from http://www.ptsd.va.gov/professional/pages/assessments/cpss.asp

Foa, E.B., Keane, T.M., Friedman, M.J., & Cohen, J.A. (2010). Treatment guidelines. In E.B. Foa, T.M. Keane, M.J. Friedman, & J.A. Cohen (Eds.), *Effective treatments for PTSD: Practice guidelines from the International society for traumatic stress studies* (2nd ed., pp. 539–616). New York: Guilford Press.

Fobair, P., Stearns, N., Christ, G., Dozier-Hall, D., Newman, N.W., Zabora, J. et al. (2009). Historical threads in the development of oncology social work. *Journal of Psychosocial Oncology, 27(2)*, 155–215.

Foster, H., & Brooks-Gunn, J. (2009). Toward a stress process model of children's exposure to physical family and community violence. *Clinical Child Family Psychology Review, 12*, 71–94.

Fowler, D.N., & Chanmugam, A. (2007). A critical review of quantitative analyses of children exposed to domestic violence: Lessons for practice and research. *Brief Treatment and Crisis Intervention, 7*, 322–344.

Freddolino, P.P., Moxley, D.P., & Hyduk, C.A. (2004). A differential model of advocacy in social work practice. *Families in Society: The Journal of Contemporary Social Sciences, 85(1)*, 119–128.

Freeman, A., & Combs, G. (1996). *Narrative therapy*. New York: W. W. Norton & Company.

Friedman, M.B. (2004). *Speak out! A guide to advocacy for improved mental health policy*. New York: The Mental Health Association of New York City and the Mental Health Association of Westchester.

Gabriel, M.A. (2007). *AIDS trauma and support group therapy: Mutual aid, empowerment, connection*. New York: Free Press.

Gallow-Silver, L. (2004). September 11th: Reflections on living with dying in disaster relief. In J. Berzoff & P. Silverman (Eds.), *Living with dying: A handbook for end-of-life healthcare practitioners* (pp. 72–93). New York: Columbia University Press.

Garfield, P. (1991). *The healing power of dreams*. New York: Simon & Schuster.

Gathanju, D. (2006).Maasai ritual of female circumcision [Electronic Version]. *Orato: Speak from Experience*. Retrieved October 3, 2012 from http://www.orato.com/world-affairs/maasai-ritual-of-female-circumcision

Gazelle, G., Buxbaum, R., & Daniels, E. (2001). The development of a palliative care program for managed care patients: A case example. *Journal of the American Geriatric Society, 49(9)*, 1241–1248.

Gelles, R. (1993). Family violence. In R. Hampton, T. Gullotta, G. Adams, E. Potter, & R. Weissberg (Eds.), *Family violence: Prevention and treatment* (pp. 1–24). Newbury Park, CA: Sage Publications, Inc.

Gelman, C.R., & Mirabito, D.M. (2005). Practicing what we teach: Using case studies from 9/11 to teach crisis intervention from a generalist perspective. *Journal of Social Work Education, 41(3)*, 479–494.

Gershater-Molko, R.M., Lutzker, J.R., & Wesch, D. (2002). Using recidivism data to evaluate Project SafeCare: Teaching bonding, safety and healthcare skills to parents. *Child Maltreatment, 7(3)*, 277–285.

Gil, E. (1991). *The healing power of play: Working with abused children*. New York: Guilford Press.

Gil, E. (2006). *Helping abused and traumatized children: Integrating directive and nondirective approaches*. New York: Guilford Press.

Giller, E. (1999). What is psychological trauma? Retrieved June 26, 2011 from http://www.sidran.org/sub.cfm?contentID=88&sectionid=4

Gillum, T.L. (2008). The benefits of a culturally specific intimate partner violence intervention for African American survivors. *Violence Against Women, 14(8)*, 917–943.

Gillum, T.L. (2009). Improving services to African American survivors of IPV. *Violence Against Women, 15(1)*, 57–80.

Gitterman, A. (1994). Developing a new group service: Strategies and skills. In A. Gitterman & L. Shulman (Eds.), *Mutual aid groups, vulnerable populations, and the life cycle* (2nd ed., pp. 59–77). New York: Columbia University Press.

Glajchen, M., Portenoy, R., Fraidin, L., Goelitz, A., Green, S., & Gregory, J. (2002). *The caregiver resource directory: A practical guide for family caregivers* (New Jersey ed.). New York: Beth Israel Medical Center.

Goelitz, A. (2001a). Dreaming their way into life: A group experience with oncology patients. *Social Work with Groups, 24(1)*, 53–67.

Goelitz, A. (2001b). Nurturing life with dreams: Therapeutic dream work with cancer patients. *Clinical Social Work Journal, 29(4)*, 375–385.

Goelitz, A. (2003a). Suicidal ideation at end-of-life: The palliative care team's role. *Palliative & Supportive Care, 1(3)*, 275–278.

Goelitz, A. (2003b). When accessibility is an issue: Telephone support groups for caregivers. *Smith College Studies in Social Work, 73(3)*, 385–394.

Goelitz, A. (2009). *The emotional content of dreams: An exploratory study of trauma survivors' dreams*. Saarbrucken, Germany: VDM Verlag Dr. Muller.

Goelitz, A., & Stewart-Kahn, A. (2006/2007). Therapeutic use of space: One agency's transformation project. *Journal of Creativity in Mental Health, 2(4)*, 31–44.

Goleman, D. (1995). *Emotional intelligence*. New York: Bantam Books.

Goleman, D. (2004). *Destructive emotions: How can we overcome them? A scientific dialogue with the Dalai Lama*. New York: Bantam Books.

Gomez, C., & Yassen, J. (2007). Revolutionizing the clinical frame: Individual and social advocacy practice on behalf of trauma survivors. *Journal of Aggression, Maltreatment & Trauma, 14(1/2)*, 245–263.

Goodman, R. (2002). *The Strengths and Difficulties Questionnaire (SDQ)*. Retrieved December 28, 2019 from https://www.sdqinfo.com/py/sdqinfo/b3.py?language=Englishqz(USA)

Goodman, R.F., & Brown, E.J. (2008). Service and science in times of crisis: Developing, planning, and implementing a clinical research program for children traumatically bereaved after 9/11. *Death Studies, 32*, 154–180.

Gordon, R. (1983). An operational classification of disease prevention. *Public Health Reports, 98*, 107–109.

Gostin, L.O. (2000). *Public health law and ethics: A reader*. Retrieved November 8, 2010 from http://www.publichealthlaw.net/Reader/docs/Tarasoff.pdf

Graber, K. (1991). *Ghosts in the bedroom*. Deerfield Beach, FL: Health Communications, Inc.

Granvold, D.K. (2005). The crisis of divorce: Cognitive-behavioral and constructivist assessment and treatment. In A.R. Roberts (Ed.), *Crisis intervention handbook: Assessment, treatment, and research* (3rd ed., pp. 650–681). New York: Oxford University Press.

Graziano, R. (1997). The challenge of clinical work with survivors of trauma. In J. Brandell (Ed.), *Theory and practice in clinical social work* (pp. 380–403). New York: Free Press.

Graziano, R. (2001). Teaching trauma: A true story. *Journal of Teaching in Social Work, 21(3&4)*, 177–185.

Graziano, R. (2003). Trauma and aging. *Journal of Gerontological Social Work, 40(4)*, 3–21.

Greenberg, L. (2004). Emotion-focused therapy. *Clinical Psychology and Psychotherapy (Special Issue), 11*, 3–16.

Greenberg, L., & Bolger, E. (2001). An emotion-focused approach to the overregulation of emotion and emotional pain. *Journal of Clinical Psychology, 57(2)*, 197–211.

Greenberg, L., & Paivio, S. (1998). Allowing and accepting painful emotional experiences. *The International Journal of Action Methods, 51(2)*, 47–62.

Greene, G.J., Lee, M., Trask, R., & Rheinscheld, J. (2005). How to work with clients' strengths in crisis intervention: A solution-focused approach. In A.R. Roberts (Ed.), *Crisis intervention handbook: Assessment, treatment, and research* (3rd ed., pp. 64–89). New York: Oxford University Press.

Greenwood, G.L., Relf, M.V., Huang, B., Pollack, L.M., Canchola, J.A., & Catania, J.A. (2002). Battering victimization among a probability-based sample of men who have sex with men. *American Journal of Public Health, 92(12)*, 1964–1969.

Greer, S. (2002). Psychological intervention: The gap between research and practice. *Acta Oncologica, 41(3)*, 238–243.

Griffith, D.M., Allen, J.O., Zimmerman, M.A., Morrel-Samuels, S., Reischel, T.M., Cohen, S.E. et al. (2008). Organizational empowerment in community mobilization to address youth violence. *American Journal of Preventive Medicine, 34(3)*, 89–99.

Gross, J.J., & John, O.P. (2003). Individual differences in two emotion regulation processes: Implications for affect, relationships, and well-being. *Journal of Personality and Social Psychology, 85(2)*, 348–362.

Haen, C. (2008). Vanquishing monsters: Drama therapy for treating childhood trauma in a group setting. In C.A. Malchiodi & B. Perry (Eds.), *Creative interventions with traumatized children* (pp. 225–246). New York: Guilford Press.

Haggis, P. (Writer and Director). (2007). *In the Valley of Elah*. Warner Independent.

Hales, T.W., Green, S.A., Bissonette, S., Warden, A., Diebold, J., Koury, S.P. et al. (2019). Trauma-informed care outcome study. *Research on Social Work Practice, 29(5)*, 529–539.

Hantman, S., & Solomon, Z. (2007). Recurrent trauma: Holocaust survivors cope with aging and cancer. *Social Psychiatry & Psychiatric Epidemiology, 42(5)*, 396–402.

Harper, F.W.K., Schmidt, J.E., Beacham, A.O., Salsman, J.M., Averill, A.J., Graves, K.D. et al. (2007). The role of social cognitive processing theory and optimism in positive psychosocial and physical behavior change after cancer diagnosis and treatment. *Psycho-Oncology*, *16(1)*, 79–91.

Harris, M., & Fallot, R.D. (2001). Envisioning a trauma-informed service system: A vital paradigm shift. In M. Harris & R.D. Fallot (Eds.), *Using trauma theory to design service systems* (pp. 3–22). San Francisco: Jossey-Bass.

Hartmann, H. (1958). *Ego psychology and the problem of adaptation* (trans. D. Rapaport). New York: International Universities Press.

Harvey, J.H., & Miller, E.D. (2000). *Loss and trauma: General and close relationship perspectives*. New York: Routledge.

Hauck, S., Schestatsky, S., Terra, L., Kruel, L., & Ceitlin, L. (2007). Parental bonding and emotional response to trauma: A study of rape victims. *Psychotherapy Research*, *17(1)*, 83–90.

Haurgrud, W., Gratch, L.K., & Magruder, V.L. (1997). Victimization and perpetration rates of violence in gay and lesbian relationships: Gender issues explored. *Violence and Victims*, *12(2)*, 173–184.

Hays, D.G., Green, E., Orr, J.J., & Flowers, L. (2007). Advocacy counseling for female survivors of partner abuse: Implications for counselor education. *Counselor Education and Supervision*, *46*, 184–197.

Heckman, T.G., Barcikowski, R., Ogles, B., Suhr, J., Carlson, B., Holroyd, K. et al. (2006). A telephone-delivered coping improvement group intervention for middle-aged and older adults living with HIV/AIDS. *Annals of Behavioral Medicine*, *32(1)*, 27–38.

Hefferon, K., Grealy, M., & Mutrie, N. (2009). Post-traumatic growth and life threatening physical illness: A systematic review of the qualitative literature. *British Journal of Health Psychology*, *14(2)*, 343–378.

Hepworth, D.J., Rooney, R.H., Rooney, G.D., Strom-Gottfried, K., & Larsen, J. (2010). *Direct social work practice: Theory and skills*. Belmont, CA: Brooks/Cole.

Herman, J. (1992). *Trauma and recovery*. New York: Basic Books.

Hesse, A.R. (2002). Secondary trauma: How working with trauma survivors affects therapists. *Clinical Social Work Journal*, *30(3)*, 293–310.

Hillman, J.L. (2002). *Crisis intervention and trauma: New approaches to evidence-based practice*. New York: Kluwer/Plenum.

Holland, J.C. (2002). History of psycho-oncology: Overcoming attitudinal and conceptual barriers. *Psychosomatic Medicine*, *64*, 206–221.

Hopper, E., Emerson, D., Levine, P.A., Cope, S., & van der Kolk, B.A. (2011). *Overcoming trauma through yoga: Reclaiming your body*. Boston: North Atlantic Books.

Horst, E.A. (2000). *Questions and answers about clergy sexual misconduct*. Collegeville, MN: Liturgical Press.

Hostler, M.J., & O'Neil, M. (2018). Reframing Sexual Violence: From #MeToo to Time's Up. *Stanford Social Innovation Review*. Retrieved August 18, 2019 from https://ssir.org/articles/entry/reframing_sexual_violence_from_metoo_to_times_up

Howard, J., & Goelitz, A. (2004). Psychoeducation as a response to community disaster. *Brief Treatment and Crisis Intervention*, *4*, 1–10.

Hudson, T. (2002, May). Support-group therapy enhances quality of life for breast cancer survivors. *Townsend Letter for Doctors and Patients*, *226*, 145.

Hussey, J.M., Chang, J., & Kotch, J.B. (2006). Child maltreatment in the United States: Prevalence, risk factors, and adolescent health consequences. *Pediatrics*, *118(3)*, 933–942.

Institute of Medicine. (1994). *Reducing risks for mental disorders: Frontiers for preventive intervention research* (Eds.: P.J. Mrazek & R.J. Haggerty). Committee on Prevention of Mental Disorders, Division of Biobehavorial Sciences and Mental Disorders. Washington, DC: National Academy Press.

Institute of Medicine. (2003). *Preparing for the psychological consequences of terrorism: A public health strategy*. Washington, DC: The National Academies Press. Retrieved December 20, 2019 from https://doi.org/10.17226/10717

Institute of Medicine. (2008). *Treatment of posttraumatic stress disorder: An assessment of the evidence*. Washington, DC: The National Academies Press.

Israelski, D.M., Prentiss, D.E., Lubega, S., Balmas, G., Garcia, P., Muhammad, M. et al. (2007). Psychiatric co-morbidity in vulnerable populations receiving primary care for HIV/AIDS. *AIDS Care, 19*(2), 220–225.

Jacob, K.S. (2013). Employing psychotherapy across cultures and contexts. *Indian Journal of Psychological Medicine, 35*(4), 323–325.

Jacobsen, L.K., Southwick, S.M., & Kosten, T.R. (2001). Substance use disorders in patients with posttraumatic stress disorder: A review of the literature. *The American Journal of Psychiatry, 158*, 1184–1190.

James, B. (1994). *Handbook for treatment of attachment-trauma problems in children*. New York: Free Press.

James, S.D. (2009). Teen commits suicide due to bullying: Parents sue school for son's death [Electronic Version]. Retrieved March 20, 2012 from http://abcnews.go.com/Health/MindMoodNews/story?id=7228335

Jaycox, L.H., Tanielian, T.L., Sharma, P., Morse, L., Clum, G., & Stein, B.D. (2007). Schools' mental health responses after hurricanes Katrina and Rita. *Psychiatric Services, 58*(10), 1339–1343.

Johnson, S. (2008). *Hold me tight*. New York: Little, Brown & Company.

Johnson, S.M., & Williams-Keeler, L. (1998). Creating healing relationships for couples dealing with trauma: The use of emotionally focused marital therapy. *Journal of Marital and Family Therapy, 24*(1), 25–40.

Jones, M.J. (1994). Speaking the unspoken: Parents of sexually victimized children. In A. Gitterman & L. Shulman (Eds.), *Mutual aid groups, vulnerable populations, and the life cycle* (2nd ed., pp. 239–255). New York: Columbia University Press.

Jones, L., Brazel, D., Peskind, E.R., Morelli, T., & Raskind, M.A. (2000). Group therapy program for African-American veterans with posttraumatic stress disorder. *Psychiatric Services, 51*(9), 1177–1179.

Jones, E., & Wessely, S.C. (2003). "Forward psychiatry" in the military: Its origins and effectiveness. *Journal of Traumatic Stress, 16*, 411–419.

Kabat-Zinn, J. (1991). *Full catastrophic living: Using the wisdom of your body and mind to face stress, pain, and illness*. New York: Dell Publishing.

Kagan, R., Douglas, A., Hornik, J., & Kratz, S.L. (2008). Real life heroes pilot study: Evaluation of a treatment model for children with traumatic stress. *Journal of Child & Adolescent Trauma, 1*, 5–22.

Kalsched, D. (1996). *The inner world of trauma*. London and New York: Routledge.

Kangas, M., Henry, J.L., & Bryant, R.A. (2002). Posttraumatic stress disorder following cancer: A conceptual and empirical review. *Clinical Psychology Review, 22*(4), 499.

Kaplan, L. (2007). Insidious trauma and the sexual minority client. In M. Bussey & J. Bula Wise (Eds.), *Trauma transformed: An empowerment response* (pp. 142–158). New York: Columbia University Press.

Kazak, A.E., Alderfer, M.A., Streisand, R., Simms, S., Rourke, M.T., Barakat, L.P. et al. (2004). Treatment of posttraumatic stress symptoms in adolescent survivors of childhood cancer and their families: A randomized clinical trial. *Journal of Family Psychology*, *18(3)*, 493–504.

Kellermann, P.F. (2000). The therapeutic aspects of psychodrama with traumatised people. In P.F. Kellermann & K. Hudgins (Eds.), *Psychodrama with trauma survivors: Acting out your pain*. London: Jessica Kingsley.

Kelley, M.L., Schwerin, M.L., Farrar, K.L., & Lane, M.E. (2005). An evaluation of a sexual assault prevention and advocacy program for U.S. Navy personnel. *Military Medicine*, *170(4)*, 320–326.

Kenardy, J.A., Spence, S.H., & Macleod, A.C. (2006). Screening for posttraumatic stress disorder in children after accidental injury. *Pediatrics*, *118(3)*, 1002–1009.

Kenny, M., Capri, V., Thakkar-Kolar, R.R., Ryan, E.E., & Runyon, M.K. (2008). Child sexual abuse: From prevention to self-protection. *Child Abuse Review*, *17*, 36–54.

Kessler, R., Sonnega, A., Bromet, E., Hughes, M., & Nelson, C. (1995). Posttraumatic stress disorder in the National Comorbidity Survey. *Archives of General Psychiatry*, *52*, 1048–1060.

Kettner, P.M., Moroney, R.M., & Martin, L.L. (2016). *Designing and managing programs: An effectiveness-based approach*. Thousand Oaks, CA: Sage.

Kiselica, M.S., & Robinson, M. (2001). Bringing advocacy counseling to life: The history, issues, and human drama of social justice work in counseling. *Journal of Counseling and Development*, *79*, 387–395.

Klein, R.J. (2008). Ready..., set..., relax! Relaxation strategies with children and adolescents. In C.A. Malchiodi (Ed.), *Creative interventions with traumatized children* (pp. 302–320). New York: Guilford Press.

Klein, S., & Alexander, D. (2011). The impact of trauma within organizations. In N. Tehrani (Ed.), *Managing trauma in the workplace: Supporting workers and organisations* (pp. 117–138). New York: Routledge.

Klingman, A., & Cohen, E. (2004). *School-based multisystemic interventions for mass trauma*. New York: Springer.

Klorer, P.G. (2006). Art therapy with traumatized families. In L. Carey (Ed.), *Expressive and creative arts methods for trauma survivors* (pp. 115–132). London and Philadelphia: Jessica Kingsley Publishers.

Knaevelsrud, C., Böttche, M., Pietrzak, R.H., Freyberger, H.J., & Kuwert, P. (2017). Efficacy and feasibility of a therapist-guided internet-based intervention for older persons with childhood traumatization: A randomized controlled trial. *The American Journal of Geriatric Psychiatry* ,*25(8)*, 878–888.

Knaevelsrud, C., & Maercker, A. (2007). Internet-based treatment for PTSD reduces distress and facilitates the development of a strong therapeutic alliance: A randomized controlled clinical trial. *BMC Psychiatry*, *7(13)*, 13.

Knox, K., & Roberts, A.R. (2005). Crisis intervention with stalking victims. In R. Roberts (Ed.), *Crisis intervention handbook: Assessment, treatment, and research* (3rd ed., pp. 483–498). New York: Oxford University Press.

Krug, E., Dahlberg, L., Mercy, J., Zwi, A., & Lozano, R. (Eds.). (2002). *World report on violence and health*. Geneva: World Health Organization.

Krysińska, K., & Lester, D. (2006). The contribution of psychology to the study of the holocaust. *Dialogue & Universalism*, *16(5/6)*, 141–156.

La Greca, A., & Silverman, W. (2009). Treatment and prevention of posttraumatic stress reactions in children and adolescents exposed to disasters and terrorism: What is the evidence? *Child Development Perspectives, 3(1)*, 4–10.

Lahad, M. (2000). Darkness over the abyss. *Traumatology, 6(4)*, 273–293.

Laird, J., & Hartman, A. (1985). *The handbook of child welfare: Context, knowledge, and practice.* New York: Free Press.

Lanche, M. (2008). Higher risk of PTSD in patients with history of mood and anxiety disorders. *Primary Psychiatry, 15(6)*, 20–21.

Lang, J.M., & Smith Stover, C. (2008). Symptom patterns among youth exposed to intimate partner violence. *Journal of Family Violence, 23*, 619–629.

Lanius, R., Williamson, P., Densmore, M., Boksman, K., Neufeld, R., Gati, J. et al. (2004). The nature of traumatic memories: A 4-T FMRI functional connectivity analysis. *American Journal of Psychiatry, 161(1)*, 36–44.

Lanius, R., Williamson, P., Hopper, J., Densmore, M., Boksman, K., Gupta, M. et al. (2003). Recall of emotional states in posttraumatic stress disorder: An fMRI investigation. *Biological Psychiatry, 53(3)*, 204–210.

Lantz, J., & Harper-Dorton, K.V. (2007). *Cross-cultural practice: Social work with diverse populations* (2nd ed.). Chicago: Lyceum Books.

Lazarus, R.S. (2006). Emotions and interpersonal relationships: Toward a person-centered conceptualization of emotions and coping. *Journal of Personality, 74(1)*, 9–46.

Lazarus, R.S., & Folkman, S. (1987). Transactional theory and research on emotions and coping. *European Journal of Personality, 1(3)*, 141–169.

Lee, J.A.B., & Swenson, C.R. (1994). The concept of mutual aid. In A. Gitterman & L. Shulman (Eds.), *Mutual aid groups, vulnerable populations, and the life cycle* (2nd ed., pp. 413–429). New York: Columbia University Press.

Lee, J.A.B., & Swenson, C.R. (2005). Mutual aid: A buffer against risk. In A. Gitterman and L. Shulman (Eds.), *Mutual aid groups, vulnerable and resilient populations, and the life cycle* (3rd ed., pp. 573–597). New York: Columbia University Press.

Lefkowitz, C., Paharia, I., Prout, M., Debiak, D., & Bleiberg, J. (2005). Animal-assisted prolonged exposure: A treatment for survivors of sexual assault suffering posttraumatic stress disorder. *Society & Animals, 13(4)*, 275–295.

Leland, J. (2010, January 31). Iraq mends a system to treat trauma. *The New York Times*, p. A6.

Lens, V. (2005). Advocacy and argumentation in the public arena: A guide for social workers. *Social Work, 50*, 231–238.

Leseho, J., & Maxwell, L.R. (2010). Coming alive: Creative movement as a personal coping strategy on the path to healing and growth. *British Journal of Guidance & Counselling, 38(1)*, 17–30.

Levenson, J.S. (2017). Trauma-informed social work practice. *Social Work, 62(2)*, 105–113.

Levine, A., & Karger, W. (2004). The trajectory of illness. In J. Berzoff & P. Silverman (Eds.), *Living with dying: A handbook for end-of-life healthcare practitioners* (pp. 273–296). New York: Columbia University Press.

Levine, E.G., Eckhardt, J., & Targ, E. (2005). Change in post-traumatic stress symptoms following psychosocial treatment for breast cancer. *Psycho-Oncology, 14(8)*, 618–635.

Levine, P.A. (1997). *Waking the tiger: Healing trauma – The innate capacity to transform overwhelming experiences*. Berkeley, CA: North Atlantic Books.

Levy, F., Ross, P., & Guthrie, T. (2008). *Enhancing safety and justice for victims of domestic violence: Voices of women in the queens integrated domestic violence Court*. New York: Vera Institute for Justice.

Levy Simon, B. (2004). *The empowerment tradition in American social work: A history.* New York: Columbia University Press.

Lew, H.L., Poole, J.H., Vanderploeg, R.D., Goodrich, G.L., Dekelboum, S., Guillory, S.B. et al. (2007). Program development and defining characteristics of returning military in a VA polytrauma network site. *Journal of Rehabilitation, Research and Development,* 44(7), 1027–1034.

Lewis, S. (2005). The crisis State assessment scale: Development and psychometrics. In A.R. Roberts (Ed.), *Crisis intervention handbook: Assessment, treatment, and research* (3rd ed., pp. 723–741). New York: Oxford University Press.

Lewis, S., & Roberts, A.R. (2001). Crisis assessment tools: The good, the bad, and the available. *Brief Treatment and Crisis Intervention, 1,* 17–28.

Lieberman, A.F., & Van Horn, P. (2004). *Don't hit my mommy: A manual for child–parent psychotherapy with young witnesses of family violence.* Washington, DC: Zero to Three.

Lightfoot, E., & Williams, O. (2009). The intersection of disability, diversity, and domestic violence: Results of national focus groups. *Journal of Aggression, Maltreatment & Trauma, 18,* 133–152.

Ligon, J. (2005). Mobile crisis units: Frontline community mental health services. In A.R. Roberts (Ed.), *Crisis intervention handbook: Assessment, treatment, and research* (3rd ed., pp. 602–618). New York: Oxford University Press.

Linehan, M.M. (1993). *Skills training manual for treating borderline personality disorder.* New York: Guilford Press.

Litz, B., Orsillo, S., Kaloupek, D., & Weathers, F. (2000). Emotional processing in posttraumatic stress disorder. *Journal of Abnormal Psychology, 109(1),* 26–39.

Logan, T.K., Walker, R., & Hunt, G. (2009). Understanding human trafficking in the United States. *Trauma, Violence, & Abuse, 10(1),* 3–30.

Lothane, Z. (1983). Reality, dream, and trauma. *Contemporary Psychoanalysis, 19(3),* 423–443.

Luebbert, K., Dahme, B., & Hasenbring, M. (2001). The effectiveness of relaxation training in reducing treatment-related symptoms and improving emotional adjustment in acute non-surgical cancer treatment: A meta-analytical review. *Psycho-Oncology, 10(6),* 490–502.

Lustig, S.L., Weine, S.M., Saxe, G.N., & Beardslee, W.R. (2004). Testimonial psychotherapy for adolescent refugees: A case series. *Transcultural Psychiatry, 41(1),* 31–45.

Mabanglo, M.G. (2002). Trauma and the effects of violence exposure and abuse of children: A review of the literature. *Smith Studies in Social Work, 72(2),* 231–251.

Mahoney, P., Williams, L.M., & West, C.M. (2001). Violence against women by intimate relationship partners. In C.M. Renzetti, J.L. Edleson & R.K. Bergen (Eds.), *Sourcebook on violence against women* (pp. 143–178). Thousand Oaks, CA: Sage Publications.

Malekoff, A. (2000). Bureaucratic barriers to service delivery, administrative advocacy, and mother goose. *Families in Society, 81(3),* 304–314.

Manfield, P., Lovett, J., Engel, L., & Manfield, D. (2017). Use of the flash technique in EMDR therapy: Four case examples. *Journal of EMDR Practice and Research, 11(4),* 195–205.

Mapp, I., & Koch, D. (2004). Creation of a group mural to promote healing following a mass trauma. In N. Webb (Ed.), *Mass trauma and violence* (pp. 100–119). New York: The Guilford Press.

Margolin, G., & Vickerman, K.A. (2007). Post-traumatic stress in children and adolescents exposed to family violence: I. Overview and issues. *Professional Psychology: Research and Practice, 38,* 613–619.

Max, W., Rice, D.P., Finkelstein, E., Bardwell, R., & Leadbetter, S. (2004). The economic toll of intimate partner violence against women in the United States. *Violence and Victims, 19(3),* 259–272.

McAlister Groves, B. (2002). *Children who see too much: Lessons from the child witness to violence project*. Boston: Beacon Press.

McAlister Groves, B., & Zuckerman, B. (1997). Interventions with parents and caregivers of children who are exposed to violence. In J.D. Osofsky (Ed.), *Children in a violent society* (pp. 183–201). New York: Guilford Press.

McBride, J., & Johnson, E.D. (2005). Crisis intervention, grief therapy, and the loss of life. In A.R. Roberts (Ed.), *Crisis intervention handbook: Assessment, treatment, and research* (3rd ed., pp. 279–290). New York: Oxford University Press.

McCann, I.L., & Pearlman, L.A. (1990a). *Psychological trauma and the adult survivor: Theory, therapy, and transformation*. New York: Brunner/Mazel.

McCann, I.L., & Pearlman, L.A. (1990b). Vicarious traumatization: A framework for understanding the psychological effects of working with victims. *Journal of Traumatic Stress, 3(1),* 131–149.

McFarlane, A.C., & Yehuda, R. (1996). Resilience, vulnerability, and the course of posttraumatic reactions. In B.A. van der Kolk, A.C. McFarlane, & L. Weisaeth (Eds.), *Traumatic stress: The effects of overwhelming experience on mind, body, and society* (pp. 155–181). New York: Guilford Press.

McPherson-Sextona, S., & Hostetler, B. (2009). How to respond to the crisis victim with PTSD symptoms: An intervener's guide. *Journal of Police Crisis Negotiations, 9(1),* 61–66.

Mickelson, J.S. (1995). Advocacy. In R.L. Edwards (Ed-in-Chief), *Encyclopedia of social work* (19th ed., Vol. 1, pp. 95–100). Washington, DC: NASW Press.

Miller, A. (1991). *The untouched key: Tracing childhood trauma in creativity and destructiveness*. New York: Anchor Books.

Miller, M. (2001). Creating a safe frame for learning: Teaching about trauma and trauma treatment. *Journal of Teaching in Social Work, 21(3&4),* 159–176.

Mindell, A. (1998). *Dreambody: The body's role in revealing the self*. Portland, OR: Lao Tse Press.

Mishna, F. (2007). Bullying and victimization: Transforming trauma through empowerment. In M. Bussey & J. Bula Wise (Eds.), *Trauma transformed: An empowerment response* (pp. 124–141). New York: Columbia University Press.

Mitchell, A., Clegg, J., & Furniss, F. (2006). Exploring the meaning of trauma with adults with intellectual disabilities. *Journal of Applied Research in Intellectual Disabilities, 19,* 131–142.

Mitchell, J.T. (1983). When disaster strikes: The critical incident stress debriefing process. *Journal of Emergency Medical Services, 8,* 36–39.

Morland, L.A., Greene, C.J., Rosen, C., Mauldin, P.D., & Frueh, B.C. (2009). Issues in the design of a randomized noninferiority clinical trial of telemental health psychotherapy for rural combat veterans with PTSD. *Contemporary Clinical Trials, 30(6),* 513–522.

Motta, R.W., Joseph, J.M., Rose, R.D., Suozzi, J.M., & Liederman, L.J. (1997). Secondary trauma: Assessing inter-generational transmission of war experiences with a modified stroop procedure. *Journal of Clinical Psychology, 53(8),* 895–903.

Murthy, R.S., & Lakshminarayana, R. (2006). Mental health consequences of war: A brief review of research findings. *World psychiatry: official journal of the World Psychiatric Association (WPA), 5(1),* 25–30.

Nader, K. (2004). Treating traumatized children and adolescents: Treatment issues modalities, timing and methods. In N.B. Webb (Ed.), *Mass trauma and violence: Helping families and children cope* (pp. 50–74). New York: Guilford Press.

Najavits, L. (2002). *Seeking safety: A treatment manual for PTSD and substance abuse*. New York: Guilford Press.

Najavits, L. (2010). FAQ – About the model. Seeking Safety website. Retrieved January 30, 2011 from http://www.seekingsafety.org/

Naparstek, B. (2005). *Invisible heroes: Survivors of trauma and how they heal*. New York: Bantam.

National Association of Social Workers. (2017). Code of ethics. Retrieved August 30, 2018 from https://www.socialworkers.org/About/Ethics/Code-of-Ethics/Code-of-Ethics-English

National Center for PTSD. (2011). Cognitive processing therapy. Cognitive processing therapy Retrieved August 13, 2011 from http://www.ptsd.va.gov/public/pages/cognitive_processing_therapy.asp

National Child Traumatic Stress Network. (n.d.b). Symptoms and behaviors associated with exposure to trauma. Retrieved February 10, 2010 from http://www.nctsnet.org/trauma-types/early-childhood-trauma/Symptoms-and-Behaviors-Associated-with-Exposure-to-Trauma

National Child Traumatic Stress Network. (n.d.c). How is early childhood trauma unique? Retrieved February 10, 2010 from http://www.nctsnet.org/content/how-early-childhood-trauma-unique

National Child Traumatic Stress Network. (2005). Facts on trauma and homeless children. Retrieved January 22, 2012 from http://www.nctsnet.org/sites/default/files/assets/pdfs/Facts_on_Trauma_and_Homeless_Children.pdf

National Coalition of Anti-violence Programs. (2009). *Lesbian, gay, bisexual, transgender, and queer domestic violence in the United States in 2008*. Retrieved December 1, 2009 from http://www.ncavp.org/

National Institute on Aging. (2016). *What are the signs of abuse?* Retrieved July 1, 2019 from https://www.nia.nih.gov/health/elder-abuse#signs

National Resource Center on Domestic Violence. (2002). *Expect Respect: A school-based program promoting safe and healthy relationships*. Retrieved September 27, 2010 from http://new.vawnet.org

Neacsiu, A.D., Rizvi, S.L., Vitaliano, P.P., Lynch, T.R., & Linehan, M.M. (2010). Dialectical behavior therapy ways of coping checklist (DBT-WCCL): Development and psychometric properties. *Journal of Clinical Psychology*, *66*(6), 563–582.

Nelson, B.S., & Wampler, K.S. (2000). Systemic effects of trauma in clinic couples: An exploratory study of secondary trauma resulting from childhood abuse. *Journal of Marital & Family Therapy*, *26*(2), 171–184.

Newgass, S., & Schonfeld, D.J. (2005). School crisis intervention, crisis prevention, and crisis response. In A.R. Roberts (Ed.), *Crisis intervention handbook: Assessment, treatment, and research* (3rd ed., pp. 499–518). New York: Oxford University Press.

Newman, E., Christopher, S.R., & Berry, J.O. (2000). Developmental disabilities, trauma exposure, and post-traumatic stress disorder. *Trauma, Violence, & Abuse*, *1*(2), 154–170.

Newmann, J.P., & Sallmann, J. (2004). Women, trauma histories, and co-occurring disorders: Assessing the scope of the problem. *Social Service Review*, *78*(3), 466–498.

Nikulina, V., Hergenrother, J.M., Brown, E.J., Doyle, M.E., Filton, B.J., & Carson, G.S. (2008). From efficacy to effectiveness: The trajectory of the treatment literature for children with PTSD. *Expert Review of Neurotherapeutics*, *8*(8), 1233–1246.

Nix, A., & Fine, S. (Writers). (2007). *War Dance*. In A. Hecht (Producer): ThinkFilm.

Norris, F. (1992). Epidemiology of trauma: Frequency and impact of different potentially traumatic events on different demographic groups. *Journal of Consulting and Clinical Psychology*, *60* 409–418.

Northen, H., & Kurland, R. (2001). *Social work with groups* (3rd ed.). New York: Columbia University Press.

Nurius, P.S., & Norris, J.A. (1996). A cognitive ecological model of women's response to male sexual coercion in dating. *Journal of Psychology and Human Sexuality, 8(1/2)*, 118–139.

Ochsner, K.N., Bunge, S.A., Gross, J.J., & Gabrieli, J.D.E. (2002). Rethinking feelings: An fMRI study of the cognitive regulation of emotion. *Journal of Cognitive Neuroscience, 14(8)*, 1215–1229.

O'Donnell, D.A., Joshi, P.T., & Lewin, S.M. (2007). Innovations: Child & adolescent psychiatry training in developmental responses to trauma for child service providers. *Psychiatric Services, 58*, 12–14.

O'Halloran, M.S., Ingala, A.M., & Copeland, E.P. (2005). Crisis intervention with early adolescents who have suffered a significant loss. In A.R. Roberts (Ed.), *Crisis intervention handbook: Assessment, treatment, and research* (3rd ed., pp. 362–394). New York: Oxford University Press.

Osborn, R.L., Demoncada, A.C., & Feuerstein, M. (2006). Psychosocial interventions for depression, anxiety, and quality of life in cancer survivors: Meta-analyses. *International Journal of Psychiatry in Medicine, 36(1)*, 13–34.

Otis-Green, S., & Rutland, C.B. (2004). Marginalization at the end of life. In J. Berzoff & P. Silverman (Eds.), *Living with dying: A handbook for end-of-life healthcare practitioners* (pp. 462–481). New York: Columbia University Press.

Ovaert, L.B., Cashel, M.L., & Sewell, K.W. (2003). Structured group therapy for posttraumatic stress disorder in incarcerated male juveniles. *American Journal of Orthopsychiatry, 73(3)*, 294–301.

Owen, J.E., Klapow, J.C., Roth, D.L., Shuster, J.L., Jr., Bellis, J., Meredith, R. et al. (2005). Randomized pilot of a self-guided Internet coping group for women with early-stage breast cancer. *Annals of Behavioral Medicine, 30(1)*, 54–64.

Pearlman, L.A., & Courtois, C.A. (2005). Clinical applications of the attachment formula: Relational treatment of complex trauma. *Journal of Traumatic Stress, 18(5)*, 449–459.

Pearlman, L.A., & Saakvitne, K. (1995). *Trauma and the therapist: Countertransference and vicarious traumatization in psychotherapy with incest survivors.* New York: W. W. Norton & Company.

Peckham, N., Howlett, S., & Corbett, A. (2007). Evaluating a survivors group pilot for women with significant intellectual disabilities who have been sexually abused. *Journal of Applied Research in Intellectual Disabilities, 20(4)*, 308–322.

Peled, E., & Davis, D. (1995). *Groupwork with children of battered women: A practitioner's manual.* Thousand Oaks, CA: Sage Publications, Inc.

Pence, E., & Paymar, M. (1993). *Education groups for men who batter: The Duluth model.* New York: Springer.

Perez Foster, R. (2001). When immigration is trauma: Guidelines for the individual and family clinician. *American Journal of Orthopsychiatry, 71(2)*, 153–170.

Perry, B.D. (2001). The neurodevelopmental impact of violence in childhood. In D. Schetky & E.P. Benedek (Eds.), *Textbook of child and adolescent forensic psychiatry* (pp. 221–238). Washington, DC: American Psychiatric Press, Inc.

Pert, C.B. (1999). *Molecules of emotion: The science behind mind-body medicine.* New York: Simon & Schuster.

Petersen, S., Bull, C., Propst, O., Dettinger, S., & Detwiler, L. (2005). Narrative therapy to prevent illness-related stress disorder. *Journal of Counseling & Development, 83(1)*, 41–47.

Pleck, E. (2004). *Domestic tyranny: The making of American social policy against family violence from colonial times to the present.* Chicago, IL: University of Illinois Press.

Pöder, U., Ljungman, G., & von Essen, L. (2008). Posttraumatic stress disorder among parents of children on cancer treatment: A longitudinal study. *Psycho-Oncology, 17(5)*, 430–437.

Posner, K., et al. (2008). *The Columbia-Suicide Severity Rating Scale (C-SSRS)*. The Research Foundation for Mental Hygiene, Inc.

PTSD Alliance. (2001a). Post traumatic stress disorder fact sheet. Retrieved July 26, 2020 from https://www.sidran.org/wp-content/uploads/2018/11/Post-Traumatic-Stress-Disorder-Fact-Sheet-.pdf

PTSD Alliance. (2001b). Who's at risk for developing PTSD? Retrieved July 1, 2011 from http://www.ptsdalliance.org/about_risk.html

Purvin, D. (1996). Child witnesses to domestic violence – common questions. Retrieved July 1, 2011 from http://www.janedoe.org/know/know_children_witnessfaq.htm

Putnam, F. (2003). Ten year research update review: Child sexual abuse. *Journal of the American Academy of Child and Adolescent Psychiatry, 42*(3), 269–278.

Raphael, B., Wilson, J., Meldrum, L., & McFarlane, A. (1996). Acute prevention interventions. In B.A. van der Kolk, A.C. McFarlane, & L. Weisaeth (Eds.), *Traumatic stress: The effects of overwhelming experience on mind, body, and society* (pp. 463–480). New York: Guilford Press.

Raymer, M., & Reese, D. (2004). The history of social work in hospice. In J. Berzoff & P. Silverman (Eds.), *Living with dying: A handbook for end-of-life healthcare practitioners* (pp. 150–160). New York: Columbia University Press.

Reichert, E. (1998). Individual counseling for sexually abused children: A role for animals and storytelling. *Child and Adolescent Social Work Journal, 15*(3), 177–185.

Reilly, I., McDermott, N., & Coulter, S. (2004). Response to community violence in Northern Ireland: A therapeutic response. In N. Webb (Ed.), *Mass trauma and violence* (pp. 304–326). New York: The Guilford Press.

Reyes, G., Elhai, J.D., & Ford, J.D. (2008). *The encyclopedia of psychological trauma*. Hoboken, NJ: John Wiley & Sons, Inc.

Roberts, A.R. (2005a). Bridging the past and present to the future of crisis intervention and crisis management. In A.R. Roberts (Ed.), *Crisis intervention handbook: Assessment, treatment, and research* (3rd ed., pp. 3–34). New York: Oxford University Press.

Roberts, A.R. (2005b). The ACT model: Assessment, crisis intervention, and trauma treatment in the aftermath of community disaster and terrorism attacks. In A.R. Roberts (Ed.), *Crisis intervention handbook: Assessment, treatment, and research* (3rd ed., pp. 143–170). New York: Oxford University Press.

Roberts, A.R., & Everly, G.S. (2006). A meta-analysis of 36 crisis intervention studies. *Brief Treatment and Crisis Intervention, 6*(1), 10–21.

Roberts, W., & Hamilton, C. (2010). "Out of the darkness into the light": A life-story from Ireland. *British journal of Learning Disabilities, 38*(2), 127–132.

Roberts, A.R., & Roberts, B.S. (2005). A comprehensive model for crisis intervention with battered women and their children. In A.R. Roberts (Ed.), *Crisis intervention handbook: Assessment, treatment, and research* (3rd ed., pp. 441–482). New York: Oxford University Press.

Roberts, A.R., & Yeager, K.R. (2005). Lethality assessment and crisis intervention with persons presenting with suicidal ideation. In R. Roberts (Ed.), *Crisis intervention handbook: Assessment, treatment, and research* (3rd ed., pp. 35–63). New York: Oxford University Press.

Rosen, C.S., Matthieu, M.M., & Norris, F.H. (2009). Factors predicting crisis counselor referrals to other crisis counseling, disaster relief, and psychological services: A cross-site analysis of post-Katrina programs. *Administration and Policy in Mental Health and Mental Health Services Research, 36*(3), 186–194.

Rosenheck, R., & Fontana, A. (1995). Long-term sequelae of combat in World War II, Korea, and Vietnam: A comparative study. In R.J. Ursano, B.G. McCaughey, & C.S. Fullerton (Eds.), *Individual and community responses to trauma and disaster* (pp. 330–359). Cambridge, UK: Cambridge University Press.

Rosenthal, E. (1993, July 20). Listening to the emotional needs of cancer patients. *New York Times*. Retrieved March 20, 2012 from http://www.nytimes.com/1993/07/20/science/scientist-work-jimmie-holland-listening-emotional-needs-cancer-patients.html

Rothschild, B. (2000). *The body remembers: The psychophysiology of trauma and trauma treatment*. New York and London: W. W. Norton & Company.

Rothschild, B.A. (2006). *Help for the helper: The psychophysiology of compassion fatigue and vicarious trauma*. New York: W. W. Norton & Company.

Rutter, M. (1988). Epidemiological approaches to developmental psychopathology. *Archives of General Psychiatry, 45*, 486–495.

Saakvitne, K. (2002). Shared trauma: The therapist's increased vulnerability. *Psychoanalytic Dialogues, 12(3)*, 443–449.

Saakvitne, K.W., Gamble, S., Pearlman, L.A., & Lev, B.T. (2000). *Risking connection: A training curriculum for working with survivors of childhood abuse*. Baltimore, MD: The Sidran Press.

Saakvitne, K., & Pearlman, L.A. (1996). *Transforming the pain: A workbook on vicarious traumatization*. New York: W. W. Norton & Company.

Sachs-Ericsson, N., Plant, E.A., Blazer, D., & Arnow, B. (2005). Childhood sexual abuse and physical abuse and the 1-year prevalence of medical problems in the national comorbidity survey. *Health Psychology, 24(1)*, 32–40.

Sandoval, J., Scott, A., & Padilla, I. (2009). Crisis counseling: An overview. *Psychology in the Schools, 46(3)*, 246–256.

Schaefer, D.S., & Pozzaglia, D. (1994). Coping with a nightmare: Hispanic parents of children with cancer. In A. Gitterman & L. Shulman (Eds.), *Mutual aid groups, vulnerable populations, and the life cycle* (2nd ed., pp. 239–255). New York: Columbia University Press.

Schiller, L.Y., & Zimmer, B. (1994). Sharing the secrets: The power of women's groups for sexual abuse survivors. In A. Gitterman & L. Shulman (Eds.), *Mutual aid groups, vulnerable populations, and the life cycle* (2nd ed., pp. 215–238). New York: Columbia University Press.

Schiraldi, G.R. (2009). *The post-traumatic stress disorder sourcebook*. Los Angeles: Lowell House.

Schneider, R.L., & Lester, L. (2001). *Social work advocacy*. Belmont, CA: Brooks/Cole Thomson Learning.

Schnyder, U., Moergeli, H., Klaghofer, R., & Buddeberg, C. (2001). Incidence and prediction of posttraumatic stress disorder symptoms in severely injured accident victims. *The American Journal of Psychiatry, 158(4)*, 594–599.

Schuhmann, E.M., Foote, R.C., Eyberg, S.M., Boggs, S., & Algina, J. (1998). Efficacy of parent–child interaction therapy: Interim report on a randomized trial with short term maintenance. *Journal of Clinical Psychology, 27(1)*, 34–45.

Schwerdtfeger, K.L., & Nelson Goff, B.S. (2007). Intergenerational transmission of trauma: Exploring mother–infant prenatal attachment. *Journal of Traumatic Stress, 20(1)*, 39–51.

Seitz, D.C.M., Besier, T., & Goldbeck, L. (2009). Psychosocial interventions for adolescent cancer patients: A systematic review of the literature. *Psycho-Oncology, 18(7)*, 683–690.

Seligman, L., & Reichenberg, L.W. (2007). *Selecting effective treatments* (3rd ed.). San Francisco: Jossey-Bass.

Shapiro, F. (2001). *Eye movement desensitization and reprocessing: Basic principles, protocols, and procedures* (2nd ed.). New York: Guildford Press.

Sharpless, B.A., & Barber, J.P. (2011). A clinician's guide to PTSD treatments for returning veterans. *Professional Psychology, Research & Practice, 42(1)*, 8–15.

Shaw, J. (2003). Children exposed to war/terrorism. *Clinical Child and Family Psychology Review, 6*, 237. Retrieved September 21, 2019 from https://doi.org/10.1023/B:CCFP. 0000006291.10180.bd

Shaw, J.A., & Harris, J.J. (1995). Children of war and children at war: Child victims of terrorism in Mozambique. In R.J. Ursano, B.G. McCaughey, & C.S. Fullerton (Eds.), *Individual and community responses to trauma and disaster* (pp. 287–305). Cambridge, UK: Cambridge University Press.

Shelby, R.A., Golden-Kreutz, D.M., & Andersen, B.L. (2008). PTSD diagnoses, subsyndromal symptoms, and comorbidities contribute to impairments for breast cancer survivors. *Journal of Traumatic Stress, 21(2)*, 165–172.

Sherraden, M.S., Slosar, B., & Sherraden, M. (2002). Innovation in social policy: Collaborative policy advocacy. *Social Work, 47(3)*, 209–222.

Shetty, S., & Kaguyutan, J. (2002). *Immigrant victims of domestic violence: Cultural challenges and available legal protections*. Harrisburg, PA: VAWnet, a project of the National Resource Center on Domestic Violence/Pennsylvania Coalition against Domestic Violence. Retrieved October 20, 2009 from http://www.vawnet.org

Shin, L., Rauch, S., & Pitman, R. (2006). Amygdala, medial prefrontal cortex, and hippocampal function in PTSD. *Annals of the New York Academy of Sciences, 1071*, 67–79.

Shirtcliff, E.A., Coe, C.L., & Pollak, S.D. (2009). Early childhood stress is associated with elevated antibody levels to herpes simplex virus type 1. *Proceedings of the National Academy of Sciences, 106(8)*, 2963–2967.

Sidran Traumatic Stress Institute. (1995–2009). Post traumatic stress disorder fact sheet. Retrieved July26. 2020 from https://www.sidran.org/wp-content/uploads/2018/11/Post-Traumatic-Stress-Disorder-Fact-Sheet-.pdf

Siegel, D. (2001). Toward an interpersonal neurobiology of the developing mind: Attachment relationships, mindsight, and neural integration. *Infant Mental Health journal, 22(1–2)*, 67–94.

Silver, R.C., Holman, E.A., McIntosh, D.N., Poulin, M., & Gil-Rivas, V. (2002). Nationwide longitudinal study of psychological responses to September 11. *JAMA: Journal of the American Medical Association, 288(10)*, 1235–1244.

Silverman, J., Raj, A., Mucci, L.A., & Hathaway, J.E. (2001). *Dating violence against adolescent girls and associated substance use, unhealthy weight control, sexual risk behavior, pregnancy, and suicidality*. Retrieved October 30, 2009 from http://jama.ama-assn.org/cgi/reprint/286/5/572

Smith, M.Y., Redda, W.H., Peyserb, C., & Vool, D. (1999). Post-traumatic stress disorder in cancer: A review. *Psycho-Oncology, 8(6)*, 521–537.

Social Solutions. (2018). *20 Alarming Domestic Violence Statistics for 2018*. Retrieved March 18, 2019 from https://www.socialsolutions.com/blog/domestic-violence-statistics-2018/

Solomon, Z., Laor, N., & McFarlane, A. (1996). Acute posttraumatic reactions in soldiers and civilians. In B.A. van der Kolk, A.C. McFarlane, & L. Weisaeth (Eds.), *Traumatic stress: The effects of overwhelming experience on mind, body, and society* (pp. 102–114). New York: Guilford Press.

Springer, K.W., Sheridan, J., Kuo, D., & Carnes, M. (2007). Long-term physical and mental health consequences of childhood physical abuse: Results from a large population-based sample of men and women. *Child Abuse & Neglect, 31*, 517–530.

Stanton, A.L. (2006). Psychosocial concerns and interventions for cancer survivors. *Journal of Clinical Oncology, 24(32)*, 5132–5137.

Stark, E. (2009). *Coercive control: How men entrap women in personal life*. New York: Oxford University Press.

Sternberg, E. (2000). *The balance within: The science connecting health and emotions*. New York: W.H. Freeman and Company.

Stover, C.S., Meadows, A., & Kaufman, J. (2009). Interventions for intimate partner violence: Review and directions for evidence based practice. *Professional Psychology: Research and Practice, 40,* 223–233.

Strand, V.C., Hansen, S., & Courtney, D. (2013). Common elements across evidence-based trauma treatment: Discovery and implications. *Advances in Social Work, 14*(2), 334–354.

Substance Abuse and Mental Health Services Administration. (2014). *SAMHSA's Concept of Trauma and Guidance for a Trauma-Informed Approach. HHS Publication No. (SMA) 14-4884*. Rockville, MD: Substance Abuse and Mental Health Services Administration.

Sullivan, C.M., & Gillum, T. (2001). Shelters and other community-based services for battered women and their children. In C.M. Renzetti, J.L. Edleson, & R. Kennedy Bergen (Eds.), *Sourcebook on violence against women* (pp. 247–260). Thousand Oaks, CA: Sage Publications.

Sumalla, E.C., Ochoa, C., & Blanco, I. (2009). Posttraumatic growth in cancer: Reality or illusion? *Clinical Psychology Review, 29*(1), 24–33.

Swan, N. (1998). Exploring the role of child abuse on later drug abuse: Researchers face broad gaps in information. *NIDA Notes, 13*(2). Retrieved March 22, 2012 from www.nida.nih.gov/NIDA_Notes/NNVol13N2/exploring.html

Sweeney, A., Fahmy, S, Nolan, F., Morant, N., Fox, Z., Lloyd-Evans, B. et al. (2014). The relationship between therapeutic alliance and service user satisfaction in mental health inpatient wards and crisis house alternatives: A cross-sectional study. *PLoS ONE, 9*(7): e100153. [PMC free article][PubMed].

Sweeney, A., Filson, B., Kennedy, A., Collinson, L., & Gillard, S. (2018). A paradigm shift: Relationships in trauma-informed mental health services. *BJPsych Advances, 24*(5), 319–333.

Taïeb, O., Moro, M.R., Baubet, T., Revah-Lévy, A., & Flament, M.F. (2003). Posttraumatic stress symptoms after childhood cancer. *European Child & Adolescent Psychiatry, 12*(6), 255–264.

Talbott, W. (2009). Early mental health interventions following disasters: What is the standard of practice? *Texas Public Health journal, 61*(2), 40–41.

Tam, D. (2007). Culturally responsive advocacy intervention with abused Chinese-Canadian women. *British journal of Social Work, 34,* 269–277.

Tarakeshwar, N., Pearce, M.J., & Sikkema, K.J. (2005). Development and implementation of a spiritual coping group intervention for adults living with HIV/AIDS: A pilot study. *Mental Health, Religion & Culture, 8*(3), 179–190.

Taylor, C.E. (1998). How care for psychological trauma in wartime may contribute to peace. *International Review of Psychiatry, 10,* 175–178.

Tedstone, J.E., & Tarrier, N. (2003). Posttraumatic stress disorder following medical illness and treatment. *Clinical Psychology Review, 23*(3), 409–448.

Teenage Research Unlimited. (2008). *Tween and teen dating violence and abuse study, Teenage Research Unlimited for Liz Claiborne Inc. and the National Teen Dating Abuse Helpline*. Retrieved October 30, 2009 from http://www.loveisnotabuse.com/pdf/Tween%20Dating%20Abuse%20Full%20Report.pdf

Tehrani, N. (2007). The cost of caring – The impact of secondary trauma on assumptions, values and beliefs. *Counseling Psychology Quarterly, 20*(4), 325–339.

Telch, C.F., & Telch, M.J. (1986). Group coping skills instruction and supportive group therapy for cancer patients: A comparison of strategies. *Journal of Consulting and Clinical Psychology*, *54*(6), 802–808.

Theodore, A., Chang, J., Runyan, D., Hunter, W., Shrikant, I., & Agans, R. (2005). Epidemiological features of physical and sexual maltreatment of children in the Carolinas. *Pediatrics*, *115*, 331–337.

Thompson, B., & Colon, Y. (2004). Lesbians and gay men at the end of their lives: Psychosocial concerns. In J. Berzoff & P. Silverman (Eds.), *Living with dying: A handbook for end-of-life healthcare practitioners* (pp. 482–498). New York: Columbia University Press.

Thornberry, C., & Olson, K. (2005). The abuse of individuals with developmental disabilities. *University of Alberta Developmental Disabilities Bulletin*, *33*(1&2), 1–19.

Tick, E. (2005). *War and the soul*. Wheaton, IL: Quest Books.

Tjaden, P., & Thoennes, N. (2000). *Extent, nature, and consequences of intimate partner violence: Findings from the national violence against women survey*. Washington, DC: U.S. Department of Justice.

Tummala-Narra, P. (2007). Conceptualizing trauma and resilience across diverse contexts: A multicultural perspective. *Journal of Aggression, Maltreatment & Trauma*, *14*(12), 33–53.

Turner, S., McFarlane, A., & van der Kolk, B.A. (1996). The therapeutic environment and new explorations in the treatment of posttraumatic stress disorder. In B.A. van der Kolk, A.C. McFarlane, & L. Weisaeth (Eds.), *Traumatic stress: The effects of overwhelming experience on mind, body, and society* (pp. 537–558). New York: Guilford Press.

Ulman, K.H. (2001). Unwitting exposure of the therapist: Transferential and countertransferential dilemmas. *The Journal of psychotherapy practice and research*, *10*(1), 14–22.

UNiTE. (2010). UNiTE to End Violence Against Women campaign. Retrieved December 27, 2009 from http://www.un.org/en/women/endviolence/about.shtml

Ursano, R.J., & Engel, C.C. (2008). Taking issue: The importance of assessing exposure to trauma. *Psychiatric Services*, *59*(3), 229.

Ursano, R.J., Grieger, T.A., & McCarroll, J.E. (1996). Prevention of posttraumatic stress: Consultation, training and early treatment. In B.A. van der Kolk, A.C. McFarlane, & L. Weisaeth (Eds.), *Traumatic stress: The effects of overwhelming experience on mind, body, and society* (pp. 441–463). New York: Guilford Press.

U.S. Department of Health and Human Services, Administration for Children and Families Administration on Children, Youth and Families, Children's Bureau. (2019). Child Maltreatment 2017. Retrieved March 18, 2019 from https://www.acf.hhs.gov/cb/research-data-technology/ statistics-research/child-maltreatment

U.S. Department of Health and Human Services, Administration on Children, Youth and Families. (2008). *Child maltreatment in 2006*. Washington, DC: U.S. Government Printing Office.

U.S. Department of Health and Human Services, Administration on Children, Youth and Families. (2009). *Child maltreatment in 2007*. Washington, DC: U.S. Government Printing Office.

U.S. Department of Justice, Bureau of Justice Statistics. (2005). *Family violence statistics*. Retrieved November 20, 2009 from http://www.ojp.usdoj.gov/bjs/pub/pdf/fvs.pdf

van der Kolk, B.A. (1989). The compulsion to repeat the trauma. Re-enactment, revictimization, and masochism. *Psychiatric Clinics of North America*, *12*(2), 389–411.

van der Kolk, B.A. (1996). The complexity of adaptation to trauma: Self-regulation, stimulus discrimination, and characterological development. In B.A. van der Kolk, A.C. McFarlane, & L. Weisaeth (Eds.), *Traumatic stress: The effects of overwhelming experience on mind, body, and society* (pp. 182–213). New York: Guilford Press.

van der Kolk, B.A. (2006). Clinical implications of neuroscience research in PTSD. *Annals of the New York Academy of Sciences, 1071(1)*, 277–293.

van der Kolk, B.A. (2009). Afterword. In C.A. Courtois, J.D. Ford, B.A. van der Kolk, & J.L. Herman (Eds.), *Treating complex traumatic stress disorders: An evidence-based guide* (pp. 166–182). New York: Guilford Press.

van der Kolk, B.A. (2014). *The body keeps the score: Brain, mind, and body in the healing of trauma*. New York: Viking.

van der Kolk, B.A., McFarlane, A., & van der Hart, O. (1996). A general approach to treatment of posttraumatic stress disorder. In B.A. van der Kolk, A.C. McFarlane, & L. Weisaeth (Eds.), *Traumatic stress: The effects of overwhelming experience on mind, body, and society* (pp. 417–440). New York: Guilford Press.

van der Kolk, B.A., McFarlane, A., & Weisaeth, L. (Eds.). (1996). *Traumatic stress: The effects of overwhelming experience on mind, body, and society*. New York: Guilford Press.

Van Minnen, A., Hendriks, L., Kleine, R., Hendriks, G.J., Verhagen, M., & De Jongh, A. (2018). Therapist rotation: A novel approach for implementation of trauma-focused treatment in post-traumatic stress disorder. *European journal of psychotraumatology, 9(1)*, 1492836. doi:10.1080/20008198.2018.1492836

Vattano, A.J. (1978). Self-management procedures for coping with stress. *Social Work, 23(2)*, 113–119.

Vermetten, E., & Bremner, J. (2002). Circuits and systems in stress. Applications to neurobiology and treatment in posttraumatic stress disorder. *Depression and Anxiety, 16(1)*, 14–38.

Vernberg, E.M., Steinberg, A.M., Jacobs, A.K., Brymer, M.J., Watson, P.J., Osofsky, J.D. et al. (2008). Innovations in disaster mental health: Psychological first aid. *Professional Psychology: Research and Practice, 39(4)*, 381–388.

Vinck, P., Pham, P.N., Stover, E., & Weinstein, H.M. (2007). Exposure to war crimes and implications for peace building in northern Uganda. *JAMA: journal of the American Medical Association, 298(5)*, 543–554.

Voices of Women Organizing Project. (2006). *Working to improve the ACS response to cases of domestic violence*. Retrieved August 20, 2010 from http://www.vowbwrc.org/

Wagnild, G., & Young, H. (1993). Development and psychometric evaluation of the resilience scale. *Journal of Nursing Measurement, 1(2)*, 165–178.

Wahler, E. (2012). Identifying and challenging social work students' biases. *Social Work Education, 31(8)*, 1058–1070.

Wainrib, B.R., & Bloch, E. (1998). *Crisis intervention and trauma response: Theory and practice*. New York: Springer Publishing Company.

Walsh-Burke, K. (2004). Assessing mental health risk in end-of-life care. In J. Berzoff & P. Silverman (Eds.), *Living with dying: A handbook for end-of-life healthcare practitioners* (pp. 360–379). New York: Columbia University Press.

Walters, K.L., & Simoni, J.M. (2002). Reconceptualizing native women's health: An "indigenist" stress-coping model. *The American journal of Public Health, 92(4)*, 520–524.

Wang, C.T., & Holton, J. (2007). *Total estimated cost of child abuse and neglect in the United States: Economic impact study*. Chicago, IL: Prevent Child Abuse America.

Weaver, A.J., Flannelly, L.T., Garbarino, J., Figley, C.R., & Flannelly, K.J. (2003). A systematic review of research on religion and spirituality in the *Journal of Traumatic Stress*: 1990–1999. *Mental Health, Religion & Culture, 6*(3), 215–228.

Webb, N. (2004). The impact of traumatic stress and loss on children and families. In N. Webb (Ed.), *Mass trauma and violence* (pp. 3–22). New York: The Guilford Press.

Weine, S., Kulauzovic, Y., Klebic, A., Besic, S., Mujagic, A., & Muzurovic, J. et al. (2008). Evaluating a multiple-family group access intervention for refugees with PTSD. *Journal of Marital & Family Therapy, 34*(2), 149–164.

Weine, S.M., Kulenovic, T., Dzubur, A., Pavkovic, I., & Gibbons, R. (1998). Testimony psychotherapy in Bosnian refugees: A pilot study. *American Journal of Psychiatry, 155*, 1720–1726.

Weingarten, K. (2004). *Common shock: Witnessing violence every day – How we are harmed, how we can heal.* New York: New American Library.

Weinstein, J. (2002). When children witness domestic violence: Expert opinion [Electronic Version]. Retrieved May 6, 2011 from http://www.nccpr.org/reports/nicholsonsummary.pdf

Weiss, D.W. (2004). Structured clinical interview techniques for PTSD. In J.P. Wilson, & T.M. Keane (Eds.), *Assessing psychological trauma and PTSD* (2nd ed., pp. 103–121). New York: The Guilford Press.

Wells, N.L., & Turney, M.E. (2001). Common issues facing adults with cancer. In M.M. Lauria, E.J. Clark, J.F. Hermann, & N.M. Stearns (Eds.), *Social work in oncology: Supporting survivors, families and caregivers* (pp. 27–43). Atlanta, GA: American Cancer Society.

Wendt, D.C., Gone, J.P., & Nagata, D.K. (2015). Potentially harmful therapy and multicultural counseling: Bridging two disciplinary discourses. *The Counseling Psychologist, 43*(3), 334–358.

West, T.M. (2007). Beyond survival: Music-evoked imagery and the cancer experience. *Journal of the Society for Integrative Oncology, 5*(4), 180.

Westover, T. (2018). *Educated: A memoir.* New York: Random House.

Whitaker, D.J., Morrison, S., Lindquist, C., Hawkins, S.R., O'Neil, J.A., Nesius, A.M. et al. (2006). A critical review of interventions for the primary prevention of perpetration of partner violence. *Aggression and Violence Behavior, 11*, 151–166.

Whitfield, C.L., Anda, R.F., Dube, S.R., & Felitle, V.J. (2003). Violent childhood experiences and the risk of intimate partner violence in adults: Assessment in a large health maintenance organization. *Journal of Interpersonal Violence, 18*(2), 166–185.

Whitlock, J., & Knox, K.L. (2007). The relationship between self-injurious behavior and suicide in a young adult population. *Archives of Pediatrics & Adolescent Medicine, 161*(7), 634–640.

Wicks, R.J. (2008). *The resilient clinician.* New York: Oxford University Press.

Wikipedia contributors. (2019, February 21). Disability abuse. In *Wikipedia, The Free Encyclopedia.* Retrieved March 17, 2019 from https://en.wikipedia.org/w/index.php?title=Disability_abuse&oldid=884348217

Wilcox, H., Storr, C., & Breslau, N. (2009). Posttraumatic stress disorder and suicide attempts in a community sample of urban American young adults. *Archives of General Psychiatry, 66*(3), 305–311.

Wilmon-Haque, S., & BigFoot, D.S. (2008). Violence and the effects of trauma on American Indian and Alaska native populations. *Journal of Emotional Abuse, 8*(1/2), 51–66.

Wolfe, D.A., Werkerle, C., Scott, K., Straatman, A., Grasley, C., & Reitzel-Jaffe, D. (2003). Dating violence prevention with at-risk youth: A controlled outcome evaluation. *Journal of Consulting and Clinical Psychology, 71*, 279–291.

Worden, J.W. (2003). *Grief counseling and grief therapy: A handbook for the mental health practitioner* (4th ed.). New York: Springer Publishing Company.

World Health Organization. (2005). *WHO multi-country study on women's health and domestic violence against women: Summary report of initial results on prevalence, health outcomes and women's responses.* Geneva: World Health Organization.

World Health Organization. (2016). *Child maltreatment fact sheet.* Retrieved March 18, 2019 from https://www.who.int/news-room/fact-sheets/detail/child-maltreatment

World Health Organization. (2017). *Violence against women key facts.* Retrieved March 18, 2019 from https://www.who.int/news-room/fact-sheets/detail/violence-against-women

World Health Organization. (2018). *Elder abuse key facts.* Retrieved March 18, 2019 from https://www.who.int/news-room/fact-sheets/detail/elder-abuse

Yorke, J., Adams, C., & Coady, N. (2008). Therapeutic value of equine–human bonding in recovery from trauma. *Anthrozoos, 21(1)*, 17–30.

Youssef, N.A., Lockwood, L., Su, S., Hao, G., & Rutten, B.P.F. (2018). The effects of trauma, with or without PTSD, on the transgenerational DNA methylation alterations in human offsprings. *Brain Sciences, 8(5)*, 83.

Ziegler, M., & McEvoy, M. (1997–2002). Hazardous terrain: Countertransference reactions in trauma groups. Retrieved March 20, 2012 from http://psybc.com/pdfs/library/Hazardous.pdf

Zielinski, D.S. (2009). Child maltreatment and adult socioeconomic well-being. *Child Abuse and Neglect, 33(10)*, 666–678.

Zimmermann, T., Heinrichs, N., & Baucom, D.H. (2007). "Does one size fit all?" Moderators in psychosocial interventions for breast cancer patients: A meta-analysis. *Annals of Behavioral Medicine, 34(3)*, 225–239.

Index

Italicized and **bold** pages refer to figures and tables respectively.

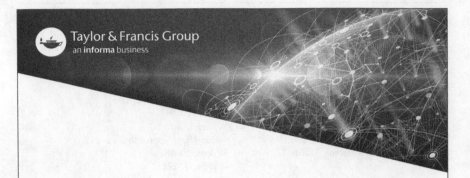

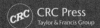

Printed in the United States
By Bookmasters